Differential Diagnosis in
Neurology

Differential Diagnosis in
Neurology

Editors

Sudesh Prabhakar MD DM FAMS FIAN
Director Neurology, Fortis Hospital
Mohali, Punjab, India
Former Professor and Head
Department of Neurology
Postgraduate Institute of Medical Education and Research
Chandigarh, Punjab, India

Gagandeep Singh MD DM
Professor and Head
Department of Neurology
Dayanand Medical College and Hospital
Ludhiana, Punjab, India

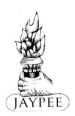
JAYPEE

The Health Sciences Publisher

New Delhi | London | Philadelphia | Panama

Jaypee Brothers Medical Publishers (P) Ltd

Headquarters

Jaypee Brothers Medical Publishers (P) Ltd
4838/24, Ansari Road, Daryaganj
New Delhi 110 002, India
Phone: +91-11-43574357
Fax: +91-11-43574314
Email: jaypee@jaypeebrothers.com

Overseas Offices

J.P. Medical Ltd
83 Victoria Street, London
SW1H 0HW (UK)
Phone: +44-2031708910
Fax: +02-03-0086180
Email: info@jpmedpub.com

Jaypee Medical Inc.
The Bourse
111 South Independence Mall East
Suite 835, Philadelphia, PA 19106, USA
Phone: +1 267-519-9789
Email: jpmed.us@gmail.com

Jaypee Brothers Medical Publishers (P) Ltd
Bhotahity, Kathmandu
Nepal
Phone: +977-9741283608
Email: kathmandu@jaypeebrothers.com

Jaypee-Highlights Medical Publishers Inc
City of Knowledge, Bld. 237, Clayton
Panama City, Panama
Phone: +1 507-301-0496
Fax: +1 507-301-0499
Email: cservice@jphmedical.com

Jaypee Brothers Medical Publishers (P) Ltd
17/1-B Babar Road, Block-B, Shaymali
Mohammadpur, Dhaka-1207
Bangladesh
Mobile: +08801912003485
Email: jaypeedhaka@gmail.com

Website: www.jaypeebrothers.com
Website: www.jaypeedigital.com

Differential Diagnosis in Neurology

First Edition: **2016**

ISBN: 978-93-5152-902-6

Printed at: Samrat Offset Pvt. Ltd.

Dedicated to

Our families who supported us all through, our teachers who still continue to inspire us, and our patients who will always form the foundation of this volume

Special mention

Jagjit S Chopra
Indu Prabhakar
Neena Johar
Amol N Singh

Contributors

EDITORS

Sudesh Prabhakar MD DM FAMS FIAN
Director Neurology, Fortis Hospital
Mohali, Punjab, India
Former Professor and Head
Department of Neurology
Postgraduate Institute of Medical Education and Research
Chandigarh, Punjab, India

Gagandeep Singh MD DM
Professor and Head
Department of Neurology
Dayanand Medical College and Hospital
Ludhiana, Punjab, India

CONTRIBUTING AUTHORS

Suvarna Alladi DM
Additional Professor, Department of Neurology
Nizam's Institute of Medical Sciences
Hyderabad, Telangana, India

Craig S Anderson MBBS FRACP PhD FAFPHM FAHMS
Professor, Stroke Medicine and Clinical Neurosciences
Head, Department of Neurology
Senior Director, The George Institute, Royal Prince Alfred
Hospital and University of Sydney
Sydney, Australia

SSK Ayyar MD DM FAAN FICP
Senior Consultant, Department of Neurology
Vijaya Health Centre
Chennai, Tamil Nadu, India

Inder D Bahia MBBS
Senior Consultant, Theriac Medical Consultancy
Bakersfield, California, United States

Kiran Bala MD DM DNB
Senior Professor, Department of Neurology
Pandit Bhagwat Dayal Sharma Post Graduate Institute of
Medical Sciences
Rohtak, Haryana, India

Amit Batla MBBS MD DM
Clinical Teaching Fellow, UCL Institute of Neurology
London, England, United Kingdom

Madhuri Behari MD DM
Professor, Department of Neurology
All India Institute of Medical Sciences
New Delhi, India

Archana Bethala MBBS MD DM
Senior Resident, Department of Neurology
Nizam's Institute of Medical Sciences
Hyderabad, Telangana, India

Kailash P Bhatia MRCP FRCP
Professor of Neurology, Sobell Department of Motor
Neuroscience and Movement Disorders
UCL Institute of Neurology
London, England, United Kingdom

Rohit Bhatia MD DM DNB
Additional Professor, Department of Neurology
All India Institute of Medical Sciences
New Delhi, India

Meghna Bhatnagar MBBS MCN
Ipswich, Suffolk, United Kingdom

Kalyan B Bhattacharyya MD DM MAMS FIAN FRCP
Professor, Department of Neuromedicine
RG Kar Medical College and Hospital
Kolkata, West Bengal, India

Sanjeev K Bhoi MD DM
Assistant Professor, Department of Neurology
Sanjay Gandhi Postgraduate Institute of Medical Sciences
Lucknow, Uttar Pradesh, India

Anirban Biswas MBBS DLO
Consultant Neurotologist, Vertigo Clinic, Belle Vue Clinic,
and Vertigo and Deafness Clinic
Kolkata, West Bengal, India

Wesley Chan MD MSc
Resident
Department of Ophthalmology and Visual Sciences
Dalhousie University
Halifax, Nova Scotia, Canada

Poodipedi S Chandra MCh
Professor, Department of Neurosurgery
All India Institute of Medical Sciences
New Delhi, India

Rima M Chaudhari DM
Post DM Research Fellow, Department of Neurology
All India Institute of Medical Sciences
New Delhi, India

Neera Chaudhry MBBS MD DM
Professor, Department of Neurology
GB Pant Hospital
New Delhi, India

Pavan K Cherukuri MD
Senior Resident, Department of Neurology
Nizam's Institute of Medical Sciences
Hyderabad, Telangana, India

Fiona E Costello MD FRCP
Associate Professor
Clinical Neurosciences/Surgery (Ophthalmology)
Cumming School of Medicine
University of Calgary
Calgary, Alberta, Canada

Chandi P Das MBBS MD DM FRACP
Senior Staff Specialist, Department of Neurology
Canberra Hospital
Faculty Australian National University
Canberra, Australia

Shyamal K Das MBBS MD DM
Professor, Department of Neurology
Burdwan Medical College
Burdwan, West Bengal, India

Deepa Dash MD DM
Assistant Professor, Department of Neurology
All India Institute of Medical Sciences
New Delhi, India

Sarita B Dave MD
Physician, New York Eye and Ear Infirmary
New York, United States

Divyaraj Gollahalli M.Phil Clinical Psychology
Senior Research Fellow, Department of Neurology
Nizam's Institute of Medical Sciences
Hyderabad, Telangana, India

Mohammed Faruq MBBS PhD
Scientist, Department of Genomics and
Molecular Medicine
CSIR-Institute of Genomics and Integrative Biology
New Delhi, India

Malay K Ghosal MBBS MD
Professor, Department of Psychiatry
Medical College, Kolkata
Kolkata, West Bengal, India

Chanchal Goyal MBBS PhD MA
Senior Research Fellow, Department of Neurology
All India Institute of Medical Sciences
New Delhi, India

Manoj Goyal MD DM
Assistant Professor, Department of Neurology
Postgraduate Institute of Medical Education and Research
Chandigarh, Punjab, India

Vinay Goyal MD DM
Professor, Department of Neurology
All India Institute of Medical Sciences
New Delhi, India

Anu Gupta MD DM
Assistant Professor, Department of Neurology
Postgraduate Institute of Medical Education and Research
Chandigarh, Punjab, India

Shakir Husain MBBS MD DM FINR
Senior Consultant
Department of Interventional Neurology and Stroke
Max Superspeciality Hospital
New Delhi, India
Director, Neurointervention Training Program
Scientific Advisor and Consultant
Interventional Neuroradiology, Department of Neurology
RKU - Universitäts- und Rehabilitationskliniken Ulm
Germany

Jayantee Kalita MD DM
Professor, Department of Neurology
Sanjay Gandhi Postgraduate Institute of Medical Sciences
Lucknow, Uttar Pradesh, India

Bhavna Kaul MD DM
Assistant Professor, Department of Neurology
Vardhaman Mahavir Medical College and
Safdarjang Hospital
New Delhi, India

Satish V Khadilkar MD DM DNB FIAN
Professor, Department of Neurology
Grant Medical College and Sir JJ Group of Hospitals
Mumbai, Maharashtra, India

Parampreet S Kharbanda MBBS MD DM
Professor, Department of Neurology
Postgraduate Institute of Medical Education and Research
Chandigarh, Punjab, India

Dheeraj Khurana MD DM
Professor, Department of Neurology
Postgraduate Institute of Medical Education and Research
Chandigarh, Punjab, India

Sudhir Kothari MD DM
Head, Department of Neurology
Poona Hospital and Research Centre
Pune, Maharashtra, India

Suresh Kumar MD DM Fellow Epilepsy (UCLA), Fellow Sleep (ISDA)
Professor and Head, Department of Neurology
Sree Balaji Medical College and Hospital
Chennai, Tamil Nadu, India

Vivek Lal MD DM
Professor and Head, Department of Neurology
Postgraduate Institute of Medical Education and Research
Chandigarh, Punjab, India

Netravathi M MBBS DM
Associate Professor, Department of Neurology
National Institute of Mental Health and Neurosciences
Bangalore, Karnataka, India

Prashant Makhija MD DM
Consultant, Department of Neurology
Seven Hills Hospital
Mumbai, Maharashtra, India

Sahil Mehta MBBS MD DM
Assistant Professor, Department of Neurology
Postgraduate Institute of Medical Education and Research
Chandigarh, Punjab, India

Usha K Misra MD DM
Professor, Department of Neurology
Sanjay Gandhi Postgraduate Institute of Medical Sciences
Lucknow, Uttar Pradesh, India

Manish Modi MD DM
Additional Professor, Department of Neurology
Postgraduate Institute of Medical Education and Research
Chandigarh, Punjab, India

Jagarlapudi M Murthy MD DM
Chief, Department of Neurology
The Institute of Neurological Sciences
Care Outpatient Centre, CARE Hospital
Hyderabad, Telangana, India

Madakasira V Padma MD DM FAMS FNASc
Professor, Department of Neurology
All India Institute of Medical Sciences
New Delhi, India

Pramod K Pal MBBS MD DNB DM FIAN
Professor, Department of Neurology
National Institute of Mental Health and Neurosciences
Bangalore, Karnataka, India

Sandip Pal DM
Professor, Department of Neurology
Medical College Hospital
Kolkata, West Bengal, India

Jeyaraj D Pandian MD DM FRACP
Professor, Department of Neurology
Christian Medical College
Ludhiana, Punjab, India

Awadh K Pandit MBBS MD DM
DBT-INCRE-Fellow, Department of Neurology
All India Institute of Medical Sciences
New Delhi, India

Abhishek Pathak MBBS MD DM
Senior Resident, Department of Neurology
All India Institute of Medical Sciences
New Delhi, India

Gunchan Paul MBBS MD IDCCM
Assistant Professor, Department of Critical Care Medicine
Dayanand Medical College and Hospital
Ludhiana, Punjab, India

Birinder S Paul MD DM
Associate Professor, Department of Neurology
Dayanand Medical College and Hospital
Ludhiana, Punjab, India

Apoorva Pauranik DM
Professor, Department of Neurology
Mahatma Medical College
Indore, Madhya Pradesh, India

Vinod Puri MBBS MD DM
Director, Professor, and Head
Department of Neurology
GB Pant Hospital
New Delhi, India

Sarbani S Raha MD
Consultant, Child Neurology and Epilepsy Clinic
KGP Children Hospital
Vadodara, Gujarat, India

Ellajosyula Ratnavalli MBBS MD DM
Consultant Neurologist, Department of Neurology
Manipal Hospital
Bangalore, Karnataka, India

K Ravishankar MD
Consultant In-charge
Dr Ravishankar's Headache and Migraine Clinic
Jaslok and Lilavati Hospitals
Mumbai, Maharashtra, India

Naveen Sankhyan DM
Assistant Professor, Department of Pediatrics
Postgraduate Institute of Medical Education and Research
Chandigarh, Punjab, India

P Satishchandra MBBS DM FAMS FICN FRCP
Director, Vice Chancellor, and Senior Professor
Department of Neurology
National Institute of Mental Health and Neuro Sciences
Bangalore, Karnataka, India

Kishore V Shetty MD DM DNB
Consultant Neurologist, Dr LH Hiranandani Hospital
Mumbai, Maharashtra, India

Simon D Shorvon MA MD FRCP
Professor, UCL Institute of Neurology
National Hospital for Neurology and Neurosurgery
London, England, United Kingdom

Garima Shukla DM
Professor, Department of Neurology
All India Institute of Medical Sciences
New Delhi, India

Rakesh Shukla MBBS MD DM MHAMS
Professor, Department of Neurology
King George's Medical University
Lucknow, Uttar Pradesh, India

Inderpal Singh MBBS MD MRCP MSc FRCP
Consultant Physician and Geriatrician
Department of Geriatric Medicine
Aneurin Bevan University Health Board
Ystrad Mynach, United Kingdom

Shaily Singh MBBS MD DM
Fellow, University of Calgary
Calgary, Alberta, Canada

Pratibha Singhi MBBS MD FIAP FAMS
Senior Professor, Department of Pediatrics
Postgraduate Institute of Medical Education and Research
Chandigarh, Punjab, India

Preeti Singla MBBS MD DM
Consultant, Department of Neurology
Ajanta hospital and IVF Centre
Lucknow, Uttar Pradesh, India

PR Srijithesh MBBS MD DM
Associate Professor, Department of Neurology
Jawaharlal Institute of Postgraduate Medical
Education and Research
Puducherry, India

Achal K Srivastava MBBS MD DM
Professor, Department of Neurology
All India Institute of Medical Sciences
New Delhi, India

Prem S Subramanian MD PhD
Professor, University of Colorado School of Medicine
Aurora, Colorado, United States

Paulin Sudhan MBBS
Research Coordinator, Department of Neurology
Christian Medical College
Ludhiana, Punjab, India

Sheetal Suresh MD Fellow Sleep Medicine (ISDA)
Senior Consultant Physician
Department of Internal Medicine
Fortis Malar Hospitals, Adyar, Apollo NOVA
Chennai, Tamil Nadu, India

Vrajesh Udani MD
Consultant, Child Neurology and Epilepsy
Department of Pediatrics and Neurology
Hinduja National Hospital
Mumbai, Maharashtra, India

Venugopalan Y Vishnu MD DM (Resident)
Senior Resident, Department of Neurology
Postgraduate Institute of Medical Education and Research
Chandigarh, Punjab, India

Jie Yang MD PhD
Associate Professor, Department of Neurology
Nanjing Medical University
Associate Chief Physician, Nanjing First Hospital
Nanjing, Jiangsu, China

Sireesha Yareeda MBBS MD
Senior Resident, Department of Neurology
Nizam's Institute of Medical Sciences
Hyderabad, Telangana, India

Zeid Yasiry MBChB MSc
Assistant Lecturer, University of Babylon
Babylon, Iraq

Preface

A multitude of thoughts came across our minds as we started writing this prelude.

Firstly, an embracing sense of satisfaction overwhelms us not just on the completion of a monumental task but because we, as editors, were able to co-ordinate the superb efforts of 81 expert contributors. All of them are tall experts in their respective fields, and so busy, that we wondered whether they would find the time to write a chapter for the book. Indeed, the hard work put in by them and their colleagues are not limited to the few weeks they put in towards writing the chapter but a lifetime applied to a particular area of clinical neurology. Suffice to mention it here, "A book is only as compelling, spirituous, and influential as its authors".

Secondly, when we began the book, there was a concern whether a book of this kind was really required. However, after two years of working on the project, we are more convinced that the publication of this book is both timely and a pressing need. Timely—because this is an era when the art of bedside clinical neurology is fading and the practice of neurology is being increasingly marginalized by a plethora of investigative approaches. The time is appropriate to systematically and rationally integrate the complexities of contemporary laboratory, imaging, and neurophysiological investigations with traditional bedside neurology. This is what this book is intended for and we do not hesitate in claiming that this book is one of its kind.

Thirdly, a curiosity—who would read the book? In this aspect too, the publication of this book is justified as we are informed of an increasing number of students pursuing postgraduate studies in neurology—every year, over 160 DM Neurology students are taken in across the country. We believe that this book targets the postgraduate students in neurology as well as internal medicine, and fosters professional competence even for the accomplished neurologists, and practicing physicians. We also hope that this number will be ever-increasing.

The book seems a befitting tribute to our teachers who taught us the fine art of bedside neurology at a time when technologies were few and far apart, and to our patients who were ever accommodating of our scholarship—all to proclaim that mastering the clinical approach is the only way forward in clinical neurology.

Finally, a resolve to continue our commitment, and we promise to come back to you with the revised edition—to keep pace with the most up-to-date information in the dynamic and expanding field of clinical neurology.

Sudesh Prabhakar

Gagandeep Singh

Acknowledgments

Many people have contributed in various ways and without their support this book would not have been possible.

First and foremost, we wish to acknowledge our great and obvious debt to more than 80 distinguished group of contributing authors who generously gave their time and expertise, and presented the material in an esoteric manner, taken from their real-life clinical experiences.

The remarkable wisdom and grace of our illustrious and eminent teachers who have always been instrumental in providing valuable direction and counsel, deserves our special gratitude.

We especially wish to recognize and never forget our patients who will always remain the foundation of all our work and knowledge. We owe tremendous thanks and appreciation to them. May we remember the words of St. Bernadette Soubirous, "Every human being is precious in God's eyes."

We were ably assisted by Dr Parveen Goel, neuropsychologist who worked with enthusiasm, alacrity, and intelligence.

Our gratitude to the Jaypee Brothers Medical Publishers for considering the publication; to the team, which supported us in the book project; and most of all to our families—who resolutely endured us as we set aside all family chores in editing the book.

Our thanks go to all those people, each of whom helped in their own unique ways in bringing this book to fruition.

Contents

Chapter 1

Clinical History and Neurologic Examination of Adult

Sudesh Prabhakar

THE NEUROLOGIC EVALUATION: HISTORY AND EXAMINATION

No textbook in clinical neurology is complete without a chapter on history taking and examination and the same is true for this one. This chapter addresses selected aspects of history taking and examination pertinent to neurological system disorders. The aim of this chapter is to familiarize, the reader with a systematic approach toward neurological evaluation. In addition, in the latter part of the chapter, noteworthy aspects of neurological examination that are frequently overlooked are discussed.

In no discipline of medicine, might the clinical diagnosis be achieved with such perfection as in neurology, yet there are several fears, and apprehensions related to neurological evaluation. Neurological evaluation is thought to be a complex process that often lacks precision and is time consuming. Furthermore, inexperienced clinicians often ask the question if clinical neurological evaluation is really required in an era of modern technology. However, with experience one learns that neurological evaluation is a straightforward process that is very precise and systemic and that any length of time spent on it is time well-spent. In addition, to avoid an investigation-based gunshot approach, detailed history, and accurate neurological examination are all the more important in modern times and will perhaps never be replaced by new technologies.[1,2]

Having said that, it is important to recognize that there are inherent difficulties with neurological evaluation. Commonly, a neurologically ill patient is brought by someone, and history might not always be reliable. To further complicate the issue, a neurologically ill patient may not be able to provide a coherent history due to alterations in level of consciousness, cognitive problems, errors of communication consequent to nervous system disease, and finally due to noncooperation. In these circumstances, history should be obtained from the primary caregivers, and should be supplemented by review of past medical records if available.[1]

The key to successful neurological evaluation is an accurate history and examination that should be focused on obtaining answers to a few key questions:[3]
1. Is there a neurological problem, or in other words, does the index patient have a neurological disorder?
2. What is the site(s) of the lesion?
3. What is the likely etiology?
4. What are the potential differential diagnoses?
5. What are the relevant investigations and the management plan?

In addition, the disease-related morbidity pertaining to social, economic, occupational, and personal factors should be noted down as these will determine the treatment.

The tools required for proper neurological examination are summarized in Box 1.1.

HISTORY (BOX 1.2)

The history is the cornerstone of medical diagnosis and neurological diagnosis is no exception. For instance, the moment a patient with classic pill-rolling tremor enters clinic, the consideration of Parkinson's disease crosses the physician's mind. However, this presentation can

---

Box 1.1: Tools required for neurological evaluation

- Predesigned protocol
- Smell: Familiar – coffee, snuff, soap, tooth paste, etc.
- Vision: Torch, bright objects, colored items/Ishihara charts, pinhole, Snellen's chart, Optokinetic tape/drum, ophthalmoscope
- Hearing: Tuning fork – 512 Hz, otoscope
- Taste: sweet, salt, bitter objects, tongue blade
- Somatic sensations: Cotton, disposable pins, hot-cold tubes, tuning fork – 128 Hz, two point discriminator, objects of different sizes, shape, weight, form, and texture, etc.
- Deep tendon reflexes: Reflex hammer
- Stethoscope
- Battery of tests/scales/scores: Glasgow-coma chart, Western aphasia battery, rating scales/scores, children's story book (especially useful in testing higher mental functions such as interpretation of visual scenes, testing for simultagnosias) among others
- Photographic/video recording

Box 1.2: History: Some important tips

Key points

- History is an important document and should be recorded in a clear logical manner
- Most of inaccuracies in neurological diagnosis result from improperly taken history
- A properly taken history not only provides pertinent clinical data, but also helps to understand patient as an individual, his expectations and his relationship to others, his feeling towards medical personal, his reactions to disease as well as social and economic consequences of disease related morbidity
- While recording history, every attempt should be made to put patient at ease. Simple gestures such as holding patient's hand, enquiring about social consequences of illness or whether he had taken food before coming to clinic often puts the patient at remarkable ease
- Usually most relevant information is obtained from patient's direct description of the symptoms
- A practical approach while obtaining history is to let the patient speak as long he is giving decent account and then assume more active role once account becomes incoherent

---

have a variety of causes, such as exposure to neuroleptic drugs, and this can be clarified only though history. Furthermore, the patient may have come for a totally different clinical problem such as foot drop superimposed on a long-standing history of Parkinsonism that can again be clarified only through accurate history. Thus,

the importance of accurate history taking cannot be undermined. In many instances, the physician learns more from history given by the patient than by any other means. A properly taken history alone may suggest the probable clinical diagnosis. Most of the inaccuracies in clinical neurology result from incomplete or inaccurate history taking. A properly taken history not only provides pertinent clinical data but also helps to understand the patient as an individual, his expectations, his relationships to others, his feelings toward the medical personnel, his reactions to disease, as well as the social and economic consequences of the disease-related morbidity.[1-3]

Taking a good history is not easy. Time, patience, compassion, and a manner that reflects interest, understanding, and empathy are critical to a good history. Every attempt should be made to put the patient at ease. Simple gestures such as holding the patient's hand, enquiring about the social consequences of illness, or whether he had his food before coming to clinic often put the patient at remarkable ease.

The history sheet is an important document and should be recorded clearly in a logical well-organized manner. Recording in a proper way is of great help to subsequent examiners and at follow-up of the patient. While recording history, it is important to note down important information keeping irrelevancies to the minimum. Patient's description of his symptoms, description given by family members/caregivers, and information from past medical records should be noted in detail. Usually, the most relevant information is obtained from the patient's direct description of the symptoms. The patient should be encouraged to provide information about his symptoms rather than giving description of what other doctors have thought at least in the beginning. This is especially true as patients often misunderstand, what they have been told by previous doctors.

In general, interviewer should intervene as little as possible while obtaining firsthand information. However, it may be necessary to take the conversation away from obviously irrelevant material. History taking varies with the type of individual. The timid, inarticulate patient requires repeated assurance, while a garrulous person may have to be interrupted several times. A depressed patient may exaggerate the complaints, while a euphoric patient may ignore a number of complaints. One patient may get offended at certain questions, while another may consider the questions commonplace. Even in a given individual, factors such as fatigue, pain, emotional conflicts, or mood fluctuations cause variation in response to questions. Thus, it is useful to keep a flexible approach while taking history. A practical approach may be to let the patient speak as long as he is giving a reasonable account and then assume a more active role if the account becomes incoherent. The patient's past medical records should always be reviewed as they may provide useful information. However, caution should be exercised in the interpretation of past medical records.[1-3]

A systematically taken history will often provide information about the presenting complaints and the present illness, past illnesses, family history, treatment details, personal information, impact of illness on the quality of life, as well as specific issues such as birth, growth, development, immunization, and travel.

CHIEF OR PRESENTING COMPLAINT (BOX 1.3)

Traditionally neurological history taking begins with the presenting complaints or the presenting illness. Most of the time spent with a new patient should be devoted to history taking and most time out of that is devoted to history of the presenting complaints. The presenting complaints provide the first clue to the etiology of the underlying illness. For instance, in a patient presenting with fever, headache, and vomiting of 15 days duration, the neurologist will be concerned with diagnosis of chronic meningitis, and further history taking will be directed to finding out the underlying etiology of the same.[2-5]

The first information about the chief or presenting complaints invariably starts with information regarding mode of onset. In this regard, it is important to note that sometimes patients with chronic disease, such as dementia, may notice symptoms suddenly (e.g., during travel) and this should not be equated with a sudden onset of disease. Onset is defined as time taken from beginning of symptoms to peak of symptoms. The onset and subsequent course of illness often helps in identifying the underlying etiology. For instance, sudden onset followed by static course or recovery will suggest

---

Box 1.3: Importance of chief complaint

Key points
- History taking usually begins with history of chief complaint and most time in history taking is devoted to that.
- Most useful information regarding history is the mode of onset
- Onset should be determined by noting time period form beginning of symptoms to peak of symptoms

---

a cerebrovascular event as an underlying cause while a course characterized by remissions and relapse with suggest a demyelinating or a neurometabolic disorder. A gradual onset and slow progression will suggest a neurodegenerative disorder or tumor. Many a times, the temporal course or the rate of progression is obtained by recording the important milestones in history, such as, when did the patient stop going for his job? When did he need one or two person's support to walk? Or, when did he require a wheelchair?

Every symptom of the presenting illness should be analyzed separately in detail. Determine the temporal course of each of the symptoms and inquire about their relationships to each other. For instance, a history of fever followed by headache will suggest intracranial infection as the cause, while a history of headache followed by fever will suggest alternate causes. For each symptom, determine the character, frequency, duration, severity, any variability (diurnal, seasonal or nocturnal), relationship to external factors as well as the response to treatment.

The patient and the clinician may use the same word to mean very different things. For instance, patients often use the word numbness to describe weakness of a limb. Similarly, the term dizziness is often used by patients to describe a variety of symptoms such as lightheadedness, confusion or weakness rather than true vertigo. It is often quite useful to try to extract detailed information regarding what the patient actually means by a particular symptom.[1,3]

REVIEW OF PATIENT-SPECIFIC INFORMATION

Every attempt should be made to obtain information about the patient's background as it may help a great deal in diagnosis. This includes information regarding current or past medical and surgical illnesses, current medications or allergies, illicit drug abuse, symptoms related to disease in other organ systems of the body, occupational history (type of job, work hours, excessive stress, occupational exposure to toxins, etc.), marital history (divorce, sexual performance and satisfaction, discordance with spouse, abuse or neglect of children or spouse, etc.), smoking or alcohol use, childhood abuse, and detailed information about disease in other family members. The chronology in which this information is obtained is not that important, but maintaining a sequence will ensure that every aspect of history is covered and adequate information is obtained.[1]

REVIEW OF SYSTEMS

In medicine, review of systems means detection of symptoms that the patient may not complain but which provide clue to the etiology of the presenting complaint. Neurological system disorders may cause dysfunction of many other systems and it is often useful to obtain neurological review of systems after obtaining detailed information about the presenting complaint. Some of the questions that may be asked while obtaining a neurological review of systems are summarized in Box 1.4. A positive response may help in clarifying the diagnosis. For instance, loss of smell in a patient, who presents with a rapidly progressive behavioral syndrome suggestive of basofrontal dysfunction will suggest the possibility of olfactory groove meningioma. Similarly, headache in a patient with paraparesis would suggest parasagittal lesion rather than cord lesion as the underlying etiology. In addition to neurological review of systems, it is also useful to obtain a general review of systems pertaining to other systems as they often provide clue to the underlying etiology. A long-standing history of diarrhea in a patient who presents with insidious-onset cerebellar ataxia points to celiac disease as the underlying etiology. The best way to obtain a detailed and coherent account of review of systems is to keep a structured questionnaire at hand at least for beginners. Gradually, with experience, one can get rid of the questionnaire. Another way to obtain review of systems is to ask the relevant questions at the time one is carrying out a detailed examination.[1,5]

Box 1.4: Functional areas commonly covered while obtaining neurological review of systems

- Cognition, behavior, personality change, mood changes, hallucinations, delusions, illusions, etc.
- Seizures/syncope/other episodic impairments of consciousness
- Headache
- Vision, smell, hearing, taste
- Speech, language (both comprehension and expression)
- Cranial nerves – diplopia, squint, visual problems, swallowing, chewing, facial functions, etc.
- Weakness in any part of the body
- Limb coordination
- Gait and stance
- Pain/other sensations
- History pertaining to bradykinesia/bradyphrenia
- Bladder, bowel, and sexual functions

PAST MEDICAL HISTORY (BOX 1.5)

Past medical history is of immense importance and very often it gives clues to the etiology of the presenting complaint. It is also of great help; especially so, as neurological symptoms are often related to an underlying systemic disorder. For example, history of headache, and seizures in a patient, who has lung cancer will immediately raise the suspicion of brain metastases. Similarly, history of long-standing asthma in a patient presenting with complaints suggestive of mononeuritis multiplex will suggest the possibility of Churg–Strauss syndrome. Usually the relevant information about past history includes history of current, chronic and past illnesses, hospitalizations, operations, trauma, information on the pregnancy, and developmental history. The past records should be assessed in detail as they may provide vital clues to the underlying etiology. The past history is very important and certain features in patient's history may raise immediate suspicion of certain disorders. Gastric surgery may cause vitamin B12 deficiency and vasculitis such as Wegener granulomatosis may present with cranial nerve palsies. At the end of the history, it is often very useful to ask the patient, "Is there any other information you want to give me, or if there is any other information you want to tell which I may not have inquired about"? One will be surprised that often the patient will come out with some new information in response to this question. The physician should not be surprised if the patient does not remember past surgeries as often patient will not give any history of past operations, while on examining one may see scars of previous operations.[1,5]

A detailed history should also be taken regarding current and past medications as a number of drugs can be associated with neurological symptoms. Many chemotherapeutic agents may be associated with peripheral neuropathy. Lithium may cause tremor as well as encephalopathy, while many neuroleptic agents may

---

Box 1.5: Drug history

Key points
- While obtaining drug history, it is extremely important to go through the old medical prescriptions. In addition whenever possible, patient should be asked to bring all the medicines at next visit and these should be checked to ensure what medicines was actually taking
- At the end of history, it is often very useful to ask the patient, "Is there any other information you want to give me or if there is any other information you want to tell which I have not enquired about"?

be associated with extrapyramidal syndromes. The use of oral contraceptive agents may be associated with chorea or it may result in cerebral venous sinus thrombosis. The use of over-the-counter medications as well as herbal medications should also be inquired for. Wherever possible, rather than going through the prescriptions, the patient should be instructed to bring all the drugs at next visit so that the physician is sure what medications the patient is taking.

FAMILY HISTORY

Many neurological disorders are hereditary. Thus, a history of consanguinity, or a history of a similar disease in the family, may provide the underlying etiology. For example, history of psychiatric disturbances or chorea in the parent of a young patient with dystonia may suggest Huntington's disease as the underlying cause. Similarly, a history of ataxia in two generations will suggest a diagnosis of spinocerebellar ataxia. In this regard, it is important to note that same gene defects may cause several different phenotypes. Thus, while obtaining history in patient with spinocerebellar ataxia, one should inquire not only about ataxia, but also about history suggestive of slow saccades (head thrusts while reading), bony abnormalities, peripheral neuropathies, or even tremor. Similarly, in a case of suspected hereditary motor sensory neuropathy, it may be useful to obtain history of bony deformities in addition to inquiries about motor or sensory deficits.[1-6]

The family history should be interpreted with caution and a negative family history may not be truly negative. Some diseases such as epilepsy are kept secret and a family history may not be forthcoming. The patient and/or relatives may not be aware of similar illnesses in the family as they may not have noticed subtle anomalies such as *pes cavus*. Finally, adoptions and disputed paternity may be another cause of negative family history. Some of the common causes for negative family history in hereditary neurological disorders are summarized in Box 1.6.

Box 1.6: Common causes of negative family history in hereditary neurological disorders

- Blanket questions such as does anybody else in the family have similar problems
- Variable expression
- Incomplete penetration
- Short survival/premature death
- Amnesia/wishful thinking
- Adoption/single parent
- Paternity issues

SOCIAL HISTORY

It is important to obtain a detailed social history. The social history includes the patient's marital status, educational status, occupation and personal habits. Marital history includes history of marital discord, interpersonal relationship, emotional stability, number of marriages, duration of the current marriage, health of the partner and the children. The reasons for divorce or marital discord, if any, should be inquired about, as these may provide important clues to the patient's behavioral and other problems.

Detailed information should be obtained about the patient's current and past employments. Information should also be obtained about the working environment, working hours, any discordance with colleagues or the employer, any occupational exposure to toxins, or illnesses in colleagues, etc. If the patient has changed his job or is not working currently, inquire about the circumstances leading to change or loss of job, such as cognitive problems, visual or hearing problems, or any other reasons. A history of occupational travel is also important, especially if an infectious disease is under consideration.

Information should be obtained about the use of tobacco, alcohol, drugs, coffee, tea, soft drinks and other similar substances. *History should also be obtained about the use of street drugs such as spray paint, glues, and gasoline.* The patient may not be forthcoming with use of drugs or alcohol. Patients often under-report the amount of alcohol they consume and while calculating the amount of alcohol consumed it may be useful to double the amount that the patient actually admits.[1-6] To obtain a more realistic data about alcohol intake, several specific questionnaires are available that may be used such as CAGE, HALT, and BUMP questionnaires.

Determining the patient's sexual behavior is very important and information should be obtained about risky sexual behavior. It is often useful to ask if the patient ever engaged in unprotected sex, how often, and whether the patient has ever had a sexually transmitted disease.

Some practical tips for history taking are summarized in Box 1.7.

EXAMINATION

After completion of the history taking, the next step is a detailed examination that includes general observations, recording of vital parameters, general physical followed by systemic examination, and finally neurological assessment.

TABLE 1.1: Glasgow coma scale

Observation	Response	Score
Eye opening	No response	1
	Response to pain	2
	Response to voice	3
	Spontaneously	4
Verbal response	No response	1
	Incomprehensible sounds	2
	Inappropriate words	3
	Disoriented conversation	4
	Oriented and appropriate	5
Motor response	No response	1
	Decerebrate posturing	2
	Decorticate posturing	3
	Flexion posturing	4
	Localizes pain	5
	Obeys commands	6

Neurological examination begins the time when the first contact with the patient is made.[3] For example, reduced facial expression or a resting pill-rolling tremor while taking the history would suggest a diagnosis of Parkinson's disease. Difficulty in articulating specific words may suggest nominal aphasia as the underlying disorder. Similarly, fluctuating bilateral ptosis would suggest diagnosis of neuromuscular junction problem, while a waddling gait when a patient enters the room would suggest proximal muscle weakness.

The nervous system is so commonly affected in systemic disorders that importance of a detailed general physical and systemic examination cannot be undermined. For example, the presence of atrial fibrillation in a patient with acute hemiparesis would suggest embolic stroke as the etiology. Similarly, concomitant findings of low heart-rate would suggest syncope rather than seizures as a cause of episodic loss of consciousness. The presence of jaundice and decreased liver span would suggest liver failure as a cause of altered sensorium rather than a primary neurological problem. The presence of characteristic rash in a patient with fever, headache and altered sensorium of short duration may suggest meningococcal meningitis.

After completion of the general physical and systemic examination, a detailed neurological assessment should be carried out that includes stepwise assessment of higher mental functions including consciousness, cranial nerves, motor and sensory systems, deep tendon reflexes, gait and stance, cerebellar functions, and finally autonomic functions. As these functions will be discussed elsewhere in the book, this chapter is not aimed at providing the detailed account of each of these functions. Instead, all these functions will be discussed briefly with emphasis on certain useful practical points.

The first step in doing a neurological assessment is an assessment of level of consciousness. A commonly used tool for assessment of sensorium is the Glasgow coma scale (Table 1.1), which is easy to administer with good intra- and inter-observer agreement. A score of <9 is suggestive of severe injury and an indication for airway support. However, it has some limitations, and is difficult to carry out in patients who are aphasic, are intubated, or are paralyzed. A better approach would be to record the entire response. For example, "the patient needed vigorous stimulation of shoulder for arousal. He woke up and asked why are you disturbing me and went back to sleep." The level of consciousness should be assessed serially as depressed sensorium may be a result of drug administration, seizures or may reflect altered sleep-wake cycle. Thus, serial monitoring may help in making therapeutic decisions.[5]

The next step in a neurological examination is testing for signs of meningeal irritation (Kerning's sign, neck stiffness, Brudzinski's sign) (see Fig. 1.1) depending on the patient's clinical condition, followed by testing for higher mental functions. Detailed higher mental function testing is time-consuming and thus is not carried out in every patient. However, the mini mental status examination (Table 1.2) may be carried out quickly in most patients depending on the clinical context. As these functions will be discussed elsewhere in the book, they are not being discussed any further in this chapter.[1,6]

Next is the assessment of cranial nerves (refer to Figs 1.2 and 1.3 for demonstration), and then

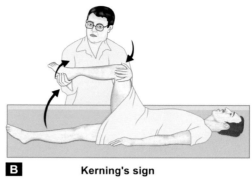

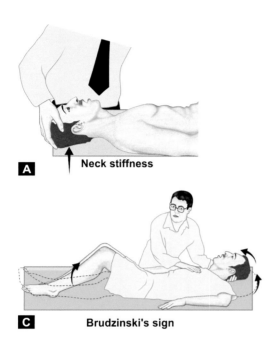

A Neck stiffness

B Kerning's sign

C Brudzinski's sign

Figs 1.1 A to C: Demonstration of meningeal signs: neck stiffness, Kerning's, and Brudzinski's sign.

TABLE 1.2: Mini mental status examination

Orientation	10
Time (date, day, season, month, year) 5	
Place (floor, hospital, state, town, country) 5	
Registration (name three objects)	3
Attention (serial 7s or reverse spell "WORLD")	5
Recall (three objects registered earlier)	3
Language (name-2, repeat-1, three-stage command-3, read-1, write-1, copy-1)	9
Total	30

follows the motor system examination that again begins with inspection. The details are summarized in Table 1.3. One should carefully observe the muscles for atrophy, hypertrophy, fasciculations, deformities, and contractures, and involuntary movements. Next, the tone is determined by gently flexing and extending the patient's elbow, wrist, fingers, ankle and knee. While testing the tone, examine for pronator catch that is elicited by rapidly alternating supination and pronation of forearm and for catch in adductors of thigh while performing abduction at hip. These two maneuvers are important in testing muscles affected earliest in spasticity. Next, while testing, the examiner should note down any confounding factors such as pain that can limit the patient's ability to exert full power. Remember that subtle weakness is often overlooked during routine examination especially while testing large muscles of trunk and legs such as the quadriceps that are very strong. For these reasons it is often useful to carry out a functional assessment of power. This is done by asking the patient to walk on toes/heels, perform a shallow knee bend on both sides, and getting up from a squatting position or from a chair. Often, the medical students measure grip strength as a toll for distal muscle strength. However, grip strength is a test for long finger flexors that are classified as intermediate muscle groups, and, therefore, the distal muscles should be tested separately in all the patients.[1-6]

After motor system examination, one can carry out either deep tendon reflexes or detailed sensory examination as per convenience. However, we prefer to perform sensory examination first as deep tendon reflexes are dependent on both motor and sensory functions. Touch, pinprick, temperature (hot-44°C and cold-30°C), vibration (128 Hz) and joint position/ kinesthetic sensations should be tested in all the limbs as well as on the face and trunk. Homologous areas on both sides of the body, as well as, the distal and the proximal parts should be compared. If an area of sensory loss is detected, try to map out the exact boundaries of this area and make an attempt to ascertain if area of sensory loss is

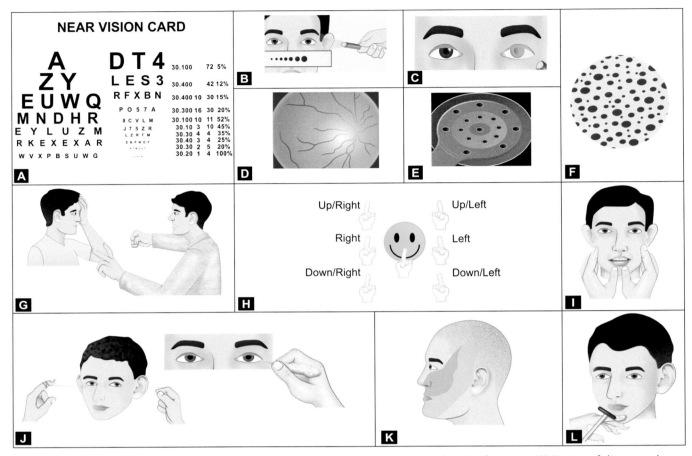

Figs 1.2A to L: Pictorial representation of optic, oculomotor, and trigeminal nerves. **The visual system, (A)** Testing of distant and near vision; **(B and C)** Pupillary reflexes; **(D)** Fundus chart; **(E)** Pinhole charts; **(F)** Ishihara chart; **(G)** Visual field examination; **(H)** Testing for ocular movements. **The trigeminal system, (I)** Testing for masseter muscles; **(J)** Corneal reflex; **(K)** Three divisions of 5th nerve; **(L)** Jaw jerk.

TABLE 1.3: **Cranial nerve examination**

Nerve	Maneuver
Olfactory nerve	Should be tested in all patients with loss of smell, Parkinson's disease, head injury; test each nostril separately using familiar substances like coffee and lemon extract; do not use noxious stimulus
Optic nerve	Test each eye separately. Test for visual acuity (near and distant vision), color vision, visual fields, fundus; use pin hole if visual acuity is suboptimal
Cranial nerves III, IV, VI	Pupillary response (both direct and consensual); test for eye movements in nine cardinal positions; observe lids for ptosis and frontalis muscles for any overactivity; look for fatigability of lids; look for nystagmus and other ocular oscillations; check both pursuit and saccades
Trigeminal nerve	Pin prick and touch in all three divisions of fifth nerve. Check for strength of jaw muscles and corneal reflex
Facial nerve	Forehead wrinkling, eyelid closure, whistle/pucker, etc.
Auditory nerve	Hearing acuity; Rinne/Weber/absolute bone conduction tests; oculovestibular reflex, Dix–Hallpike maneuver and cold caloric tests for vestibular component
Glossopharyngeal and vagus nerves	Palate lifts (say aah); gag reflex
Spinal accessory nerve	Trapezius and sternocleidomastoid muscle testing
Hypoglossal nerve	Tongue protrusion and tongue strength; right hypoglossal nerve protrudes tongue to left side

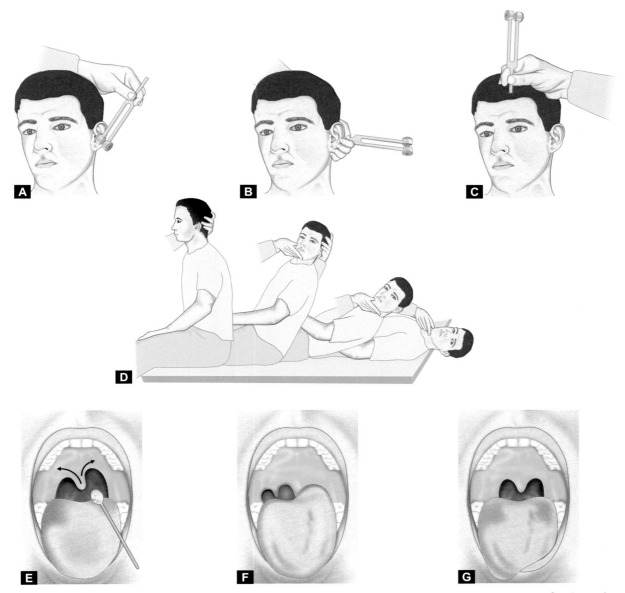

Figs 1.3A to G: Testing of cranial nerves. **(A and B)** Rinne test; **(C)** Weber test; **(D)** Dix–Hallpike test; **(E)** Gag reflex (note that the right side is moving less); **(F and G)** Testing for lingual functions (note the atrophy on right side of the tongue and its deviation to the right side on protrusion).

in distribution of a nerve or a root or if there is a sensory level consistent with cord disease. After testing for primary sensations, which, if intact, one should also test for cortical sensations that include precise localization, discrimination, stereognosis (size, shape, form, texture, etc.), barognosis, graphesthesia/figure writing, and finally double simultaneous stimulation. The sensory examination is summarized in Figure 1.4.

Next, deep tendon reflexes should be tested and the observations noted down. The deep tendon reflexes can be graded from 0 to 4 depending upon the response:

0   Absent
1   Present but with reinforcement
2   Normal
3   Exaggerated
4   Clonus

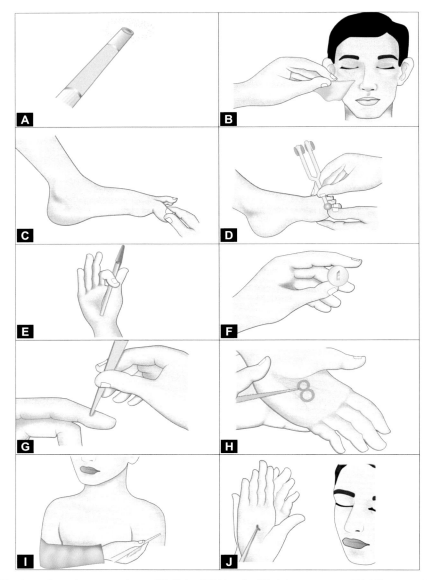

Figs 1.4 A to J: Testing of routine sensations. **(A)** Pain; **(B)** Touch; **(C)** Joint position; **(D)** Vibration. **Testing for cortical sensations. (E and F)** Stereognosis; **(G)** Tactile discrimination; **(H)** Graphesthesia; **(I)** Double simultaneous stimulation; **(J)** Note the patient's eyes should always be closed while performing the sensory examination. The facies should not be identifiable.

Also, superficial reflexes including corneal, gag, abdominal, cremasteric, plantar, anal, and bulbo-cavernosus reflexes should be tested[1-6] (Fig. 1.5).

Testing for cerebellar and extrapyramidal functions that are often assessed by examination of tone, abnormalities of posture, scanning/hypophonic quality in speech, examining eyes for evidence of nystagmus, square wave jerks, saccadic dysmetria, slow saccades, saccadic pursuit, etc., asking the patient to perform rapid alternating movements, finger-to-nose and heel-to-shin test and finally by noting down gait and asking him to walk in a straight line. Remember that in cerebellar lesions, there may be dissociation between affection of limb coordination and affection of gait and stance depending on the site of lesion in the cerebellum. Then test for gait and stance (Fig. 1.6). This is done by asking the patient to rise from sitting position, do a shallow knee-bend, walk in a straight line and turn around, walk heel-to-heel in a

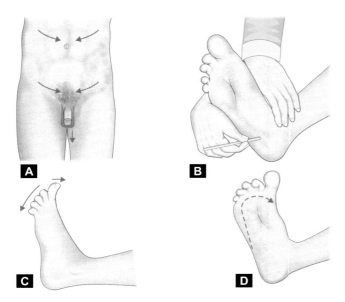

Figs 1.5A to D: Demonstration of superficial reflexes. (A) Abdominal and cremasteric reflexes; and (B–D) Plantar responses.

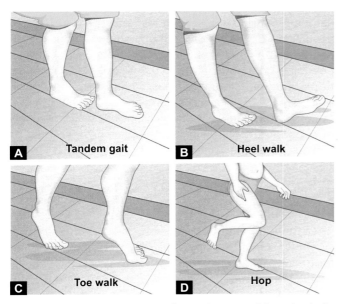

Figs 1.6A to D: Examination of gait. Some useful methods for elicitation of minimal abnormalities during gait examination.

straight line, walk on toes/heels, hop on each foot, and finally perform the pull test. In addition, the Romberg's test is performed by asking the patient to stand with feet together and eyes closed, and any deviations from normal are recorded.[1-6] The autonomic nervous system should also be evaluated as summarized in Box 1.8.

The neurological examination as explained above need not be performed in the above-said sequence. Every physician develops his own routine for the examination. However, it should be recorded in a uniform method that begins with mental status followed by cranial nerves, motor system, sensory system, deep tendon reflexes, cerebellar function, gait, and stance, and other signs in that order.

The extent to which a neurological assessment is carried out varies according to the given clinical situation. Examination done in a patient with headache alone is different from that done in a patient who presents with cognitive decline. If a patient is in pain or otherwise unstable, it may be wiser to do a brief examination with focus on the initial area of complaint followed by a more comprehensive assessment later. Similarly, a complete examination may be impossible in a comatose patient. Thus, the examination should be tailored as per the demands of the clinical situation. For patients with minor complaints, it may be better to carry out a rapid screening examination (Box 1.9) rather than a detailed neurological assessment that may be carried out later depending on the results of the screening examination.

ASSESSMENT OF THE SITE OF LESION—ANATOMICAL LOCALIZATION

Anatomical localization means determining from patients symptoms and signs, which site in the neuraxis is affected by the disease in question. The patients' symptoms and signs offer important clues to localization. The initial question is whether the disease is in the brain, spinal cord, peripheral nerve, neuromuscular junction or muscle. Then, an attempt should be made to determine if the disorder is focal, multifocal, or systemic.

The first step in localization is to determine if the site of lesion is in a nucleus or in a tract or in a part of the nervous system. For example, loss of pain, and temperature on one side of the body and other side of the face in association with Horner's syndrome and vagus nerve palsy would localize the site of lesion to lateral medulla. Similarly, a combination of sixth cranial nerve palsy with Horner's syndrome would localize the lesion to the cavernous sinus. A patient, who presents with tingling and paresthesias in both feet will immediately arouses suspicion of peripheral neuropathy. However, if examination reveals hyper-reflexia including brisk ankle jerks, one would think of a lesion in the spinal cord lesion rather than peripheral neuropathy.[1-4,6]

In addition, an attempt should be made to determine if all the symptoms, and signs can arise from a single lesion or there have to be multiple lesions. The principle of parsimony or Occam's razor requires that the physician try to hypothesize one lesion. In clinical practice, at times it is possible to fit all the symptoms into one lesion, at other times, it may not be possible. For example, a patient with bilateral primary optic atrophy, and paraparesis with sensory level on trunk along with slurring of speech is most likely suffering from multifocal disease. In such a patient, further details such as remitting relapsing course would suggest diagnosis of multiple sclerosis.

DIFFERENTIAL DIAGNOSIS

Once the likely site of lesion has been identified, the next step is to formulate differential diagnosis or to generate a list of possible diseases. The most likely causes are listed first depending on specific patient characteristics, sites of nervous system affected, and relative frequency of each disease. Remember the aphorism that uncommon manifestations of common diseases are more common than common manifestations of uncommon diseases. In addition, one should keep diagnoses in the list that if missed could have a significant morbidity. Thus, it is

---

Box 1.10: Occam's Razor

• Though it is strongly recommended to follow principle of parsimony or Occam's razor while determining site of anatomic localization and listing differential diagnoses, remember that nature does not always follow principle of parsimony

---

important to list both the most common diseases and the ominous ones.[1,3]

Even in differential diagnosis, the principle of parsimony or Occam's razor should be followed. For example, a patient with paraparesis of 2-month duration with sensory level who develops sudden onset slurring of speech may be considered to have a small stroke superimposed on a progressive spinal cord lesion. However, according to Occam's razor, one should try to find out a single etiology and on applying this principle the most likely consideration with be a malignancy with both spinal and cranial metastases. However, remember that nature does not always follow the principle of parsimony (Box 1.10).[1,3]

The differential diagnosis generally begins with pathological diagnoses such as stroke, abscess, and neoplasm. However, an attempt should be made to determine the exact etiology. For example, it may be possible to differentiate the type of stroke into embolic, thrombotic, or hemorrhagic based on history and clinical signs. Treatable disorders should always be kept in mind even if they are unlikely. This is especially true when they may mimic a potentially untreatable disorder such as amyotrophic lateral sclerosis.

LABORATORY INVESTIGATIONS AND MANAGEMENT

After the differential diagnosis is enlisted, the clinician carefully chooses appropriate investigations, and formulates a management plan. These aspects will be covered in subsequent chapters in this book and will not be discussed in detail here.

Toward the end, an attempt should be made to ascertain that all the relevant questions have been answered:
1. Is there is neurological problem or in other words does the index patient has a neurological disorder?
2. What is the site(s) of lesion?
3. What is the likely etiology?
4. What are the potential differential diagnoses?
5. What are the relevant investigations and management plan?

Where and why do mistakes occur in clinical practice and what can be done to overcome these?[7]

Despite all the recent advances, it is often surprising how frequently mistakes occur in clinical practice. Some of the commonly given explanations for the decision errors are as follows:

1. The correct diagnosis never crossed my mind.
2. I paid too much attention to an isolated finding of laboratory results.
3. I did not listen enough to the patient's story.
4. I was in too much of a hurry.
5. I did not know enough about the disease.
6. I did not reassess the situation when things did not fit.
7. The patient had too many problems at once.
8. I was influenced by a recent similar case.
9. I could not convince the patient to get further investigations.
10. I was in denial of an upsetting diagnosis (Box 1.11).

The clinical mistakes can occur during the basic history taking or during the examination, while generating the differential diagnosis, while selecting or validating a diagnosis from the list, and finally in formulating the plan of action. In fact, most errors in clinical diagnosis are not due to incompetence or inadequate knowledge but due to frailty of human thinking under conditions of complexity, uncertainty, and time constraints.

In fact, by using simple principles, most of these errors can be avoided at the bedside. Some of these principles are as follows:

Box 1.11: Some of the common causes of bedside mistakes are:

- Ignorance about the disease
- Too much focus on laboratory results
- Not listening properly to history
- A hurried examination
- Not reassessing the clinical situation, even though clinical findings did not fit
- Denial of an upsetting diagnosis
- No performing appropriate laboratory diagnostic tests
- Always remember that aim of clinical evaluation is to manage the patient appropriately and aim of laboratory tests is both to ensure proper management of patient as well as ascertaining that patient does not suffer due to mistakes made by clinician on examination

---

Box 1.12: Some common methods by which clinical errors can be avoided include

- Apply epidemiology: Uncommon manifestations of common diseases are more common than common manifestations of uncommon diseases
- Use principle or parsimony or Occam's razor as described previously
- Use logic: When you hear hoof beats, think of horses and not of zebras
- Use Sutton's law: Go where the money is i.e. favor a diagnosis which explains all the findings and choose the diagnostic tests that are most likely to verify diagnosis

---

1. Apply epidemiology: uncommon manifestations of common diseases are more common than common manifestations of common diseases.
2. Use the principle of parsimony or Occam's razor.
3. Use logic: when you hear hoof beats, think of horses, and not zebras.
4. Use Sutton's law: go where the money is, i.e., favor a diagnosis that explains all the findings and choose the diagnostic tests that are most likely to verify the diagnosis.
5. Treat patients and not numbers (Box 1.12).

REFERENCES

1. Campbell WW. History, physical examination and overview of the neurological examination. In: Campbell WW (Ed). DeJong's the Neurological Examination, 7th edition. New Delhi: Lippincott Williams and Wilkins, South Asian Edition; 2013. pp. 5-46.
2. Lowenstein DH, Martin JB, Hauser SL. Approach to the patient with neurological disease. In: Longo DL, Fauci AS, Kasper DL, Hauser SL, Jameson JL, Loscalezo J (Eds.). Harrison's Principles of Internal Medicine, 18th edition. New York: McGraw-Hill Companies; 2012. pp. 3233-9.
3. Brazis PW, Masdeu JC, Biller J. General principles of neurologic localization. In: Brazis PW, Masdeu JC, Biller J (Eds). Localization in Clinical Neurology, 5th edition. New Delhi: Lippincott Williams and Wilkins, South Asian Edition; 2007. pp. 1-26.
4. Prasad K, Yadav R, Spillane J. Approaching a neurological problem. In: Prasad K, Yadav R, Spillane J (Eds). Bickerstaff's Neurological Examination in Clinical Practice, 7th edition. New Delhi: Wiley India; 2013. pp. 3-5.
5. Daroff RB, Fenichel GM, Jankovic J, Mazziotta JC. Diagnosis of neurological disease. In: Daroff RB, Fenichel GM, Jankovic J, Mazziotta JC (Eds). Bradley's Neurology in Clinical Practice, 6th edition, Vol 1, Principles of diagnosis and management, Philadelphia: Elsevier publishers; 2012. pp. 2-9.
6. Ropper AH, Samuels MA. Approach to the patient with neurologic disease. In: Ropper AH, Samuels MA (Eds). Adams and Victor's Principles of Neurology, 9th edition. New York: McGraw-Hill Companies; 2009. pp. 3-12.
7. Scott IA. Errors in clinical reasoning, causes and remedial strategies. BMJ. 2009;339:22-25.

Chapter 2

Historical Aspects of Neurological Examination

Kalyan B Bhattacharyya

INTRODUCTION

Seldom in any other branch of medicine is clinical information of greater importance than in neurology. A detailed and appropriate inquiry into the problems of the patient, coupled with a thorough, and relevant clinical examination and apposite investigations is of paramount importance for arriving at the etiological, anatomical, and pathological diagnosis of a neurological disorder. Indeed, there is no short-cut approach to diagnose a neurological ailment.

In order to understand the historical evolution of clinical neurology, it should be remembered that the neuroscientists of the earlier generations, who, by their painstaking efforts tried to unravel the mysteries of the structure and functions of the nervous system in the normal and the diseased state, are to be studied in the beginning. In fact, the process of evolution is spread over several centuries.

Though Leonardo da Vinci (1452–1519), the multi-faceted genius of the Renaissance period in Italy, is often accredited with the first description of the structure of the nervous system, the palm goes unhesitatingly to Andreas Vesalius (1514–1564) (Fig. 2.1.1), a professor of anatomy at the university of Padua, Italy, who virtually spent days and nights with corpses, utterly decomposed, and stinking, and as the story goes, even wrote to the local court judge to fix a certain time of the day for execution of convicts so that he could reach there on time to collect the corpses for anatomical dissection.[1,2] His detailed study of the human nervous system did much to do away with the older doctrines of neural spirit, devised at the time of the

Greek physician, Galen (129–200) (Fig. 2.1.2), and it took many centuries to dispel such myths. His classic book, *De humani corporis fabrica*, is universally acknowledged as one of the greatest documents written in the history of medical sciences.[1] Thereafter, Thomas Willis (1621–1675) (Fig. 2.1.3), from England, worked on the anatomy of the circulation in brain and described the circle, named after him and wrote his observations in the magnificent treatise, *Cerebri Anatome* in 1664. Interestingly, Willis got the clue from studying a patient suffering from carcinoma of the stomach whose left carotid artery was occluded and yet he did not suffer from stroke since his right carotid artery was hugely dilated. Willis felt that the two carotid arteries from the two sides must have some sort of communication.[3]

Soon after the microscope was introduced in the 1640s, Antonie van Leeuwenhoek (1632–1723), a Dutch scientist, used it extensively. Thereafter, a variety of stains became available for identifying various cells in the human body. Camillo Golgi (1843–1926) (Fig. 2.1.4), an Italian pathologist, devised the silver stain, and it was profitably put to use by Ramon y Cajal (1852–1934) (Fig. 2.1.5) from Spain.[4] This revolutionized the understanding of the neurocellular microarchitecture and thenceforth emerged the *neuron theory* for which Golgi and Cajal jointly received the Nobel Prize in 1906, in spite of the fact that they did not see eye to eye, and openly debated the relevance of the neuron theory in their Nobel Lectures. Cajal accurately described the distinguishing features of the neuron and the glial cells and characterized their local organizations based on the description and drawings by Golgi. He also perfected Golgi's method of staining, rejected the reticular theory of neural organization by showing the variability of dendritic arborization and axon terminations, established that the free ends of axons make contacts, and conceived the idea that neural impulse is conducted between axons, dendrites, and the cell body of the nearby neurons.[4,5] Many historians believe that Cajal is the most influential neuroscientist of the twentieth century.[3]

The understanding of the functions of the nervous system grew side by side and Thomas Willis felt that muscular contraction was like the explosion of gun powder, whereby new spirits were supplied to the muscles by the circulating blood.[3] William Croone (1633–1684), in *De Ratione Motus Musculorum, postulated* an interaction of spirits from the nerves, and blood agitating the space between the muscle fibers and, therefore, transmitting to them, a force that increased their width, and shortened their length.[3] However, a truly significant advancement in the understanding of neural functions was advanced by Robert Whytt (1714–1766) of Edinburgh, who consolidated the reflex theory, and thus settled once for all, the debate between René Descartes (1596–1650) of France, who described the first reflex in man, the *menace reflex*, and Thomas Willis, who argued about the dependence of the integrity of peripheral nerve plexus for the causation of reflex actions. His experiments on frogs, performed in 1751, established the fact that reflex activity depended on the segmental integrity of the spinal cord, and he also described the pupillary reflex. Charles Bell (1774–1842) (Fig. 2.1.6) of England described the reflex arc but wrongly attributed both the motor and sensory functions to the anterior root, which was corrected by François Magendie (Fig. 2.1.7) from France in 1822, and this doctrine of the anterior and posterior nerve roots carrying motor and sensory impulses, respectively, came to be known as *Bell-Magendie law*.[4] Marshall Hall (1790–1857) (Fig. 2.1.8) from England, coined the term, *reflex arc,* and Hughlings Jackson (1835–1911) (Fig. 2.1.9), universally regarded as the *Father of British Neurology*, provided the organizational principles of cerebral functions. He postulated that in the brain lies a three-layer organizational stratum, the lowest layer carrying out the primitive, and vegetative functions that operate through the spinal reflexes, the second one, like the striatum cortex, and the long tracts controls movements and sensations, while the highest level being the premotor cortex, which provides the components of higher mental functions. He was influenced by the evolutionary theory of Herbert Spencer (1820–1903), the British philosopher, and his views were subsequently studied in detail by

Sigmund Freud (1856–1939), the French neurologist, and psychoanalyst.[7-9] Henry Head (1861–1940) (Fig. 2.1.10), the British neurologist, concluded that function is not localized normally but is dependent on a complex, and complicated network, even though lesions at certain sites lead to some specific deficits.[4,10] Jackson's pronouncements were experimentally studied by David Ferrier (1843–1928), the British physiologist, who by means of electrical stimulation of the primate and canine cortex, and the subsequent clinical developments, concluded that certain areas of the brain do possess defined, and definite functions and lesions resulting from lesions in these areas were largely predictable and reproducible.[4] Charles Sherrington (1857–1952) (Fig. 2.1.11), of Oxford and Liverpool, the co-sharer of the Nobel laureate of 1932 along with Edgar Adrian from Cambridge, was a doyen of neurophysiology, who claimed wordwide fame for his demonstration of the spinal reflex arc and the inhibitory influence of the long tracts in the spinal cord.[4,11] He coined the term, *synapse*, and he stated that nowhere in physiology was the cell theory of paramount importance than in neurosciences. He formulated ideas on the propagation of neural impulse through the synapse, defined afferent and efferent properties of muscles and nerves, and characterized the properties of the tendon stretch reflex. He also introduced the concept of reciprocal innervation of muscles and the final common pathway in the nerves, apart from contributing to the physiology of the postural reflexes. He was appropriately called the *Harvey of Neurology* and his book, *The Integrative Action of the Nervous System,* published in 1905, remains a classic.[11]

In this backdrop, let us now discuss some of the important high watermarks in the historical evolution of clinical neurology.

Despite the fact that Thomas Willis described the cranial nerves, ciliary ganglion, thalamus, lentiform bodies, corpus striatum, and intercostal nerves and distinguished between cerebral and meningeal inflammation, and James Parkinson, in 1817, in his book, *An Essay on the Shaking Palsy*, described the disease that goes by his name, but neither did actually examine the patients. Their accounts were dependent entirely on historical evaluation.[6] Physical examination as a tool for clinical diagnosis came into practice with time and celebrated textbooks were compiled that recorded in detail, systematic clinical signs. The first such book published was by Moritz Heinrich Romberg (1795–1873) (Fig. 2.1.12), of Germany and was entitled, "*Lehrbuch der Nervenkrankheiten des Menschen,*" meaning, *A Manual of Nervous Diseases of Human Beings.* For sixteen long years, he was preoccupied with writing this book, which he conceived long ago, and ultimately it was published in parts, from 1840 to 1846 and three editions were exhausted by 1857. In the preface to this book, he criticized his predecessors for the inadequacy of their contributions, "The blame lies, in a measure, with the distinguished members of our profession who have been deterred by a fear that pathological investigations would fail to cope with the advanced state of physiological inquiry; in others, the fault is to be attributed to that mental indolence that gives the preference to the easy path of tradition, and with foolish skepticism rejects everything that is new".[4,6] William Gowers (1845–1915) (Fig. 2.1.13) of the National Hospital, Queen Square, England, wrote a magnificent book, entitled, "Manual of Diseases of the Nervous System," published in two volumes in 1886 and 1888 and acclaimed universally as *"The Bible of Neurology."* Importantly, Gowers provided line drawings of patients, and pathological specimens in this book and many of the accounts are valid even to this day. It was often said that when in doubt, Gowers only consulted his own manual and nothing else![7] Other compilations were Carl Wernicke's (1848–1905), "Der Aphasische Symptomenkomplex. Eine Psychologische Studie auf Anatomischer Basis" and Hermann Oppenheim's (1858–1919) (Fig. 2.1.14), "Lehrbuch der Nervenkrankheiten für Ärzte und Studierende," both from Germany, and Jules Dejerine's (1849–1917) (Fig. 2.1.15), *Dans les maladies du système nerveux*, from Salpêtrière, France.[6] Wernicke wrote his book when he was only 26 years of age. Samuel Alexander Kinnier Wilson (1878–1937) (Fig. 2.1.16) wrote a magnificent treatise, entitled, "Textbook of Neurology," published posthumously in 1938.[4] Gordon Holmes (1876–1965) (Fig. 2.1.17), of Queen Square, England published a system of examination of the sensory and motor system, cerebellar signs, vision, ocular movements, aphasia, mental state, and the autonomic nervous system in 1946, which is still used by neurologists throughout the world.[6] Lord Walter Russell Brain (1895–1966) (Fig. 2.1.18) of Eynsham wrote a classic in 1933 when he was only 37 years of age, and since 1969, the onus fell on Lord John Walton of Detchant, who ultimately relinquished the charge to Michael Donaghy since 2001.[3] The book is read avidly by neurologists all over the world even today.

The art of clinical examination and the subject of pathological anatomy reached their zenith at the Hôpitaux de Paris, Salpêtrière, in France and the chief architects for this development were Alfred Vulpian (Fig. 2.1.19) and his younger duumvir, Jean Martin

Charcot (1825–1893)[4] (Fig. 2.1.20). The tradition was, thereafter, followed by their legendary pupils like Joseph Babinski (1857–1932) (Fig. 2.1.21), Pierre Marie (1853–1940), Jules Dejerine (1849–1917), Gilles de la Tourette (1857–1904), Sigmund Freud (1856–1939), and others. It is generally felt that Vulpian did not get his due recognition since the imperious and omniscient Charcot had possibly stolen the show. Augusta Dejerine, an estimable neurologist by her own right and the wife of the brilliant Jules Dejerine of Salpêtrière, Paris, recorded how Vulpian demonstrated before her, the extension of the big toe in paraplegics long before Babinski's description of this extraordinary sign.[4] JMS Pearce, the noted medical historian from Leeds, United Kingdom, wrote in the *Journal of Neurology, Neurosurgery and Psychiatry* in 2002 that,

"The name of Charcot has outstripped all other distinguished founders of contemporary neurology whose development can be traced to the Salpêtrière. Yet, even a cursory reading of Vulpian's texts shows that none exceeded him in brilliance, originality and meticulous clinical prowess".[4]

Patrick Jucker-Kupper from Switzerland felt that Vulpian was perhaps even more learned than his great friend Charcot, an experimenter and a fine teacher, though somewhat retiring and restrained and, therefore, greatly overshadowed by the latter.[4] Walter Freeman, from California, the United States of America, wrote,

"How much of Vulpian there was in Charcot's achievements, is hard to know, given their daily cooperation... Vulpian's influence upon his many followers in several fields of knowledge made him the intellectual leader of his day and his probity and kindness were much revered."[4]

However, Charcot has, quite justifiably, been labeled as the "Father of Clinical Neurology" and his seminal works like, Charcot's triad in multiple sclerosis, Charcot-Bouchard aneurysm, Charcot's joint in syringomyelia and other conditions, description of Charcot–Marie–Tooth disease and Charcot's disease or motor neuron disease, and a myriad other conditions attest to the versatility of his genius and unparalleled clinical acumen. Later, the name of Joseph Juan Felix Francois Babinski, possibly the most gifted student of Charcot, illumined the field of clinical neurology for ages to follow, for the description of a superficial reflex that remains unequivocally, the most incontrovertible clinical sign of pyramidal tract dysfunction. His description of the "plantar reflex" shall be discussed in some detail when we shall examine the evolution in the understanding of human reflexes[4,12] (Fig. 2.2).

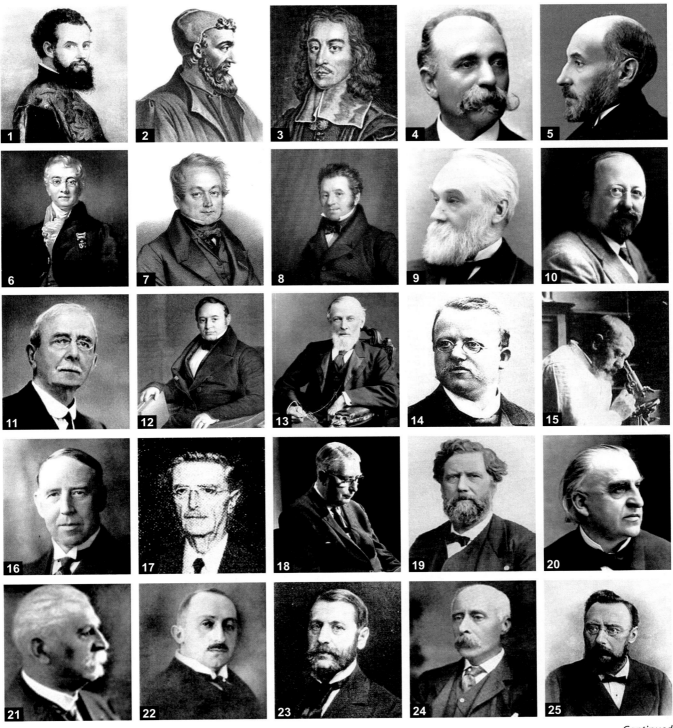

Continued

Continued

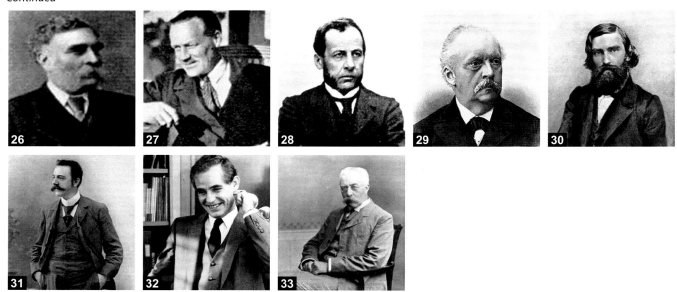

Figs 2.1.1 to 33: Pioneers in neurology. **(1)** Andreas Vesalius (1514–1564); **(2)** Galen (129–200); **(3)** Thomas Willis (1621–1675); **(4)** Camillo Golgi (1843–1926); **(5)** Ramon Y Cajal (1852–1934); **(6)** Charles Bell (1774–1842); **(7)** Francois Megendie (1822); **(8)** Marshall Hall (1790–1857); **(9)** Hughlings Jackson (1835–1911); **(10)** Henry Head (1861–1940); **(11)** Charles Sherrington (1857–1952); **(12)** Moritz Heinrich Romberg (1795–1873); **(13)** William Gowers (1845–1915); **(14)** Hermann Oppenheim (1858–1919); **(15)** Jules Dejerine (1849–1917); **(16)** Samuel Alexander Kinnier Wilson (1878–1937); **(17)** Gordon Holmes (1876–1965); **(18)** Lord Walter Russell Brain (1895–1966); **(19)** Alfred Vulpian; **(20)** Jean Martin Charcot (1825–1893); **(21)** Joseph Babinski (1857–1932); **(22)** Ludwig Edinger (1855–1918); **(23)** Carl Westphal (1833–1890); **(24)** Robert Marcus Gunn (1850–1909); **(25)** Johann Friedrich Horner (1831–1896); **(26)** Douglas Marie Cooper Lamb; **(27)** William John Adie (1886–1935); **(28)** Henri Perinaud (1844–1905); **(29)** Ferdinand von Helmholtz (1821–1894); **(30)** Albrecht von Graefe (1828–1870); **(31)** Van Gehuchten (1861–1914); **(32)** Charles David Marsden (1938–1999); **(33)** Adolph Strumpell (1853–1925).

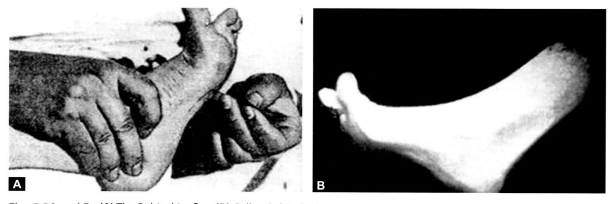

Figs 2.2A and B: (A) The Babinski reflex; **(B)** Collier Babinski sign.

CLINICAL NEUROLOGY AND CRANIAL NERVES

Reference to the cranial nerves first appears in the rudimentary remains of the writings of Herophilus (335–280 BC) of Greece, often deemed to be the first anatomist, and his close associate Eristratus (304–250 BC), although it is doubted if they believed in the continuity between the cranial nerves, spinal cord, and the brain.[6] Rufus of Ephesus, Greece, in the first century AD, first conceived of this continuity, but it was left to Claudius Galen in the second century, to comment on the structure and function of cranial nerves described in his series of 15 volumes, "On Anatomic Procedures." He identified seven pairs of cranial nerves, the optic, oculomotor, sensory, and motor parts of the trigeminal, facial-vestibulocochlear, glossopharyngeal-vagus-accessory, and the hypoglossal. It is possible that the trigeminal motor root that he described could actually be the abducent nerve or the combined trochlear–abducent nerve. The trochlear nerve was possibly described by Alessandro Achillini (1463–1512), from Italy, while Gabriele Fallopius (1523–1562) from the same country, identified the trochlear, and the abducent nerves separately. Thomas Willis of England identified 10 pairs of cranial nerves of which the first 6 conform to the present day terminology.[1,6] He felt that the seventh nerve was the facial-vestibulocochlear, the eighth was the glossopharyngeal-vagus-accessory, and the tenth was the first cervical nerve. Samuel Thomas von Sömmering (1755–1830) of Germany separated the facial nerve from the vestibulocochlear nerve, and the glossopharyngeal and the vagus from the spinal accessory, and excluded the first cervical nerve from the list.[6] Fallopius gave a detailed account of the innervation of oculomotor nerve in 1561 in his treatise, *Observationes Anatomicae*, and identified the innervation of the superior rectus, inferior rectus, medial rectus, inferior oblique, and the levator palpebrae superioris muscles.[1,2,6] He also described the termination of the abducent nerve, while his predecessor, Realdo Colombo (1516–1559) who took over from the immortal Andreas Vesalius described the innervation of the superior oblique by the trochlear nerve. Charles Bell demonstrated the precise anatomy of the facial nerve for the first time and separated its motor root from the sensory part. Capavacci, a physician in Padua, Italy, differentiated between nerve deafness and conductive deafness; and the modern tuning fork was devised by the flutist, John Shore from England, in 1711.[6] In 1546, Giovanni Filippo Ingrassia (1510–1580) of Italy discovered bone conduction by observing that if the vibrating tuning fork was pressed against the teeth, it could be heard. Air and bone conduction were compared by Friedrich Rinne (1863–1933) of Freiburg, Germany, in 1864.[1,6]

Visual acuity has been studied over ages. The Persian scientists described the concept of *minimum separabile*, that is, the minimal distance required between two dots to be perceived by the eyes as separate.[6] In the nineteenth century, the Viennese physician Eduard Jaeger Ritter von Jaxthal (1818–1884) published a chart of various rows of numbers of increasing size, known even to this day as the *Jaeger Chart*. Franciscus Cornelis Donders (1818–1889), the Dutch professor of physiology at Utrecht but also interested in ophthalmology, summoned Hermann Snellen (1834–1908), the ophthalmologist, who took over from Donders, to work further on this issue, and Snellen published his observations in a book in 1862, which contained the chart named after him.[6]

The pupillary reflex was extensively studied by Robert Whytt (1714–1766) of Edinburgh, Scotland, and he described a hydrocephalic child with fixed pupils that did not react to light.[4,11] He had been suffering from a cyst compressing the lateral geniculate body and Whytt concluded that fibers subserving the route for the light reflex were interrupted. He also described the pupillary changes on accommodation. In 1885, Ludwig Edinger (1855–1918) (Fig. 2.1.22) of Frankfurt, Germany, identified that the midbrain was involved in the mediation of the light reflex and Carl Westphal (1833–1890) (Fig. 2.1.23), his colleague from Berlin, confirmed this observation in 1887 and the nucleus has been assigned the name, *Edinger-Westphal nucleus*.[4,6] Robert Marcus Gunn (1850–1909) (Fig. 2.1.24), the Scottish ophthalmologist, described the afferent pupillary defect in 1902 and wrote,

"The eye must also be kept under direct stimulation of light and the pupil watched as to whether or not it shows that secondary dilatation under continued exposure that is found associated with the amblyopia of retro-ocular neuritis."[6]

Johann Friedrich Horner (1831–1896) (Fig. 2.1.25) from Zurich, Switzerland, described the eponymous syndrome in 1869 by observing incomplete ptosis in a 40-year-old lady. He wrote:

"Lacking the usual accompanying signs of oculomotor paralysis... the upper lid covers the right cornea to the upper edge of the pupil... The pupil of the right eye is considerably more constricted than that of the left, but reacts to light... the right side of her face became red and warm... while the left side remained pale and cool... the right side had never perspired."

Douglas Marie Cooper Lamb Argyll Robertson (1837–1909) (Fig. 2.1.26), the handsome Scottish ophthalmologist with a demure walk and a gray frock-coat and the cynosure of all ladies, described the pupil, immortalized after his name, in five patients. William John Adie (1886–1935) (Fig. 2.1.27), the Australia-born neurologist, who worked most of the time in Queen Square, London, and was associated with Sir Gordon Homes, his mentor, described meiosis and absent tendon reflexes in 15 patients.[4,6] Henri Parinaud

(1844–1905) (Fig. 2.1.28), the ophthalmologist with Charcot at Salpêtrière, Paris, realized that the center for disorders of conjugate eye movements must be located centrally. In a paper published in the journal *Brain* in 1925, he described in great detail the condition that goes by his name.[6] Bernhard Kayser (1869–1954), a German ophthalmologist from Tübingen, described the corneal ring in Wilson's disease in 1902, 10 years before Samuel Alexander Kinnier Wilson published his monumental paper in the journal *Brain*.[6,7] Initially, he felt that it was a congenital abnormality. Then, Bruno Fleischer (1874–1965) another ophthalmologist from Stuttgart, Germany, again observed the ring in 1903. The ring that he described goes by the name, "butcher's ring," presumably because Fleischer was appointed as a butcher's assistant in the department of ophthalmology in 1909.[6] Kinnier Wilson, however, thought it to be a highly inconsistent sign.[4,7]

The invention of the ophthalmoscope is, in general, attributed to Hermann Ludwig Ferdinand von Helmholtz (1821–1894) (Fig. 2.1.29) of Berlin, Germany. Albrecht von Graefe 1828–1870) (Fig. 2.1.30), also from Germany, was the first physician to apply this instrument in his clinical practice.[4,6] William Gowers from England wrote a classic monogram, *A Manual and Atlas of Medical Ophthalmoscopy*, and he used the instrument extensively in the wards of the National Hospital for the Paralyzed and the Epileptic, Queen Square.[4,7] His mentor, John Hughlings Jackson took profound interest in ophthalmoscopy and examined many patients in the famous Moorefield Eye Hospital in London.[7] Gower's book ran into several editions and he stated that the ophthalmoscopy is of use to the physician because it gives information, often not otherwise obtainable, regarding the existence of disease elsewhere than in the eyes.[13] Robert Foster-Kennedy (1884–1952), an associate of Gowers, with the aid of the ophthalmoscope first described a syndrome that goes by his name.[4,5]

CLINICAL EXAMINATION FOR SENSORY SYSTEM

In 1838, Johannes Müller (1808–1858), an outstanding physiologist from Germany, formulated the idea of "specific energy" and "specific irritability" and stated that the same stimulus could produce different sensations if it was applied to nerves supplying different sensory modalities.[4,5] Henry Head (1861–1940) of England, suggested that there were two specialized types of cutaneous sensory nerves and formulated the concept of "specific fiber theory."[4-6] He defined "epicritic"

and "protopathic" sensibility and postulated that the former was concerned with fine discrimination of touch and temperature sensation and had localizing ability, whereas the latter, detected changes in temperature and pressure, without the ability to localize any abnormality. Van Gehuchten (1861–1914) (Fig. 1.1.31) of Belgium, in a case of syringomyelia, observed that pain and temperature sensations were impaired though fine touch was preserved and this led to the hypothesis that there were two different pathways for sensation, one travelling anterolaterally in the spinal cord, while the other was placed posteriorly.[6] In 1826, Charles Bell of England, alluded to the existence of "*a sixth sense*," which later was recognized as the proprioceptive function.[6]

Charles-Edouard Brown-Séquard (1817–1894), the first physician appointed to Queen Square, London, in 1860, described a classic syndrome that goes by his name. In patients with injury to the spinal cord, he observed that there was dissociation of sensory loss in these subjects. There was loss of pain and temperature in the contralateral side, whereas position and vibration sense were impaired in the ipsilateral side.[4-6] Jean-Martin Charcot, the first ever professor of neurology, tested cutaneous pain sensation by pin-prick, pinching or by electrical stimulation of the skin, and developed a temperature perception device by utilizing a heated thermometer on the skin.[6] Charles Scott Sherrington created dermatomal maps of the peripheral nerves in monkeys, while Henry Head studied the same in man, particularly by observing the distribution of the rash in herpes zoster. Interestingly, he was frustrated at the inconsistent answers from patients' observations and severed his own superficial radial nerve in order to study its distribution and the subsequent changes with time.[4-6] Otfried Foerster (1873–1971), the neurosurgeon from Germany and famed for carrying out rhizotomy and anterolateral cordotomy for the relief of intractable pain also contributed towards the understanding of the dermatomal concept of sensory system by observing the effects of injury in soldiers at the time of the World War I. Gordon Holmes utilized the pin prick test proximally and distally for localization of the lesion.[4]

William Gowers provided a detailed description of the clinical examination of the sensory system for the first time in his classic book, "A Manual of Diseases of the Nervous System." However, there was no account of examination of the vibration sense in his treatise. By 1920, four functions were being tested at bed-side, namely, tactile sensibility, temperature sensation, pain sensation and deep sensibility. Gowers wrote:

"In examining the tactile sensibility, it is important to ascertain, not only whether the patient can feel, but whether he is able to recognize the place touched, whether he can correctly localize the sensation… It may be tested by prick or pinch. For a prick, too fine a point must not be used not only because a sharp point may inflict a needless wound, but because, in the less sensitive part of the skin, where the terminal nerve plexus is wide, a fine point may here or there be unfelt, although it penetrates the skin. Hence a somewhat blunt point should be employed."[13]

For testing temperature sensation, most examiners used metallic substances, since they were good conductors of heat. Gowers wrote that for coarse examination, hot and cold spoons were excellent tools whereas, to detect the power of differential discrimination, test tubes containing water would be the ideal substance.[6] As already stated, Charcot used a thermometer to detect temperature sensation, and he showed that patients with epilepsy suffered from raised cutaneous temperature while hysterical subjects could sustain several clinical attacks in a single day without such elevation.[6] Two-point discrimination was first used by Ernst Heinrich Weber (1795–1878), a German physiologist. He wrote a book in 1846, entitled, "Handwoerterbuch der Physiologies" and he described the use of a compass for this test.[6] Additionally, he described the concept of "just noticeable difference" (JND) and worked with discrimination of weights, in which case, JND is the minimum amount of difference between two weights necessary to tell them apart. This was later named, *"Weber's law."*[1,2,6] Later, in 1927, Gordon Holmes described the use of the compass for the diagnosis of cortical lesions causing sensory loss. He wrote about a case:

"On the dorsum of the left foot she was always correct when the points were separated by 3 cm, but on the right foot she frequently failed to recognize them, even when they were 5 cm apart."

In 1889, Heinrich Theodor Rumpf (1851–1923) from Germany used the tuning fork for testing vibration sense in the limbs.[6] Vibration sense was not considered valid till the early years of the twentieth century, when it was generally agreed that it was a separate and distinct sensory function of the brain and the loss of vibration sense was referred to as *pallanesthesia*. Soon, the test made its appearance in textbooks like, Max Lewandowsky's (1876–1916) *Handbook of Neurology* and Robert Bing's (1878–1956) *Compendium of Regional Diagnosis* and the loss of vibration sense was referred to as *pallanesthesia*. Later, in

1927, Gordon Holmes described the use of the compass on cortical lesions that caused sensory loss by studying two cases of endotheliomas of the falx and in one case of glioma where the compass test was the only positive diagnostic test.[6]

In the 1970s, Peter Dyck and his colleagues developed another method for testing sensation by using an automated system to test touch, pressure, vibration and thermal sensation. The system had 21 stimulus levels and scoring was by computer analysis. However, the system did not find widespread acceptance.[6,14]

In the 19th and the 20th century it was felt that lesions in the posterior columns of the spinal cord, rather than the spinothalamic tract would impair tactile sensibility and lesion in the posterior and lateral columns would completely abolish tactile sensation. Additionally, it was erroneously felt that the pyramidal tract and other descending pathways played a role in the production of pain. Pinprick testing during this time provided an excellent way for localizing pain and this led Joseph Erlanger and Herbert Gasser to perform localized nerve blocks and much of the knowledge garnered from nerve blocking contributed to the development of the concept of local anesthesia.[4,5]

CLINICAL EXAMINATION FOR POSTURAL INSTABILITY

In the first half of the nineteenth century, European physicians described the loss of postural impairment in darkness in patients with disturbed proprioception. Later, this sign universally came to be known as the "Romberg's sign," although Moritz Heinrich Romberg was not the first neurologist to describe the sign. Balance is maintained by a coordinated combination of vision, proprioceptive sensation, vestibular input, intact cerebellar control, and sensory input from the cervical bones and ligaments. In case of loss of one of these components, the body can compensate for the deficiency and postural instability is not observed. However, if two or three of these inputs are compromised, the subject reels or sways from side to side and eventually falls. This is the basis of the phenomenon, *Romberg's sign*, where the posterior column, subserving the proprioceptive sensations, is jeopardized, and on closing the eyes, the patient falls like a log of wood. Marshall Hall, more renowned for the formulation of the concept of the reflex arc, described this phenomenon in his book, "Lectures on the Nervous System," published in 1831 and he wrote:

"I have seen this day a patient with a slight degree of paralysis of feeling and of voluntary motion of the lower limbs. He walks safely while his eyes are fixed upon the ground, but stumbles immediately if he attempts to work in the dark. His own words are, "my feet are numb; I cannot tell in the dark where they are, and I cannot poise myself."[5]

Hall recognized that proprioception, as well as vision, were important for postural control and vision could partially compensate for inadequate proprioceptive sensation.[4] Furthermore, he felt that in darkness, where vision was impaired, postural control was grossly impaired. However, Hall did not pursue this observation further and did not use it as a clinical test for diagnosing proprioceptive pathology. It was left to Romberg in 1851, who in the second edition of the classic "Lehrbook der Nervenkrankheiten des Menschen," in 1851, drew attention to this phenomenon in patients with tabes dorsalis. He worked on Hall's observation and devised the famous clinical test that goes by his name. He wrote,

"Lässt man ihn in aufrechter Stellung die Augen schliessen, so fängt er sofort an zu schwanken und zu taumeln….,"

which almost literally means that "If he is ordered to close his eyes while in the erect posture, he at once commences to totter or swing from side to side; the insecurity of his gait also exhibits itself more in the dark."[5] In the English translation of his book by Edward Sieveking in 1853, it reads,

"If the patient is told to shut his eyes while in the erect posture, he immediately begins to move from side to side, and the oscillations soon attain such a pitch that unless supported he falls to the ground… The eyes of such patients are their regulators, or feelers; consequently in the dark… the helplessness is extreme."[5]

He further added:

"… the patient has the sensation as if they were covered with a fur… he does not feel the tread to be firm, he puts down his heels with greater force. From the commencement of the disease the individual keeps his eyes on his feet to prevent his movements from becoming still more unsteady. If he is ordered to close his eyes while in the erect posture, he at once commences to totter and swing from side to side; the insecurity of his gait also exhibits itself more in the dark."[5]

Bernardus Brach, another German physician in the nineteenth century, described similar symptoms in 1840. He wrote:

"It is known that people with tabes dorsalis have unusual gait…While other paralytics drag their legs, a patient with tabes dorsalis lifts his leg with a straight knee… With fearful eyes he watches his every step. With tests such as cold and warm, pressure, pinching, scratching with a needle tip, or a hair, the patients responded just like a healthy person. Thus, one cannot say that they do not have any sensation."[5]

William Alexander Hammond (1828–1900), working in New York, wrote the first ever textbook of neurology from the United States of America in 1871 entitled "A Treatise on Diseases of the Nervous System" and gave an account of tabes dorsalis. He emphasized the absence of weakness of the limbs in this condition and wrote about the significance of distinguishing tabes dorsalis from cerebellar pathology by applying this sign.[5,15] William Osler (1849–1919), while working at the University of Philadelphia, wrote his celebrated textbook, "The Principles and Practice of Medicine" in 1892 and described the importance of Romberg's "symptom" for diagnosing tabes dorsalis and also mentioned the presence of muscle power in this condition. William Gowers also alluded to this sign in his classic textbook, "A Manual of Diseases of the Nervous System."[5,13] However, there is no consensus on certain matters pertaining to this sign. There is no unanimous agreement on what should be considered a positive test like, increased sway, a step to the side, fall, and the like. It is not clear whether the hands should be kept by the side or extended forward. The position of the feet like, as close as possible, in tandem position, use of footwear, is also debated. Later neurologists used terms like, exaggerated Romberg's sign, where the patient stands on one leg, or sharpened Romberg's sign, where the patient stands on his toes or stands on foam rubber to further reduce proprioceptive input from the feet. It has also been suggested that Romberg's sign may be positive in involvement of spinocerebellum and bilateral vestibular nerve pathology.[5] And lastly, it is worth remembering that though William Osler referred to Romberg's "symptom," another condition goes by the name, "Romberg-Howship symptom," a variety of referred pain to the knee joint due to a compressive lesion in the groin, usually an inguinal hernia, which presses upon the obturator nerve. The pathogenesis is explained by the fact that the obturator nerve pierces the popliteal fascia and ends by supplying the cruciate ligaments of the knee joint.[4]

TESTING THE CEREBELLAR FUNCTIONS

Luigi Rolando (1773–1831), the Italian anatomist from the University of Turin, first indicated that following a lesion in the cerebellum, consciousness was retained, and involuntary movements do not appear. He further noted that partial removal of the median lobe of cerebellum leads an animal to sway from side to side.[5] Marie-Jean-Pierre Flourens (1794–1867), the French physiologist, ablated the cerebellum of a pig and a dog and found that they tended to be clumsy and fell frequently. Flourens hypothesized that cerebellum was responsible for regular and coordinated movements.[4,5] John Call Dalton (1825–1889), the American physiologist, removed part of the cerebellum of pigeons and observed that the degree of in-coordination was proportional to the amount of tissue lost. He further noted that with time, the pigeons recovered if the medulla was kept intact. He sacrificed the pigeons later and found that there was no growth of cerebellum that could have accounted for the improvement in functions and, therefore, he concluded that the remaining portion of the cerebellum could make up for the lost functions.[5]

William Alexander Hammond, the celebrated American neurologist, developed criteria for distinguishing locomotor ataxia from cerebellar ataxia. He said that the movements of a patient of a cerebellar disorder were like that of a drunken person, whereas in posterior column involvement they were jerky, and exaggerated. He further stated that in cerebellar lesions, the sensation remained unimpaired, while in locomotor ataxia, loss of position, vibration, and temperature sensation were consistent features. He recorded features like titubation, muscle weakness, uncertain gait, festination, broad-based gait, and optic atrophy in a patient of cerebellar tumor. He observed that staggering gait was due to lesion of the vermis and believed that nystagmus was a constant sign in cerebellar diseases.[6] William Richard Gowers of England also noticed reeling and swaying of the trunk in midline lesions of the cerebellum. He also noticed that in lesions of the middle cerebellar peduncle, the eyes assumed an abnormal position, one being at a lower plane than the other.[13] Charles Karsner Mills (1845–1933), an American neurologist and famed for his book, *The Nervous System and Its Diseases*, observed that lesions in the anterior vermis led to fall backward, while the reverse was true for posterior lesions.[15] Joseph François Felix Babinski of Paris, France described *dysdiadochokinesia* in 1902 and later, in 1933, introduced the term *asynergia*.[4]

One of the leading figures in the study of cerebellar disorders was Gordon Morgan Holmes of England, who spent most of his life in the hallowed precincts of Queen Square, London. He served in the battlefields of France during World War I and came across many soldiers with traumatic lesions in the cerebellum. He wrote:

"The opportunity of making uncomplicated clinical observations is rare in civil life, since acute lesions of the cerebellum comparable with those produced by physiologists are uncommon; …In warfare, wounds limited to the cerebellum and injuries of it … can be frequently observed."[6]

Holmes noted that acute lesions of the cerebellum led to ipsilateral hypotonia and the speed of movement was also lessened. Grainger Stewart (1877–1957) along with his resident physician, in 1904, described the *rebound phenomenon,* and later in the same year described *rubral tremor.* He also wrote on the direction of the fast component of nystagmus and adduced proof for dysdiadochokinesia in his famed Croonian lecture on the functions of the cerebellum. He further confirmed the observation of Robert Bárány (1876–1936) that if the arms are outstretched and the eyes closed, the limbs ipsilateral to the side of the lesion will deviate toward that side. By using a kymograph, he showed that the affected limb fell faster when outstretched than the other one.[6]

Following World War II, Harry Boterell (1906–1997), the neurosurgeon from Canada and John Fulton (1899–1960), the neurophysiologist from Harvard, USA, provided experimental evidence of the signs produced by cerebellar lesions. By ablating one half of the neocerebellum they could provide evidence for ipsilateral hypotonia, gait disturbance, and fall to the same side. If the dentate nucleus was damaged, unilateral limb tremor, and ataxia were observed.[6] Importantly, these features disappeared with time, and thus the view held by John Call Dalton that recovery with time was the rule, was further vindicated. That the cerebellum has a role to play in cognition is a later development, though Gordon Holmes, and others had hinted at this association long ago. This has been explained by the extensive connections between the cerebellum and the frontal and parietal lobes and many patients with degenerative cerebellar ataxia display various degrees of cognitive decline.

CLINICAL EXAMINATION OF REFLEXES

René Descartes (1596–1650) of France who spent the major part of his life in Holland, described the first reflex in man, the *menace reflex*, often known as *Descartes reflex*, and he felt that the seat of the reflex was in the pineal gland.[10] Stephen Hales (1677–1761) of England first indicated the spinal origin of reflex by being able to elicit the action following pinching the skin of decapitated frogs and showed that it disappeared following resection of the spinal cord.[11] Robert Whytt of Edinburgh, Scotland, confirmed the spinal nature of reflex, and described the light reflex. Marshall Hall of England described the gag reflex and introduced the terms *reflex and nervous arc.*[11] Charles Scott Sherrington of Oxford, England, introduced the term *stretch reflex* and advanced the theory of final common pathway in the mediation of the reflex.[4,12] Much later, Charles David Marsden (1938–1999) (Fig. 1.1.32) of England carried out an elegant experiment in 1973 and showed that at least the upper limb reflexes had a cortical component. He showed that the longer latency of the biceps jerk, as compared to the knee jerk, could be reduced if the spinal cord was transected at the cervical level. This indicates a transcortical component to the biceps jerk and this was a considerable departure from the classical Sherringtonian concept that deep tendon reflexes are mediated through the spinal cord and that they are monosynaptic in nature.[4,18]

Two reflexes, one superficial, and one deep, deserve some detailed discussion. On the 22nd of February, 1896, Joseph Juan Felix Francois Babinski from Paris, France, presented a paper before the "Société de Biologié titled", "phenomenon des orteils," simply meaning "phenomenon of the great toe." Later, his publication ran into 28 lines only. It reads:

> On the cutaneous plantar reflex in certain organic disorders of the nervous system,
>
> I have observed that in a certain number of cases of hemiplegia or lower limb monoplegia, related to an organic disorder of the central nervous system, there is a disturbance of the cutaneous plantar reflex that I shall describe in a few words.
>
> On the healthy side, pricking of the sole provokes.flexion of the thigh on the pelvis, of the leg on the thigh, of the foot on the leg, and of the toes upon the metatarsus.
>
> On the paralyzed side, the toes instead of flexing execute a movement of extension upon the metatarsus.
>
> I have also observed that in paraplegia due to organic lesion of the spinal cord, an extensor movement of the toes occurs following a pinprick in the sole.
>
> In summary, the reflex movements following a pinprick in the sole of the foot may, in paralysis of the lower limbs, be attributable to an organic disorder of the central nervous system.[4,16]

Babinski's own photograph demonstrated the sign appeared first in the medical literature in 1900, while James Collier (1870–1935), of the Institute of Neurology, Queen Square, London, and famed for first providing evidence for false localizing signs in cerebral disorders,

published the first photograph of Babinski's sign in the celebrated English journal *Brain* in 1902 and called it "extensor plantar reflex."[16] Charles Gilbert Chaddock (1861–1936) demonstrated the same sign in the United States of America in 1911,[4] and with the passage of time, many eminent neurologists started describing various alternative methods of scratching or pressing other areas in the lower limb in order to see the great toe going up. However, as written by van Gijn, an estimable medical historian, who wrote an incomparable treatise at the time of the centenary year of Babinski's description of *Phenomenon des Orteils*, the often discussed fanning of the toes while eliciting plantar response was, in fact, demonstrated by Dupré, and thus, it was wrongly attributed to Babinski, though others still maintain that this sign also was described by him (*signe de l'éventail*).[16] Babinski published his observations in "Semaine Medicale" in 1898 with accounts of cases of hemiplegia, Jacksonian epilepsy and strychnine poisoning and also explained its significance in detail. He concluded that the sign was to be explained by affection of the pyramidal tract and he also noticed that it was found in healthy infants as well. He further wrote that the sign did not appear in hysteria and thus elicitation of this sign could differentiate the two conditions.[16]

It is worth remembering that the phenomenon of upgoing toe was known long before Babinski described it and van Gijn and Peter Ziffling gave excellent accounts of its chronological evolution.[4,16] Additionally, an admirable account of the Babinski response, entitled, '*The Babinski Response: A Review and New Observations*' has been written by P W Nathan and M C Smith from Queen Square, London, which appeared in the *Journal of Neurology Neurosurgery and Psychiatry* in 1955.[4,20] Alfred Vulpian had observed the same feature in certain types of brain damage almost fifty years ago and even demonstrated it before his pupil, Auguste Marie Klumpe.[4] Furthermore, this was adequately depicted in the paintings in the medieval age, Renaissance and Baroque period, while the Raphael's painting of Christ in the arms of Madonna incontrovertibly shows the upgoing great toe.[21] Carl Wernicke from Germany reported it in hemiparetic conditions in 1874, Adolph Strümpell (1853–1925) (Fig. 2.1.33), again from Germany in amyotrophic lateral sclerosis in 1876 and Robert Remak (1815–1865), a Polish-German, observed it in cases of transverse myelitis in 1893, though none wrote anything about its significance. Hermann Oppenheim from Germany challenged the importance of the reflex and stated that in spite of his recognizing the reflex, he did not attach much importance to it, since he felt that it was too inconsistent to be of any clinical value; on the contrary, he demonstrated that pressing the anterior border of tibia downwards, one could elicit the same response, which goes by his name. Van Gehuchten of Belgium however, independently published his observations on this reflex and Babinski sent him a piquant letter claiming his primacy in regard to its description. Gehuchten, in his magnanimity, accepted Babinski's view and in his graciousness, preferred to call it 'Babinski reflex'. For some unknown reasons, in the Netherlands the reflex is known as the 'Plantar response according to Strümpell'.[17]

Charles Gilbert Chaddock's contribution needs some detailed description. In 1911, he read his paper, entitled, "A preliminary communication concerning a new diagnostic nervous sign," where he said,

"I have found the extension of one or more or all the toes with or without fanning of them when the external inframalleolar skin is irritated in cases of organic disease is a spinal cortical reflex path. I shall call it the external malleolar sign."[4,16]

The few issues where Chaddock, in a way, outshone Babinski include his demonstration that in unilateral lesions also, one could observe both the great toes moving upward on scratching, most probably due to involvement of uncrossed corticospinal fibers, innervating the lateral aspect of the foot and the sign described by him appeared and persisted, even when Babinski's sign could no longer be elicited. Withdrawal responses were also less frequently observed. And importantly, he described an equivalent sign in the upper extremity as well. He propounded that stimulating the ulnar side of palmaris longus or flexor carpi radialis led to the rather abnormal response of wrist flexion with the fingers spreading in involvement of the corticospinal tract. Incidentally, Babinski acknowledged his description of the alternate sign though he never mentioned this reflex in his later works.[16] However, it is on record that Kisaku Yoshimura (1879–1945) from Japan alluded to this sign much earlier in 1906.[4] Babinski's observations were later verified by experiments in chimpanzees by John Fulton (1899–1960) of United States of America and Eric Kugelberg (1913–1983) from Sweden.[4]

The tendon hammer was first devised by Ernst Trömner (1868–1930) from Germany.[1] Many modifications of the hammer exist that often go by the names of Taylor, Queen Square, Babinski, and Buck. The significance of the patellar tendon reflex was identified more or less at the time by two German neurologists, Wilhelm Heinrich Erb (1840–1921) and Carl Friedrich Otto Westphal (1833–

1890).[4,6] Interestingly, Erb sent his paper to *Archiv für Psychiatrie und Nervenkrankheiten* for publication and it was being reviewed by Karl Westphal who, along with Bernhard von Gudden (1824–1886) and Theodor Meynert (1833–1892), was the editor of the journal at that time.[4,6] Both Westphal and Erb published their work in the same January 1875 issue of the journal, where Westphal wrote the editorial. Westphal used the term *"the lower limb phenomenon,"* while Erb called it "patellar tendon reflex." Westphal wrote:[4,6]

"During the preparation of this essay for publication, I received the preceding manuscript of Professor Erb. To my surprise, I saw that my honored friend was reporting facts that, in part, were virtually identical to those to be published by myself."

Since then, the phenomenon is known as *Erb-Westphal symptom*. Westphal further wrote that he had been aware of the reflex since 1871 and Erb noticed it in 1870 and that the account provided by Erb was in greater detail. He wrote:

"In 1871, a patient who consulted me because of motor weakness in a leg and certain cerebral symptoms informed me that, when he sat on a chair and lightly tapped the area below the knee cap of that affected leg, it moved forward with a sudden jerk. Because the complaints of the patient were sometimes difficult to interpret, one might have been inclined to regard this peculiar symptom as the outcome of hypochondriacal imagination. However, I easily convinced myself that I was dealing here with a phenomenon that had nothing to do with imagination and which could not be duplicated in the other leg."[4,6]

This is in short, the story of the growth and evolution of the subject of clinical neurology. We often marvel at the percipience and perspicacity of the minds of the great masters of the past who burning the midnight oil and toiling hard went on bravely expanding the mental horizons of our knowledge of neuroscience. And we, the torchbearers, simply carry forward the message they have left for us.

REFERENCES

1. www.wikipidea.com
2. www.whonamedit.com
3. Michael Donaghy (Ed). Brain's Diseases of the Nervous System. Oxford University Press. 12th edition, 2009.
4. Bhattacharyya KB. Eminent neuroscientists: their lives and works. Academic Publishers. 2011.
5. Webb Haymaker, Francis Schilller (Eds). Founders of Neurology. Charles C Thomas, 1970.
6. Elan D Louis (Ed). Seminars in Neurology. The Neurological Examination (with an emphasis on the Historical Underpinnings). Thieme Medical Publishers, Inc. New York, USA. 2002.

7. Wilson SAK. Neurology. Edward Arnold & Co, London, Vol I. 1940.

8. Queen Square and the National Hospital (1860-1960). Edward Arnold Publishers Ltd.

9. Firkin BG, Whiteworth JA (Eds). Medical Eponyms. Pub: The Parthenon Publishing Group Ltd, UK, 1987.

10. William Pryse-Phillips (Ed). Companion to Clinical Neurology. Oxford University Press, 2003.

11. F Clifford Rose (Ed). A Short History of Neurology. The British Contribution. Butterworth-Heinemann, Linacre House, Jordan Hill, Oxford, UK, 1999.

12. F Clifford Rose (Ed). Twentieth Century Neurology. The British Contribution. Imperial College Press, Covent Garden, London, UK. 2001.

13. Gowers WR. Manual of diseases of the nervous system. London. J & K Churchill. 1888.

14. Stephen Ashwal (Ed). Founders of Child Neurology. Norman Publishing and the Child Neurological Society, 1990.

15. Some Aspects of History of Neurosciences (Vols 1-4). Eds: KK Sinha, DK Jha. Association of Neuroscientists of Eastern India. 2001-2004.

16. The Babinski Sign: A centenary. By J. van Gijn. Utrecht, Heidelberglaan, the Netherlands, Universiteit Utrecht, 1996.

17. www.jnnp.bmj.com

18. www.bmj.org

19. www.ncbi.nlm.nih.gov/pubmed

20. Nathan PW, Smith MC. The Babinski response: a review and new observations. J Neurol Neurosurg Psychiatry. 1955;18:250-9.

21. Nair RK. Evolution of Neurosciences in India: Biographical sketches of some Indian Neuroscientists. St. Joseph's Press, Thiruvanananthpuram, India, 1998.

Chapter 3

Transient Loss of Consciousness

Jagarlapudi M Murthy

INTRODUCTION

Consciousness is "the state of awareness of self and the environment." Consciousness has two components: the arousal and cognition. Arousal is a primitive function sustained by deep brain stem and medial thalamic structures. Cognitive functions require an intact cerebral cortex and major subcortical nuclei.

Consciousness depends on interaction between the ascending reticular activating system (ARAS) and the cerebral cortex (Fig. 3.1). The ARAS is a system of fibers that arise from the reticular formation of the brain stem that lies in the paramedian tegmental region of the posterior part of midpons and midbrain. Ascending reticular activating system projects fibers to the paramedian, parafascicular, centromedian, and intralaminar nuclei of the thalamus, which in turn sends projections diffusely to the cerebral cortex. Loss of consciousness results from either the dysfunction of the ARAS or the diffuse involvement of the cerebral cortex bilaterally.

TRANSIENT LOSS OF CONSCIOUSNESS

Transient loss of consciousness (TLoC) is a very common symptom and can be defined as "a self-limited transient short-lived loss of consciousness not due to head trauma." The recovery of consciousness is always complete.[1] The important neurologic causes of TLoC include (1) syncope, (2) epileptic seizures, and (3) steal or vertebrobasilar transient ischemic attack (TIA).

Loss of consciousness due to brain concussion injury is usually transient with variable duration. Unconsciousness associated with other brain disorders is not always transient. If they are, they are not necessarily self-limited, or short-lived (e.g., metabolic disorders and intoxications).[1] Other differential diagnoses of TLoC include other attacks with apparent unconsciousness that are commonly misdiagnosed as syncope conditions (Box 3.1)[1,2]

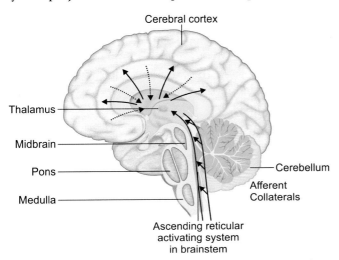

Fig. 3.1: Diagrammatic representation of brain structures involved in consciousness.

Box 3.1: Causes with apparent unconsciousness

- Falls
- Cataplexy
- Drop attacks
- Psychogenic pseudosyncope
- Transient ischemic attacks of carotid origin

CLINICAL EVALUATION OF TLoC

The reliability of the diagnosis of the first TLoC is surprisingly low.[3] History is the best diagnostic tool in the evaluation of a patient with TLoC. Gather detailed information about the initial event (TLoC). This includes circumstances of the event and the duration of event, person's posture immediately before loss of consciousness, prodromal symptoms, posture-related change, presence or absence of limb movements during the attack, tongue-biting, whether eyes were open or shut, event-related injuries, presence or absence of confusion during the recovery period, and weakness down one side during the recovery period, medical history and any family history of cardiac disease or an inherited cardiac condition.[4] Such a detailed account of the event helps to differentiate various causes of TLoC.

Physical Examination and Diagnostic Evaluation of TLoC

A supine blood pressure and pulse after the patient has remained prone for at least 10 minutes, and then standing for 3 minutes should be performed almost in all the patients with history of syncope. In older patients, the causes for syncope may be multifactorial, and the evaluation should include heart disease, arrhythmia, medication effects, and orthostatic hypotension (OH).

In patients with neurally mediated syncope, clinical examination is usually normal except in patients with carotid sinus syncope in whom massage of carotid sinus may precipitate syncope. However, auscultation for a carotid artery bruit prior to carotid sinus message is essential. In patients with atypical neurocardiogenic syncope and also in patients with no apparent specific cause for syncope, tilt-table testing[5] is indicated.

In patients with suspected seizures, awake, and sleep EEG, and neuroimaging to detect a structural lesion are the investigations to establish the diagnosis and to institute the appropriate antiepileptic drug therapy. Patients with OH need detailed work to define the clinical syndrome.

In patients with cardiogenic syncope, cardiac examination for any cardiac structural lesions and 12-lead ECG are essential components of clinical evaluation. The ECG is not only important for diagnostic purpose but also for stratifying the patient into a high- or low-risk group for serious morbidity and mortality. The other investigations should include two-dimensional echo and Holter monitoring. Invasive electrophysiologic evaluation may be required to identify the arrhythmia so that appropriate therapy can be started.

SYNCOPE

Syncope, often referred as "fainting," "passing out," or "block out," is defined "as a transient, self-limited loss of consciousness, usually leading to falling."[2] Syncope is a symptom, not a disease.

In the Framingham study, the cumulative incidence of syncope was estimated at 3–6% over 10 years and the recurrence rate was 9–22%.[6,7] Neurally mediated syncope is the most common cause of syncope.[7-9] Syncope accounts for 3–5% of emergency department visits and 1–6% of hospital admissions.[10-12] The prevalence and incidence of syncope increase with advancing age.[13]

Neurally Mediated Syncope

Neurally mediated syncopal syndrome includes neuro-cardiogenic (vasovagal) syncope, situational syncope, and carotid sinus syndrome (Box 3.2).

Neurocardiogenic Syncope

Neurocardiogenic syncope is the most common cause of syncope both in children and adults with a mean prevalence of 22% in the general population[14] and accounts for 50–60% of unexplained syncope.[14,15] Pathophysiology of neurocardiogenic syncope involves stimulation of cardiac C fibers resulting in vasodilatation and increased vagal tone, with consequent reduction in the cardiac filling, and bradycardia, with ensuing syncope (Fig. 3.2).[16]

Diagnosis of neurocardiogenic syncope can fairly be made by the detailed history of the event (Box 3.3). Prolonged standing or sitting, prodromal symptoms such as blurring of vision, dizziness, sweating, feeling warm or hot, light headedness, headache, abdominal pain, nausea, fatigue, pallor before the event, and presence of provoking factors such as pain or a medical procedure, smell or

---

Box 3.2: Neurally mediated syncope

- Neurocardiogenic syncope
- Situation-related syncope: micturition, cough, defecation, swallowing
- Syncope associated with glossopharyngeal/trigeminal neuralgia
- Carotid sinus hypersensitivity

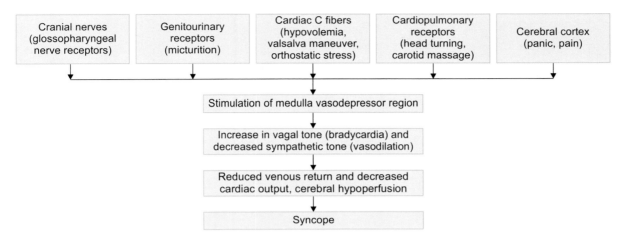

Fig. 3.2: Pathophysiology of syncope.

Box 3.3: Features of neurocardiogenic syncope

- Usually occurs in younger patients
- Usually occurs while standing
- Prodromal symptoms often present
- Consciousness regained almost immediately after falling
- Physical examination normal
- Positive tilt-table test

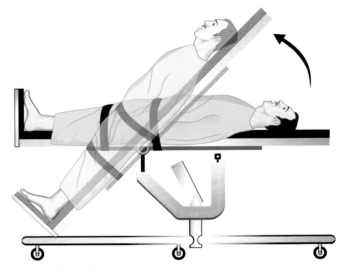

Fig. 3.3: Tilt-table testing.

fear suggest neurocardiogenic syncope.[4,16-20] Absence of classic prodromal symptoms may suggest other causes of syncope. However, in the study by Graham, and Kenny,[16] over one-third of the patients had atypical presentation, syncope episodes without prodromal features.

Orthostatic stress has been suggested as a common prerequisite for the triggering of a neurally mediated response.[21-23] Neurocardiogenic syncope tends to occur in standing position due to gravitational effect and is uncommon in supine position because of the absence of orthostatic stress and presence of gravitational effects that maintain adequate cerebral perfusion.[24] However, neurocardiogenic syncope can occur in sitting and supine positions and also in more than one position, though rarely.[20] This fact should be considered while evaluating (Fig. 3.3, Table 3.1) a patient with neurocardiogenic syncope.

Situational Syncope

Situational syncope can be defined as temporary loss of consciousness in a particular kind of situation. Syncope after cough, defecation, sneezing, and micturition suggests situational syncope and syncope associated with

throat (glossopharyngeal neuralgia) or facial (trigeminal neuralgia) pain is indicative of neurally mediated syncope with neuralgia.

Micturition syncope typically occurs during or shortly after micturition. While urinating, the mechanoreceptors in the contracting bladder wall are stimulated to produce reflex bradycardia, and vasodilation. Standing adds an orthostatic component to the hypotension and contributes to loss of consciousness. In cough or tussive syncope, the increase in the intrathoracic pressure brought on by intense coughing intensifies the hypotensive response by impairing venous return, and decreasing cardiac output. Vigorous coughing may induce a gag response, leading to reflex bradycardia, and vasodilation.

TABLE 3.1: **Tilt-table testing**

Indications	An unexplained, single syncopal episode in high-risk settings (e.g., occurrence of, or potential risk of physical injury or with occupational implications) or recurrent unexplained episodes in the absence of organic heart disease, after cardiac causes of syncope have been excluded
Contraindications	• Morbid obesity (technicians cannot tilt safely) • Unable to stand for long periods due to pain • Pregnancy • Recent (within 6 months) myocardial infarction or stroke/transient ischemic attack • A known tight stenosis anywhere (e.g., heart valve, left ventricular outflow obstruction, coronary or carotid/cerebrovascular artery)
Procedure	The patient is strapped to a tilt-table lying flat and then tilted or suspended at an angle of 60–80 degrees. If the test remains nondiagnostic, pharmacologic provocation may be used
Monitoring	Continuous noninvasive beat-to-beat blood pressure • Intermittent blood pressure (manual) every 5 minutes • Continuous 3-lead ECG • Continuous end-tidal CO_2 using nasal cannulae and a capneograph
End points	Systolic blood pressure falls below 80 mmHg – or is falling rapidly • Heart rate falls below 50/min – or is falling rapidly • Heart rate rises above 170/min • Acute arrhythmia • Hyperventilation leading to an end-tidal CO_2 of <20 mmHg if not able to bring it under control • Patient distress or discomfort
Interpretation	A "positive" tilt test is when the patient's syncopal or presyncopal symptoms are reproduced and accompanied by hypotension, bradycardia (relative or otherwise) or both. Heart rate and blood pressure changes in isolation should not prompt a diagnosis of neurally mediated or orthostatic hypotension syncope

Carotid Sinus Syncope

Carotid sinus hypersensitivity (CSH) is an exaggerated response to carotid sinus baroreceptor stimulation, which leads to bradycardia or vasodilatation resulting in hypotension, presyncope, or syncope (carotid sinus syncope). Carotid sinus syncope is an under-recognized cause of recurrent syncope. Carotid sinus hypersensitivity predominantly affects elderly males. A central degenerative process likely underlies the pathophysiology, but this is as yet unproven.[25]

Carotid sinus syncope should be suspected when syncope is precipitated by rotation or turning of head or pressure (tight collars) on the carotid sinus. Carotid sinus hypersensitivity may occasionally occur without any stimulation. The hemodynamic changes following carotid sinus stimulation are independent of body position. Carotid sinus hypersensitivity documented by carotid sinus massage may be only indicating the possibility of carotid sinus syncope as the cause of syncope [26] (Fig. 3.4, Table 3.2). Auscultation for a carotid artery bruit prior to carotid sinus massage is essential in the evaluation of

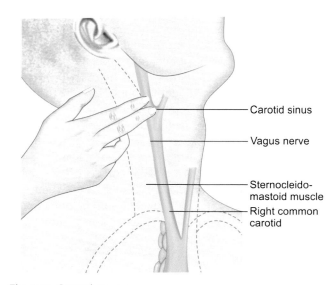

Fig. 3.4: Carotid sinus massage

Labels: Carotid sinus; Vagus nerve; Sternocleido-mastoid muscle; Right common carotid

carotid occlusion. Carotid sinus syncope is an important cause of unexplained falls and syncope in the elderly.

TABLE 3.2: Carotid sinus massage

Indications	A procedure that is used to investigate unexplained dizziness, falls or faints in older individuals
Procedure	It involves gently massaging the carotid artery for 5 seconds on one side of the neck, while monitoring the heart rhythm and blood pressure
Contraindications	• Presence of carotid bruit • Acute myocardial infarction or stroke in the preceding 3 months • History of serious disturbances of the heart rhythm (e.g., ventricular fibrillation or ventricular tachycardia) • Adverse reaction to previous carotid sinus massage

NEUROGENIC ORTHOSTATIC HYPOTENSION

Orthostatic hypotension is a drop in blood pressure on assuming an upright position and is defined as a fall of systolic blood pressure of at least 20 mmHg or a fall of diastolic blood pressure of at least 10 mmHg within 3 minutes of standing.[27] In addition to the commonly recognized OH form between 1 and 3 minutes, there are two other forms of OH, "initial orthostatic hypotension" (IOH)[28] and "delayed orthostatic hypotension" (DOH).[29] Initial orthostatic hypotension occurs immediately upon standing and is detectable only by beat-to-beat blood pressure monitoring.[30] Delayed orthostatic hypotension develops between 5 and 45 minutes. This emphasizes the need to observe for changes in blood pressure on standing for a longer period. Neurogenic OH is a disorder of noradrenergic neurotransmission. Upon standing without noradrenergic release from postganglionic sympathetic terminals, vascular resistance does not increase to compensate for the gravitational volume shift, and blood pressure falls and resultant compromise of blood supply to brain.[31]

Syncope immediate after standing up or prolonged standing or after exertion suggests that the syncope may be related to postural drop in blood pressure. A temporal relation with start of medication leading to hypotension or changes of dose also suggests syncope due to OH.[2] Patients with neurogenic OH have other features of dysautonomia that include impaired papillary function, dry eyes, supine hypertension, reduced gastrointestinal motility, gastroparesis, constipation or diarrhea, bladder

Box 3.4: Clinical characteristics of neurogenic orthostatic hypotension

- Syncope immediate or within few minutes on standing or when making postural changes to a more upright position
- Most common cause of syncope in the elderly
- May be associated with prodromal symptoms of blurred vision, nausea, and disequilibrium
- Consciousness regained almost immediately after falling
- Often associated with other features of dysautonomia
- May have neurologic deficits

Box 3.5: Neurological disorders associated with orthostatic hypotension

- Autonomic neuropathy
- Pure autonomic failure
- Parkinson's disease
- Multiple system atrophy
- Dementia with Lewy bodies
- Dopamine b hydroxylase deficiency
- Brain stem lesions
- Spinal cord injury

dysfunction, erectile dysfunction in males, and impaired sweating (Box 3.4). The neurological disorders associated with OH are given in Box 3.5.

POSTURAL ORTHOSTATIC TACHYCARDIA SYNDROME

Postural orthostatic tachycardia syndrome is defined by excessive heart rate increments, an increase of 30 minutes or more per minute upon standing and/or an increase to 120 beats or more per minute upon standing.[32] The tachycardia response is sometimes accompanied by a decrease in blood flow to the brain and a wide variety of symptoms associated with cerebral hypoperfusion. Syncope is one of the symptoms related to cerebral hypoperfusion. Postural orthostatic tachycardia syndrome is common in women (75–80%) and in the menstruating age group. Diagnosis can be established from the clinical features and measurement of patient's heart rate and blood pressure lying and standing. Tilt-table test[5] is vital to establish the diagnosis (Fig. 3.3, Table 3.1).

CARDIAC SYNCOPE

Medical history and any family history of cardiac disease or inherited cardiac condition, family history of sudden death and syncope occurring in all positions (supine, standing, sitting) and in more than one positions, syncope occurring during exertion, and syncope preceded by palpitation or accompanied by chest pain suggest cardiac syncope.[2,4,15] Potentially confusing features such as palpitations, chest pain, and shortness of breath can also occur in a significant number of patients with neurocardiogenic syncope.[17] Patients with the following characteristics: male gender, age >54 years, two or less episodes of syncope, and duration of warning five seconds or less should be evaluated for cardiac syncope due to atrioventricular block or ventricular tachycardia.[32]

EPILEPTIC SEIZURES

Sometimes, it will be difficult to distinguish between syncope and epileptic seizures. The diagnosis of an epileptic seizure is dependent on the detailed account of the event by the patient and a reliable eye witness. Prolonged aura, a prodromal déjà vu, opened eyes, up rolling of eyes, deviation of eyes to one side, or jerking eye movements, prolonged automatisms, forced head deviation to one side, unusual posturing of limbs, prolonged limb jerking, confusion following the event, a bitten tongue, and amnesia to the event are suggestive of epileptic seizures.[4,31] Upward turning of the eyes, asynchronous myoclonic jerks, and brief automatisms occur frequently during syncope. Urinary incontinence is uncommon in syncope but frequent in epileptic seizures.[31] Sheldon et al.[19] developed a five-point scoring system that distinguishes syncope from seizures (Table 3.4). The point score based on symptoms alone correctly classified 94% of patients, diagnosing seizures with 94% sensitivity and 94% specificity. Including symptom burden did not significantly improve accuracy, indicating that the symptoms surrounding the loss of consciousness accurately discriminate between seizures and syncope. A score of 1 provides a sharp demarcation between the diagnoses of syncope and seizures and a score > 1 suggests diagnosis of epileptic seizure.

STEAL OR VERTEBROBASILAR TRANSIENT ISCHEMIC ATTACK

Brain stem ischemia can result in a syncopal attack. This can occur with subclavian steal syndrome and very rarely

TABLE 3.4: Diagnostic questions to determine whether loss of consciousness is due to seizures or syncope

Symptoms	Points
At times do you wake with a cut tongue after your spell?	2
At times do you have a sense of déjà vu or jamais vu before the spells?	1
At times is emotional stress associated with losing consciousness?	1
Has anyone ever noted your head turning during a spell?	1
Has anyone ever noted that you are unresponsive, have unusual posturing or have jerking limbs during your spells, or have no memory of your spells afterwards? (Score as yes for any positive response)	1
Has anyone ever noted that you are confused after spell?	1
Have you ever had lightheaded spells?	-2
At times do you sit before your spells?	-2
Is prolonged sitting or standing associated with your spells?	-2

TABLE 3.5: Red flag symptoms in syncope diagnosis

Chest pain, palpitations, dyspnea	Cardiac syncope
Syncope during or following exertion	Cardiac syncope
Family history of cardiac disorder	Cardiac syncope
Tongue bite, urinary incontinence, limb jerking	Seizure
Preceding headache	Neurological disorder
Use of hypoglycemics	Hypoglycemia

with TIA in the vertebrobasilar territory. Other features of brain stem ischemia such as dizziness, diplopia, dysarthria, dysphagia, and ataxia help in suspecting vertebrobasilar TIA or steal. Syncope due to subclavian steal syndrome typically presents with exercise-induced arm pain on the side of subclavian stenosis or occlusion and other features of brain stem. Sometimes syncope may be the only presenting feature. Physical examination may reveal low amplitude radial artery pulse and subclavian bruit.

Finally, when the cause of syncope could not be established by detailed history, neurologic, and cardiac examination, and appropriate investigations, a workup for the uncommon causes of TLoC should be considered. This should include psychiatric evaluation (Table 3.5). The reader is referred to chapter on psychogenic epilepsy. Source: Ref Sheldon et al. (2002).

REFERENCES

1. Colman N, Naham K, van Dijk JG, et al. Diagnostic value of history taking in reflex syncope. Clin Auton Res. 2004;14(Suppl 1):37-44.
2. The Task Force on Syncope, European Society of Cardiology. Guidelines on management (diagnosis and treatment) of syncope – update 2004. Europace. 2004;6:467-537.
3. Hoefnagels WAL, Padberg CW, Overweg J, et al. Syncope or seizure? A matter of opinion. Clin Neurol Neurosurg. 1992;94:153-6.
4. NICE Clinical Guidelines- 109: Transient loss of consciousness ("blackout") management in adults and young people. National Institute of Health and Clinical Excellence, UK, 2010.
5. Kenny RA, Ingram A, Bayliss J, et al. Head-up tilt test: a useful test for investigating unexplained syncope. Lancet. 1986;1(8494):1352-5.
6. Savage DD, Corwin L, McGee DL, et al. Epidemiologic features of isolated syncope: the Framingham study. Stroke. 1985;16:626-9.
7. Soteriades ES, Evans JC, Larsen MG, et al. Incidence and prognosis of syncope. N Engl J Med. 2002;347:878-85.
8. Blitzer ML, Saliba BC, Ghantous AE, et al. Causes of impaired consciousness while driving a motorized vehicle. Am J Cardiol. 2003;91:1373-4.
9. Ammirati F, Colivicchi F, Santini M. Diagnosing syncope in clinical practice: implementation of a simplified diagnostic algorithm in a multicenter prospective trial the OESIL 2 study (Osservatorio epidemiologico della Sincope nel Lazio). Eur Heart J. 2000;21:935-40.
10. Day SC, Cook EF, Funkenstein H, et al. Evaluation and outcome of emergency room patients with transient loss of consciousness. Am J Med. 1982;73:15-23.
11. Morichetti A, Astorino G. Epidemiological and clinical findings in 697 syncope events (in Italian). Minerva Med. 1998;89:211-20.
12. Doherty IU, Pembrook-Rogers D, Grogan EW, et al. Electrophysiological evaluation and follow-up characteristics of patients with recurrent unexplained syncope and presyncope. Am J Cardiol. 1985;55:703-8.
13. Kenny RA. Neurally mediated syncope. Clin Geriatr Med. 2002;18:191-210.
14. Kapoor WN. Syncope. N Engl J Med. 2000;343:1856-62.
15. American Heart Association. Syncope www.americanheart.org/, accessed on 23 June, 2013
16. Chen-Scarabelli C, Scarabelli TM. Neurocardiogenic syncope. Br J Med. 2004;329:336-41.
17. Graham LA, Kenny RA. Clinical characteristics of patients with vasovagal reactions presenting as unexplained syncope. Europace. 2001;3:141-6.
18. Sorajja D, Nesbitt GC, Hodge DO, et al. Syncope while driving: clinical characteristics, causes, and prognosis. Circulation. 2009;120:928-34.
19. Sheldon R, Rose S, Ritchie D, et al. Historical criteria that distinguish syncope from seizures. J Am Coll Cardiol. 2002;40:142-8.
20. Khadilkar SV, Yadav RS, Jagiasi A. Are syncopes in sitting and supine position different? Body positions and syncope: a study of 111 patients. Neurol India. 2013;61:239-43.
21. Brignole M, Alboni P, Benditt DG, et al. for the Tasks Force on Syncope. European Society of Cardiology. Guidelines on management (diagnosis and treatment) of syncope – update 2004 executive summary. Eur Heart J. 2004;25:2054-72.
22. Therneau T, Sicks JR, Bergstralh E, et al. Expected survival based on hazard rates. Rochestr. Minn: Department of Health Sciences Research 2000. Technical report series No 52.
23. Fenton AM, Hammil SC, Rea RF, et al. Vasovagal syncope. Ann Intern Med. 2000;133:714-25.
24. Iskos D, Shultz JJ, Benditt DG. Recurrent supine syncope: an unusual manifestation of the neurally mediated faint. J Cardiovasc Electrophysiol. 1998;9:441-4.
25. Seifer C. Carotid sinus syndrome. Cardiol Clin. 2013;31:111-21.
26. Healey J, Connolly SJ, Morillo CA. The management of patients with carotid sinus syndrome: is pacing the answer? Clin Auton Res. 2004;14(Suppl 1): 80-86.
27. Schatz IJ, Bannister R, Freeman RL, et al. Consensus statement on the definition of orthostatic hypotension, pure autonomic failure, and multiple system atrophy. Neurology. 1996;46:1470.
28. Wieling W, Krediet CT, van DN, et al. Initial orthostatic hypotension: review of a forgotten condition. Clin Sci (Lond). 2007;112:157-65.
29. Gibbons CH, Freeman R. Delayed orthostatic hypotension: a frequent cause of orthostatic intolerance. Neurology. 2006;47:28-32.
30. Krediet CT, Go-Schon IK, Kim YS, et al. Management of initially orthostatic hypotension: lower body muscle tensing attenuates the transient arterial blood pressure decrease upon standing. Clin Sci (Lond). 2007; 112:157-65.
31. Kaufmann H, Wieling W. Syncope: a clinically guided diagnostic algorithm. Clin Auton Res. 2004;14(Suppl 1):87-90.
32. Grubb BP. Orthostatic intolerance. National Dysautonomia Research Foundation Patient Conference. Minneapolis, Minnesota. July, 2000.
33. Calkins H, Shyre Y, Frumin H, et al. The value of the clinical history in the differentiation of syncope due to ventricular tachycardia, atrioventricular block, and neurocardiogenic syncope. Am J Med. 1995;98:365-73.

Chapter 4

Approach to Patients with New Onset Seizures

Zeid Yasiry, Simon D Shorvon

INTRODUCTION

A seizure, according to the International League Against Epilepsy (ILAE) is defined as the "transient occurrence of signs and/or symptoms due to abnormal excessive or synchronous neuronal activity in the brain."[1] Seizures are associated with both systemic and central nervous system (CNS) conditions that can be transient or more permanent. Seizures, in other words, may be engendered by reversible causes such as an electrolyte disturbances with no risk of recurrence once the culprit cause is corrected; these are referred to as a provoked seizures (or sometimes an acute symptomatic seizure although this is a term we prefer not to use). However, seizures can have no identifiable precipitating factor on clinical assessment and preliminary investigations; these are referred to as unprovoked seizures. Over 50% of these unprovoked seizures will have a recurrence in the first year, and 73% of those patients will have a third seizure, and of the latter, 76% will have a fourth one.

The term epilepsy is used to denote an enduring propensity to seizures. It can be therefore diagnosed from the second seizure onward.

Acute provoked seizures have an incidence of 20–39 per 100,000 people per year and constitute 40–50% of all afebrile seizures. A single unprovoked seizure, however, has an incidence of 11–24 per 100,000 people per year, while all unprovoked seizures have an incidence of 42–61 per 100,000 per year.[2] To add up, 5% of the people have at least one seizure in their lifetime; the risk is highest in those below 1 year and those above 65 years of age. Epilepsy, however, affects around 0.5–1% of worldwide population at any given point of time.[3] This difference highlights the fact that not every seizure amounts to epilepsy.

When facing a patient who presents with manifestations suggestive of an epileptic seizure, the first priority is to make sure that it is, indeed, an epileptic seizure. At the same time, the semiology of the seizure should be determined, and a short list of potential differential diagnoses be recalled with emphasis on the most common differentials first. Clinical assessment combined with electroencephalography (EEG) constitutes the most essential part of the diagnostic process, while neuroimaging is indicated in a significant fraction, but not all, of circumstances.

This chapter will concentrate on the major possible clinical presentations of seizures, their main differential diagnoses and clues to help differentiate them. Also, it will outline the essential investigative protocols and necessary laboratory or radiological tests required to reach an etiological diagnosis.

SEMIOLOGY OF SEIZURES

By definition, semiology refers to the field of linguistics involved in the study of symptoms and signs (here, of seizures).[4] The aim is to draw up a phenotype of the relevant clinical event that fits into an established clinicopathological or more commonly, a syndromic diagnosis. When dealing with a patient with a new-onset seizure, an attempt should be made to designate the event into a semiological category in order to phenotype, to synthesize a list of potential differential diagnoses, and lastly to a arrive at a diagnosis that is amenable to confirmation by further neurophysiological, imaging, or molecular techniques.

FOCAL MOTOR ACTIVITY

The term motor seizure is defined by the ILAE as involving musculature in any form. The motor event could consist of an increase (positive) or decrease (negative) in muscle contraction to produce a movement. The motor seizure might be generalized or focal, depending on whether the networks of the seizure originated from or engaged into are bilaterally distributed or not.[5] For the purpose of this chapter, a focal motor seizure will be defined as an abnormal motor activity (or lack thereof) that is not generalized, or at least asymmetric, with no, or very subtle, impairment of consciousness, caused by abnormal excessive or synchronous electrical activity in the brain.

The majority of focal motor seizures originates from the motor cortices (primary motor cortex, supplementary sensory motor cortex, and premotor cortex) but have variable etiologies. Box 4.1 gives a brief description of the semiological varieties of focal motor seizures.

Age of onset is a useful indicator of possible etiology. The implications and clinical and therapeutic approaches to a focal motor seizure affecting the corner of mouth in a child differ from a similar seizure in an adult. Childhood focal motor seizures are often of idiopathic etiology in comparison to adult-onset seizures. Older patients might be able to describe the seizure and any preictal and postictal states, unless a secondary generalization of the seizure ensues. In focal clonic seizures, the patients might describe a constellation of sensory phenomena that are often not stereotypic enough to be labeled as auras. Auras may occur in association with tonic seizures of parieto-occipital origin.[8] Paroxysmal tonic attacks during sleep are likely to arise from the supplementary sensorimotor cortex, and are unlikely to be either psychogenic or a movement disorder. They should also be differentiated from parasomnias by their stereotypy and shorter duration. Certain clues for the localization of focal motor seizures can be found in Table 4.1.

Box 4.1: Semiological types of focal motor seizures

- *Focal clonic with or without march/hemiclonic seizures*: it refers to regularly repetitive brief (<100 ms) contractions of a muscle or group of muscles at a frequency of 2–3 Hz with an overall seizure duration of 1–2 minutes.[4,6] The seizures usually begin in the hand or face due to their large representation in the motor cortex. They may remain focal or they may recruit further muscles, i.e., march, secondary to sequential ictal firing in the motor strip. This phenomenon was described by Jackson 150 years ago, hence these seizures are eponymously named, "Jacksonian seizures"[7]

- *Focal tonic seizures*: sustained muscle activity of 5–10 seconds duration that affects a muscle or group of muscles only on one side of the body. The supplementary sensorimotor cortex in the mesial frontal cortex (area 6), rostral to the primary motor (leg area) cortex, is the symptomatogenic zone (with or without being the epileptogenic zone) in the majority of tonic seizures[8]

- *Focal myoclonic seizures*: a myoclonus is a single or repetitive, involuntary, sudden, and brief (<100 ms) contraction of a muscle or group of muscles.[4] Focal myoclonic jerks can be epileptic in origin when myoclonus is the result of synchronous electrical activity in the cerebral cortex,[9] in contrast to subcortical or peripheral origin of myoclonus. The synchronous activity is localized to a hyperexcitable zone, usually within the primary motor cortex.[10] Focal myoclonic seizures, when compared to clonic seizures are arrhythmic, more stereotyped, and less likely to march. Focal epileptic myoclonia occurs in symptomatic or cryptogenic primary motor cortex epilepsies, and very rarely in few idiopathic epilepsies. Epilepsia partialis continua (EPC) is an unremitting focal myoclonus that carries on incessantly. Rasmussen's encephalitis is the most common cause of EPC in many series; however, other vascular, metabolic, inflammatory, and degenerative causes have been reported to cause EPC[11]

- *Versive seizures*: These are "unquestionably forced, involuntary extreme deviations of head and eyes to one side resulting in sustained unnatural positioning of the head and eyes."[11] These seizures result from abnormal discharges in the contralateral premotor cortex, anterior to the primary face, and arm motor cortex. However, version may be seen in seizures originating in temporal or occipital lobes, in which consciousness is often impaired[12]

- *Phonatory/vocalization seizures*: The seizures result from ictal discharges involving supplementary sensory motor area or primary motor cortex below the lip/tongue area. A useful clinical tip would be that in the former, the vocalization is more or less sustained while in the latter the vocalization is interrupted[13,14]

- *Gelastic seizures*: These are involuntary epileptic laughter with or without mirth, and with mild autonomic alterations. The typical association is with hypothalamic hamartomas in infants and neonates, although tumors, vascular anomalies and cortical dysplasia in the mesial frontal, cingulate, or fusiform cortices[15] have all been reported[16]

TABLE 4.1: Localizing features in focal motor seizures

Features	Localized to
Version of head and eye with preserved consciousness	Contralateral frontal lobe focus[12]
Rapid version (<18 seconds) from onset	Extratemporal focus[17]
Tonic component as the initial seizure manifestation	Frontal lobe focus[8]
Aura preceding tonic seizure	More likely to have parieto-occipital focus[8]
Sustained phonatory seizure	Supplementary sensorimotor cortex[13]
Postictal (Todd's) paresis	Contralateral to the epileptogenic zone,[18] especially in clonic seizures of motor cortex origin[19]
Sustained ictal vocalization	Supplementary sensorimotor cortex[13]
Interrupted ictal vocalization	Primary motor cortex[14]

Differential Diagnosis

Focal motor seizures with retained consciousness have a broad spectrum of differential diagnoses, mainly related to subcortical localization, e.g., movement disorders, or psychogenic disorders. The main differentials are outlined in Table 4.2.

GENERALIZED MOTOR ACTIVITY

This falls into several semiological categories:
- Generalized tonic–clonic seizures (GTCS)
- Generalized tonic
- Generalized clonic
- Generalized myoclonic
- Focal hypermotor seizures of frontal lobe origin
- Epileptic spasms.

Generalized Tonic–clonic Seizures

Referred to historically as "grand mal" seizures, these seizures should be easy to differentiate from other nonepileptic paroxysmal disorders. Other conditions may, however, be mistaken for GTCS because of the presence of one or more of the elements of the latter.

Some Features are Virtually Pathognomonic of GTCS

- Head injury secondary to fall
- Severe lateral tongue bite
- Posterior shoulder dislocation
- Bilateral positive Babinski responses in the immediate postictal period.[21]

Generalized tonic–clonic seizures might occur in the context of idiopathic generalized epilepsies (IGEs), various

TABLE 4.2: Differential diagnoses of focal motor seizures

Differentials		Differences from focal motor seizures (besides normal EEG and abnormal basal ganglia functional imaging)	Similarities to focal seizures
Primary paroxysmal dyskinesia			
	Paroxysmal kinesigenic dyskinesia	• Triggered by a kinetic precipitant (although reflex epilepsies may rarely be precipitated by tactile and kinetic triggers) • The duration can extend up to minutes • The frequency of attacks can be as high as hundreds per day • Nonstereotyped movement, in contrast to seizures • Spontaneous resolution or marked reduction in attacks frequency around the third decade • Good response to small doses of sodium channel blockers • Prominent male predominance	• Consciousness is never lost • Coexistent personal or family history of seizures may be present • Dystonic movements may resemble focal tonic seizure • Sensory aura (anticipatory) in the form of tingling, crawling, numbness, warmth or tightness (in the affected limb or in the epigastrium) immediately precede the attack in at least 50% of cases
	Paroxysmal nonkinesigenic dyskinesia	• Triggered by exercise, caffeine, alcohol • Onset of symptoms typically after an hour from the triggering factor, symptoms may take up to 10 minutes to reach their peak • Duration of attacks from minutes to hours • Frequency of attacks are 2–3 per day • Symptoms are relieved by sleep (definite association with familial cases)	

Continued

Continued

Differentials	Differences from focal motor seizures (besides normal EEG and abnormal basal ganglia functional imaging)	Similarities to focal seizures
Paroxysmal exercise-induced dyskinesia	• Long duration exercise triggers the attacks • Duration is 5–30 minutes	• Same as above
Secondary paroxysmal dyskinesia[20]		
Tonic spasms of multiple sclerosis	• Painful spasms, may be triggered by sudden movements • Other neurological symptoms and signs may be present interictally • Remissions may be seen in relapsing remitting disease • Abnormal MRI with areas of demyelination is the usual accompaniment	
Cerebrovascular disorders (limb shaking TIA and orthostatic paroxysmal hemidystonia)	• Vascular risk factors are usually present • Usually triggered upon assuming sudden upright posture • Side or both upper and lower limb are affected simultaneously, rather than gradually or in a marching pattern • Face and trunk are usually spared • Associated with high degree of stenosis or occlusion of the internal carotid artery • Ictal SPECT shows hypoperfusion rather than hyperperfusion	• Unilateral, upper and/or lower limbs shaking, mimicking clonic seizures, or dystonic posturing
Metabolic causes (hypoglycemia, hyperglycemia and hypocalcemia)	• Biochemical abnormality is detected by routine/targeted testing • In hyperglycemia, abnormal neuroimaging may be seen • Other signs and symptoms may be present such as alternating weakness	• Neuroglycopenic symptoms may resemble sensory/autonomic aura • In hypocalcemia and hypoglycemia, genuine seizures may coexist with the less common movement disorders
Episodic ataxia type 1	• Dysarthria is prominent • Typical description is that the limbs is not obeying the commands rather than experiencing a volley of involuntary movements • Association with perioral or periorbital myokymia is common	• Marching from caudal to rostral (leg, arm, and trunk then face) is common • Electroencephalography might be abnormal with sharp-slow-wave complexes bitemporally
Psychogenic (functional) paroxysmal focal motor phenomena	• Lack of stereotypy • Enhancement/precipitation by suggestion • Incongruent/nonanatomical distribution of movements • Relative absence of symptoms during lack of observation • When compared to focal tonic seizures, association with pain is common with lack of task specificity as a trigger when compared to frontal lobe seizures, less associated with tonic posturing and prone position; the duration is usually >2 minutes	
Focal dystonias	• Presence of interictal clinical background abnormalities • Slower and gradual onset • Duration of minutes to days • Response to anticholinergics and botulinum toxin injections	
Nonepileptic myoclonus	• Polygraphy criteria (see text) can differentiate epileptic from nonepileptic cortical myoclonus	• Could be cortical or reticular myoclonus, bilateral or unilateral

Continued

Continued

Differentials	Differences from focal motor seizures (besides normal EEG and abnormal basal ganglia functional imaging)	Similarities to focal seizures
In early childhood and infancy		
Benign infantile myoclonus of sleep	• Normal otherwise neonates • Exclusively nocturnal, myoclonic jerks of upper limbs • Does not interfere with sleep • Spontaneous resolution	
Sandifer's syndrome	• Within 1 hour of meals, due to gastroesophageal reflux disease • Usually associated with hiatal hernia • Paroxysmal dystonia of neck and arching of the back	
Self-gratification behavior	• More likely when the child is relaxed, or attending a certain activity • Distractibility from the behavior is possible, but resumption is usual	• Tonic posturing of the back or legs, shaking, rocking movements may be mistaken for seizures
Childhood		
Tics, mannerism, and stereotypies		
Nocturnal events		
Parasomnias	• Longer duration • Patients have no tonic/versive components • Offset of episode is not abrupt • Complex behavior, associated walking or standing, if present, is against epilepsy • Abnormal polysomnography	• Violent, hyperkinetic movements with or without vocalization may resemble nocturnal frontal lobe epilepsy
Periodic limb movement of sleep	• Affected patients suffer daytime somnolence, although they seldom report being awakened by the movements during night • Movements are distal rather than proximal, mostly involving the lower limbs and of simple semiology (flexion/extension) • Good response to dopaminergic medications or clonazepam	

EEG, electroencephalography; SPECT, single proton emission computerized tomography.

syndromes of focal seizures evolving to generalized seizures, and also in the setting of drug intoxication, traumatic brain injuries, cerebrovascular events, or acute encephalopathy due to inflammatory, infectious or metabolic/electrolyte disturbances. Two conditions most commonly confused with GTCS are syncopal attacks and psychogenic nonepileptic seizures (Table 4.3).

Hypermotor Seizures

This is typically manifestations of focal symptomatic (or rarely, idiopathic as in autosomal dominant nocturnal frontal lobe epilepsy) epilepsy localized to frontal cortex. These are characterized by very brief (15–60 seconds) bizarre, generalized movement involving proximal limb musculature with or without tonic deviation of the head or pedaling/cycling movements of the lower limbs. Consciousness is usually preserved unless, not uncommonly, secondary generalization ensues. These seizures often occur in sleep and therefore cause diagnostic confusion with parasomnia, especially when the interictal EEG is normal.[28]

Because of their bizarre nature, retained consciousness, and nocturnal preponderance, hypermotor seizures are often confused with psychogenic nonepileptic attacks, parasomnia rapid eye movements (REM) and non-rapid eye movements (NREM), and movement disorders (Table 4.4).[29,30]

TABLE 4.3: Differential diagnoses of generalized tonic–clonic seizures

Differential diagnoses	Suggestive features
Syncope (10 times more common than epileptic seizures, 50% lifetime incidence of syncope)	**Interictal[22]** • Palpitations, paroxysmal, or orthostatic dizziness • Cardiac baseline structural lesion or rhythm/conduction defect • Past medical history of diabetes, cardiovascular, or valvular heart diseases • Concurrent drug history of antihypertensives, antipsychotics, antiparkinsonian, and diuretics • Family history of sudden death • Electrocardiogram may show the cardiac rhythm abnormality or hint to structural abnormality • Echocardiography can show abnormal structure or movements of cardiac muscles or valves • Electroencephalography is normal or show bilateral synchronous slow wave activity during the loss of consciousness and muscle atonia[23] **Ictal[24]** • Classical and well-defined precipitating/triggering event is usually present, including exercise, pain, venipuncture, strong emotional trauma, sight of blood, prolonged standing, straining, and coughing, warm, and humid environment. Events occurring during rest do not exclude the possibility of syncope (e.g., cardiac syncope) • A prodrome with characteristic patient and witness-based account is usually present; sweatiness, nausea, palpitations, muffling of sounds, visual whitening, darkening or graying, and pallor • The onset is gradual, taking few seconds to cause fall • Brief myoclonic jerks after the fall are the rule in syncope, rather than the exception (90% of cases) • Lateral tongue bite is rare, and urinary incontinence is uncommon • Offset is usually quick, once the patient is level on the floor • No postictal confusion
Psychogenic nonepileptic convulsive attacks[25] (20% of "new onset seizures" are dissociative, 10% of cases of status epilepticus[26]	**Interictally** • Age of onset under 10 years is uncommon • High female to male ratio; 8:1 • History of multiple complaints is common • History of psychiatric treatment, suicidality, and/or physical or sexual abuse is common • High frequency of attacks is common • Interactional clues include avoidance of the patient to describe the details of the events or the exact account of the confinements of memory loss during the events. Also the patient is reported to prefer using lay terms to describe his symptoms rather than the elaborate and medical terms used by epileptic patients • EEG is normal by definition or may show nonspecific normal variants, or discordant finding with the semiology, as does neuroimaging **Ictally[27]** • Common precipitants include emotional stress, quarrels, or inpatient stay/outpatient doctor's visit inducibility by suggestion • Unlikely to occur during sleep, or after waking; the patient may however has pseudosleep, where the eyes are closed when the attack takes place • Usually occurs in the presence of a witness • Onset is sudden, with no preceding events; however, psychogenic seizures may be preceded by a period of sympathetic overactivity (sweating, tachycardia, and tremor, dry mouth) • Duration is usually more prolonged than seizures or syncope (typically >2 minutes) • Waxing and waning, nonstereotyped, out-of-phase, asynchronous movements; highly suggestive patterns include thrashing, flailing, pelvic rocking, jactitation, and back-arching (opisthotonus) • **Normal consciousness and verbal interaction in the presence of generalized convulsive seizure** • **Absence of tachycardia and cyanosis in presence of generalized convulsive seizure** • Biting of tip of tongue is not uncommon, incontinence is rare but possible • Offset is usually rapid, recovery is less associated with postictal symptoms than in seizures, anterograde amnesia for the event is commonly lacking • **During the seizures and in the immediate postictal phase eyes are closed, with resistance to attempts to passively open the eyes** Serum prolactin is typically normal 20 minutes after the attack

TABLE 4.4: **Differential diagnosis of hypermotor seizures**

Differential diagnoses	Suggestive features
Psychogenic nonepileptic attacks	• Teenage or adult onset • Nonstereotyped • No usual pattern of occurrence • The attacks is usually prolonged, typically >5 minutes • History of psychogenic trauma or psychiatric comorbidity may be present
Parasomnia	• Typically childhood onset • Nonstereotyped • Nocturnal (first one-third of the night for NREM and last half of the night for REM parasomnia) • Amnesia for the event is usual • EEG-polysomnography is crucial (NREM: arousal from slow sleep, REM: REM sleep with EMG normotonia)
Tics	• For primary tic disorders, onset below 18 or 21 years is a diagnostic criterion • Nonstereotyped, semi-purposeful • Suppressible, diurnal (nocturnal events rule out a diagnosis of any movement disorder) • Differing complexity and multiple types are possible • Association with obsessive compulsive disorder and attention deficit hyperactivity disorders is common

NERM, non-rapid eye movements; REM, rapid eye movements; EMG, electromyography; EEG, electroencephalography.

Epileptic spasms are part of catastrophic epilepsy syndromes (epileptic encephalopathies) and are beyond the scope of this chapter.[31-33]

TRANSIENT LOSS/ALTERATION OF CONSCIOUSNESS

Paroxysmal transient loss/alteration of consciousness (TLOC, henceforth) can be a manifestation of abnormal electrical activity in the brain, a seizure, or alternatively can result from several other conditions such as transient cerebral hypoperfusion as in syncope.

Transient loss/alteration of consciousness can be the sole manifestation of epileptic seizures of generalized type; more commonly, it is an accompaniment of GTCS, focal complex (complex partial) seizures, or focal seizures with secondary generalization. This section will deal with TLOC as the primary or first manifestation of seizures with no fall or conspicuous motor activity.

Epileptic seizures presenting with loss or impairment of consciousness are of three main types: typical absence seizures, atypical absence seizures, and complex partial seizures.[14,34]

The approach to these seizures entails excluding the most common differentials and, then, to confirm neurophysiologically the presence, localization, and distribution of epileptic discharges. The latter may not be easily achieved via scalp EEG though. Attaining a specific etiology is required later in patients with focal seizures. A simplified clinical algorithm can be followed when assessing episodes of epileptic TLOC (Fig. 4.1).

Typical absence seizures are divided into simple and complex according to the presence and absence of mild motor activity, respectively.[35] Atypical absences are characterized by slower and less monomorphic EEG patterns, failure of reproducibility by hyperventilation and being part of severe epileptic syndrome(s), and abnormal background developmental status.[14]

The following points are essential for a diagnosis of a typical absence seizure versus complex focal seizures and other nonepileptic causes of vacant spells and impaired consciousness.

Features Suggesting Typical Absences

• Young onset: usually typical absences are part of IGE, typically presenting in childhood or adolescence; they may, however, continue or even present de novo in adulthood[36,37]
• Family history: significant clinical (70%) and EEG (84%) concordance in twin studies and in first-degree relatives (15–44%)[37]
• Ictal manifestations: abrupt onset and offset, often with a vacant stare, interruption of activity with occasional subtle reduction of tone, eyelid twitching with or without simple oral automatism (the longer the absence, the more likely is the automatism.[38] Patients report no prodrome, no aura, no post ictal confusion, and they are unaware of the ictal events. They may estimate the time their spells took.[39] The duration is typically <30 seconds and can occur from tens to hundred times daily[40]
• Reproducibility/inducibility: hyperventilation for 3–5 minutes induces absences in >90% of untreated patients.[9] Photic stimulation and watching television reproduce absences in up to 15% of older patients[41]

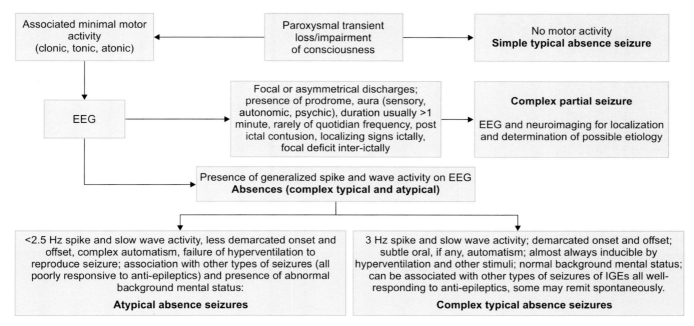

EEG, electroencephalography; IGEs, idiopathic generalized epilepsies.

Fig. 4.1: Algorithm for clinical approach to patients presenting with epileptic TLOC.

- Patients are usually of normal neurological and mental development and performance
- Electroencephalography is essential for the diagnosis: bilateral, symmetrical, 3–4 Hz spike, and waves are characteristic.[35,42] They are monomorphic with highest amplitude in the frontocentral leads. A negative EEG in a patient with typical absence-like semiology, and 5 minutes of hyperventilation, argues strongly against a diagnosis of absence seizures.[9]

Features Suggesting a Complex Partial Seizure

- Ictal manifestations: gradual onset and offset, frequently associated with aura and complex automatism, prominent postictal confusion (especially if originated from the temporal lobe,[43] hardly if ever quotidian and more prolonged than absences (typically minutes)
- Patients may have focal signs interictally or abnormal neurological or mental status[14]
- Electroencephalography: focal interictal discharges or slowing; can be normal ictally and interictally[9]
- Neuroimaging: can show focal lesions (congenital, acquired or developmental) (Table 4.5)[44,45]

TABLE 4.5: **Differential diagnoses of epileptic TLOC**

Differential diagnoses	Suggestive features
Behavioral staring episodes (day dreaming)	• No interruption of play • Preserved responsiveness to touching • Initial identification by professionals (teachers, health care providers)[46]
Attention-deficit hyperactivity disorder	• History of learning difficulties, may be on the autistic spectrum • Hyperactive states, restlessness, fidgety state
Psychogenic staring spells	• History of psychiatric problem • Possibly drug induced • Spells brought up by suggestion[47]
Acute confusional state	Metabolic or infectious precipitant is common

PAROXYSMAL SENSORY EVENTS

Recurrent isolated sensory disturbances due to ictal activity are known as focal sensory seizures or sensory auras; these can involve somatosensory or the special sensations.[34] Visceral sensations, such as epigastric rising, despite being associated with temporal lobe seizures will also be considered with sensory seizures.

General characteristics of focal sensory seizures[48] include the following:

- No loss of consciousness
- They may exhibit marching phenomenon, similar to motor Jacksonian march, causing larger sensory deficit or spread to the motor cortex to cause focal motor seizures
- They cause both positive and negative symptoms although positive phenomena tend to predominate

- Negative postictal phenomena may be seen, analogous to Todd's paresis with focal motor seizures.

Focal sensory seizures fall into the following types[34,49] outlined in Table 4.6.

Differential Diagnosis

Focal sensory seizures are commonly misdiagnosed for other conditions, due to close resemblance of some of its types, such as visual or occipital seizures, to other neurological and psychiatric conditions. The main differentials for each type are outlined in Table 4.7.[50-52]

TABLE 4.6: **Clinical features of sensory seizures**

Type of seizures	Examples	Localization	Associated features	Etiology and syndromic association
Somatosensory				

Localized, elementary sensory symptoms	Tingling, numbness, electrical sensation	• Primary sensory cortex
		• Supplementary sensorimotor cortex
		• Posterior insular cortex
			• Marching to proximal sensory areas or to cause focal motor seizures
			• Ten percent have postictal sensory loss
				• Idiopathic such as benign childhood epilepsy with centrotemporal spikes
				• Symptomatic
				  ○ Vascular
				  ○ Tumors

Diffuse, bilateral sensory symptoms	Warmth, coldness, pressure, vague indescribable somatosensory phenomena	• Supplementary sensorimotor cortex
		• Mesial parietal and temporal cortex
				○ Developmental (focal cortical dysplasia, malformation of cortical development)
				  ○ Neurocutaneous syndromes
				  ○ Infection

With experiential symptoms	• Limb agnosia
	• Feeling of distorted posture or limb position
	• Alien or abnormal/absent limb
		Sensory association cortex, usually nondominant		○ Inflammation/autoimmune
				  ○ Neurodegenerative disease
				  ○ Mitochondrial diseases
				  ○ Metabolic diseases
				• Cryptogenic

Pain	Cephalic	• Temporal lobe cortex
		• Occipital cortex
			May be migrainous but more demarcated onset and offset and sharp and steady quality	• Idiopathic: childhood occipital epilepsy
				• Symptomatic:
				  ○ Temporal lobe epilepsy
				  ○ Occipital calcification and Lafora disease

	Abdominal	Mesial temporal structures but can be induced by electrical stimulation of several other locations	More likely to be epigastric rising or discomfort, may be experienced as pain	Symptomatic mesial temporal lobe epilepsy
	Somesthetic	• Primary and secondary somatosensory cortex • Insula		

Continued

Continued

Type of seizures	Examples	Localization	Associated features	Etiology and syndromic association
Visual				

Positive simple (phosphenes)	Dots, circles, simples shapes, mostly colored, but monochrome or black and white phosphenes have been described	Primary visual cortex (calcarine cortex)	Presence of eye signs:
			• Deviation in up to 52%
			• Blinking in up to 56%
			• Nystagmus in up to 12%
			• Pulling sensation in up to 16%
			• With phosphenes, peripheral field onset with progression to opposite visual field can progress to focal sensorimotor or generalized convulsive seizures (supracalcarine focus) or to focal complex or psychomotor seizures (infracalcarine focus)
				• Idiopathic (late-onset benign childhood occipital epilepsy–Gastaut type; early onset childhood occipital epilepsy–Panayiotopoulos type)
				• Symptomatic: all causes including vascular, inflammatory, traumatic, but in particular:
				  ○ Tumors
				  ○ Encephalomalacia
				  ○ Focal cortical dysplasia
				  ○ Neurocutaneous syndromes with meningeal angiomas (Sturge–Weber syndrome)
				  ○ Neurodegenerative diseases
				  ○ Occipital calcification in coeliac disease
				  ○ Lafora disease
				• Cryptogenic

Positive complex				
Hallucinations	• Objects, scenes, faces • Autoscopy (seeing self-image)	• Visual association cortex • Posterior temporal cortex		
Illusions	• Micropsia • Macropsia • Palinopsia (persistence of visual image after actual disappearance) • Objects nearer or farther • Objects clearer or fainter			
Negative	• Scotomas • Amauroses • Visual field defects	Visual association cortex		
Auditory				
Simple	Buzzing, humming, drumming, chirping, machine like	Primary auditory cortex (transverse temporal gyrus of Heschel)	• Contralateral or bilateral • Ear plugging or covering is said to be localizing to contralateral primary auditory cortex	• Mostly symptomatic causes • Genetic: autosomal dominant partial epilepsy with auditory features
Complex	Voices, music	Auditory association cortex (superior temporal gyrus)	Usually evolve to or associated with other experiential phenomena and may progress to dyscognitive seizures	

Continued

Continued

Type of seizures	Examples	Localization	Associated features	Etiology and syndromic association
Olfactory				
Elementary	• Usually unpleasant odor, or vaguely familiar, yet unrecognizable • Burning rubber, chemical, acrid, putrid	• Mesial temporal structures, amygdala is the most common site of ictal activation • Olfactory bulb (on stimulation), • Orbitofrontal cortex	Usually associated with gustatory seizures	Symptomatic mesial temporal lobe epilepsy due to • Hippocampal sclerosis • Focal cortical dysplasia • Vascular malformation • Malformation of cortical development • Infection • Trauma
Gustatory				
Elementary	Usually unpleasant taste, metallic, bitter, rusty, rotten food	• Parietal and/or Rolandic operculum • Superior insular cortex	• May be associated with relevant/ similar olfactory hallucination(s) • May propagate to suprasylvian structures with further sensorimotor seizures, or to temporal structures to cause psychomotor seizures	Symptomatic mesial temporal lobe epilepsy for isolated gustatory or combined gustatory and olfactory seizures
Vestibular (vertiginous) seizures				
Elementary	• Illusion of rotation around vertical or sagittal axes • Horizontal/vertical movements or tilting	• Posterior superior temporal gyrus (close to Heschel gyrus) • Parietal lobe • Other temporal structures		Lateral temporal lobe epilepsy

TABLE 4.7: **Differential diagnoses of sensory seizures**

Seizure type	Differential(s)	Suggestive features
Somatosensory seizures	Transient ischemic attacks	• Only negative features • Facial and trunk involvement in the sensory loss • No march, all areas affected simultaneously • Offset of symptoms is not as abrupt as in sensory seizures • Duration is usually longer, minutes to hour, typically 10–20 minutes • Vascular risk factors may be readily detectable
	Migrainous aura[53]	• Marching takes typically minutes • Duration from 4 minutes up to 1 hour • Followed by migrainous type headache
	Peripheral neuropathy	• Bilateral symptoms • Continuous symptoms (but with paroxysmal worsening) • Numbness and tingling usually worse at night • Usually acral, in glove, and stoking pattern • The underlying pathology is usually already diagnosed

Continued

Continued

Seizure type	Differential(s)	Suggestive features
Auditory	Psychogenic	• Nonstereotyped • Longer duration • Charged with emotional content/significance • Pre-existing psychiatric diagnosis
Olfactory	Chronic sinusitis	Clinical signs and symptoms of infection
	Psychogenic	• Nonstereotyped • Longer duration • Charged with emotional content/significance • Pre-existing psychiatric diagnosis
Gustatory	Drug induced dysgeusia	Precipitating agent
	Psychogenic	• Nonstereotyped • Longer duration • Charged with emotional content/significance • Pre-existing psychiatric diagnosis
Visual	Migraine aura	• Longer in duration (4–30 minutes) • Less likely to recur at daily basis • Achromatic or black and white linear phosphenes • Onset from center of visual field to the periphery • Not associated with eye signs (deviation, nystagmus) • Postictal headache and vomiting more likely than in occipital epilepsy • Not associated with or evolving to other types of seizures nor loss of consciousness
	Basilar migraine	• Longer in duration (4–30 minutes) • Associated with brainstem signs/symptoms • Central-to-peripheral expansion of phosphenes • Loss of consciousness may follow • Postictal blindness may follow • Not associated with or evolving to other seizures
	Psychogenic	• Nonstereotyped • Longer duration • Simple or complex, and usually charged with emotional content • Pre-existing psychiatric diagnosis
	Neurodegenerative diseases (Alzheimer, Parkinson, dementia with Lewy bodies, and others)	Other baseline neurological or cognitive deficit present
Vertiginous	Vestibular/vestibulonuclear and vestibulocerebellar vertigo	• A paroxysmal attack may be triggered with change in head position • May be associated with residual hearing deficit • Other brain stem signs may be present

DROP ATTACKS

Drop attacks are episodes of falling that occur without warning, with no loss of consciousness, or postictal abnormalities. They are thought to be caused by abnormal postural tone affecting mainly the axial and lower limbs musculature. Classically, power, coordination, and autonomic function should be preserved; however, it is quite difficult to ascertain whether these elements are actually momentarily impaired or not. There are several categories of conditions that are reported to cause drop attacks (Table 4.8). Epileptic drop attacks refer to falls that are caused by abnormal excessive or synchronous electrical activity in the brain. The falls should be the main clinical manifestation and most importantly, from the semiological standpoint, devoid of lapses of consciousness.

Epileptic seizures that can manifest solely as drop attacks, also known as astatic seizures, are defined by the ILAE as "loss of erect posture that results from an atonic, myoclonic or tonic mechanism."[4] They should be differentiated though from falls caused by epileptic autonomic dysfunction leading to syncope[54] or epileptic akinetic seizures in which both consciousness and muscle tone as preserved but the patient's inability to do corrective movements (secondary to epileptic negative phenomenon) can result in falls.[55]

Although, epileptic drop attacks can develop at any age,[56] they are mainly a childhood phenomenon. Astatic seizures are not only a frequent component of generalized epileptic encephalopathies but also can be seen in patients with IGE.[14] The two relevant examples are Lennox–Gastaut syndrome and Epilepsy with myoclonic–astatic seizures of Doose, respectively. These two condition share borderlines, may overlap, and each can be a chameleon for the other. For example, seizures, in both, develop at an approximate age of 2–5 years; both are characterized by more than one seizure type; lastly, both can be associated with cognitive decline at certain points of course.

In a patient with suspected epileptic drop attacks, it is quite essential to perform a video-EEG/EMG/ECG (polygraphy) monitoring in order to document peri-ictal and ictal EEG changes (spike, polyspike, slow wave, fast activity, flattening) and EMG to show atonia or myoclonic jerks. ECG would be important to exclude epileptic and nonepileptic cardiac syncope (Table 4.9).[62]

TABLE 4.8: The main differential diagnoses of visual or occipital seizures

Lennox–Gastaut syndrome[57-59]	Doose syndrome[60,61]
Age of onset: 1–7 years	Age of onset: 2–5 years
In up two-thirds of cases, abnormal developmental background is present, up to one-third progressed from West syndrome	Develops in previously normal children
Family history is uncommon	Strong family history is usually present
Most common seizure types: tonic (up to 100% of patients), atypical absences, atonic, and myoclonic	Most common seizure types: myoclonic, atonic, and myoclonic-atonic seizures. Presence of tonic seizure is against the diagnosis
Interictal EEG is always abnormal, with generalized slow spike-wave discharges as the hallmark feature; episodic fast wave activity is also characteristic but not sensitive	Interictal EEG is typically normal, but generalized spike-wave discharges may be seen especially during sleep.
Neuroimaging is almost always abnormal	Neuroimaging is typically normal
Refractory to polytherapy, with 5% mortality and up to 92% have significant behavioral and cognitive impairment	Prognosis is relatively good if recognized early and started treatment early, especially in the idiopathic form

EEG, electroencephalography.

TABLE 4.9: Differential diagnoses of epileptic drop attacks

Differential	Suggestive features
Vascular	
Vertebrobasilar insufficiency[63]	• Vascular risk factors and history of previous strokes/TIAs might be present • Usually precipitated by neck extension or head turning • Usually associated with other features of brain stem dysfunction, such as diplopia, dysarthria
Bilateral anterior cerebral artery ischemia[54,64]	• Vascular risk factor might be present • Limb shaking (TIAs) may be a recognized antecedent[65]
Vestibular dysfunction, otolithic catastrophe, or Tumarkin attacks[66]	• A diagnosis of Meniere's disease may have already been made • Sensorineural deafness is usually present[67] • Patients usually describe being "knocked down" or "thrown," or describe a tilt in the environment[68] • No associated nausea, vomiting, aural fullness, or vertigo • The patient is able to stand up immediately after fall

Continued

Continued

Differential	Suggestive features
Acute hydrocephalus due to third/fourth ventricular mass (choroid plexus papilloma, colloid cyst, intraventricular cysticercosis)[69-71]	• Sudden head turning or neck flexion brings out the attack (Bruns' sign)[54] • Usually associated with and temporally related to position-induced headaches
Posterior fossa mass lesions[72,73] or malformations, e.g., Chiari malformation	Sudden neck flexion can precipitate drop attacks
Cataplexy (stimulus sensitive loss of tone)	
Narcolepsy[74]	• Presence of other features of narcolepsy: day time somnolence and sleep attacks, hypnagogic and hypnopompic hallucinations, and sleep paralysis • Cataplexy is usually sensitive to emotional stimuli, most strongly to laughter
Hereditary cataplexy[75]	Autosomal dominant, family history of cataplexy with no other findings of narcolepsy
Niemann–Pick disease C[76]	• Autosomal recessive family history, consanguinity might be a clue • Vertical supranuclear gaze palsy, ataxia, progressive dementia • Organomegaly • Bone marrow showing foam cells
Coffin–Lowry syndrome[77]	• Dysmorphic features, skeletal abnormalities, and mental retardation • Cataplexy is tactile and auditory stimuli-sensitive; exaggerated startle response may also overlap with cataplexy
Hyperkeplexia[78] (major form)	• Autosomal-dominant condition, sporadic cases reported • Childhood-onset falls, first signs of exaggerated startle detected after birth, resistant to habituation, generalized hypertonia in flexion with normal tone during sleep (normal tone by age of three years), exaggerated DTR[79] • Difficult to differentiate from startle-induced epileptic falls without combined EEG-EMG recording

EEG, electroencephalography; EMG, electromyography; DTR, deep tendon reflexes.

PAROXYSMAL BEHAVIORAL, PSYCHIC, DYSMNESTIC, AND CONFUSIONAL STATES (DYSCOGNITIVE SEIZURES)

There is a wide range of symptoms and experiences that all are reported in complex partial seizures, Expectedly, different seizures localize to different areas of cortex; however, temporal, and frontal lobes seem to be the most commonly described epileptogenic foci.[80]

Seizures may involve differing combinations of abnormal perception of self (depersonalization), environment (derealization), time (slowing, fasting, stand still), decreased or rarely increased attention, awareness or concentration, abnormal emotion (ictal fear, euphoria, depression), abnormal memory (flash backs or recurrence of past event), or abnormal executive function with impaired anticipation, selection, and monitoring of complex motor activities as praxis or speech function. EEG and MRI are useful in establishing an epileptic basis for these disorders. The main differential diagnoses of dyscognitive seizures are outlined in Table 4.10.[81,82]

PAROXYSMAL AUTONOMIC DYSREGULATION

Autonomic disturbances are commonly encountered in seizures, yet these are, usually, an accompaniment to more florid GTCS or complex partial seizures rather than being the initial or most dominant feature.[84] When subjective or objective autonomic disturbances constitute the principal manifestation of the seizures, the terms, autonomic auras, and autonomic seizures are used.

The most common types of autonomic seizures are those related to gastrointestinal tract (rising epigastric sensation, pain, nausea, vomiting, urge to defecate) and cardiorespiratory systems (tachycardia, bradycardia, asystole, arrhythmia, hyperventilation, apnea, chest pain, dyspnea, bronchospasm, increased bronchial secretions). Pilomotor, vasomotor (flushing, pallor), pupillary (mydriasis, miosis, hippus), and genitourinary (incontinence, sexual/orgasmic)-related seizures are all less common phenomena. Most of the autonomic seizures arise from mesial temporal, insular, and opercular cortices.

TABLE 4.10: **Differential diagnoses of dyscognitive seizures**

Semiology	Differential	Suggestive features
Prolonged confusional state	• Acute encephalopathy: ○ Metabolic (hypoglycemia, electrolytes, renal, or hepatic failure) ○ Infection (systemic, CNS) ○ Inflammation (autoimmune, vasculitic) ○ Urea cycle disorders, acute intermittent porphyria • Drug intoxication • Head trauma • Vascular insults • Intermittent psychosis	Relevant symptoms, signs, and lab results
	Confusional migraine	• Prolonged for hours • Resolves by sleep • Association with hyperactivity, variable amnesia, impaired responsiveness, and vomiting • Association with migraine aura (visual), headaches • EEG shows nonspecific regional slowing
Fear[83]	Panic attacks	• Anticipatory anxiety, hyperventilation, tingling sensation • Onset is gradual over minutes • Duration of attacks is commonly 5 minutes • Association with sweating, tremor, palpitation, choking, chest pain, and feeling of impending doom • There should be no loss of consciousness nor postictal confusion • Association with other features of anxiety disorders such as agoraphobia
Memory loss	Transient global amnesia	• Longer than a seizure (median of 4 hours, up to 24 hours) • Middle age to elderly, usually men • Anterograde amnesia, variable retrograde amnesia • Repeatedly questioning about the whereabouts • Preserved personal identity, remote memory and attention • Spontaneous resolution
	Dissociative fugue state	• Brief, self-limited inability to remember the past • Loss of self-identity or formation of new one • Association with sudden unplanned distant travel
Memory of past events, dreamy states	• Drug-induced flashbacks • Psychosis	

CNS, central nervous system; EEG, electroencephalography.

Panayiotopoulos syndrome is a prototype epileptic syndrome in which autonomic seizures/autonomic status epilepticus is the cornerstone feature. The typical patients are children with average age of onset of 4–5 years, who will have infrequent, mainly nocturnal, seizures (total of 1–5) on a normal developmental background. The seizures are emetic in nature and can be severe; there may be associated headache and abdominal pain. In almost all of the patients, there is subsequent variable alteration of consciousness and more than half of the patients will have motor features such as eyes and head deviation. In 80% there is interictal EEG abnormality manifested as

TABLE 4.11: **Differential diagnoses of autonomic seizures**

Differential diagnoses	Suggestive features
Hypoglycemia	• Episodic hunger pain, sweating, tachycardia, tremor, confusion • Relation to skipping meals, or insulin or oral hypoglycemic agent intake • Resolution with glucose intake • Low random blood sugar; further testing in nondiabetic patients for nesidioblastosis or insulinoma (insulin, proinsulin, C-peptide, glucose in a 72-hour supervised fast)
Pheochromocytoma	• Episodic hypertension, tachycardia, sweating, tremor • Plasma and urine catecholamine metabolites/metanephrines • Clonidine suppression test • Imaging for localization • Increased chromogranin A
Carcinoid syndrome	• Flushing, bronchospasm, diarrhea • Urinary 5-HIAA • Increased chromogranin A and platelet serotonin • Imaging studies (MRI, CT, octreotide scan) for localization of primary tumor and extent of pulmonary and cardiac metastases
Menopausal symptoms (hot flushes)	Typical signs and symptoms
Panic attacks	See Table 4.10
Acute intermittent porphyria	• Association of episodic abdominal pain, constipation, hypertension, tachycardia with other feature, such as fever, peripheral nerve palsy, hallucination, delirium, and even psychosis • Genuine seizures may also coexist • A history of acute precipitant such as newly prescribed drug is usually present • A positive family history (AD) may be present • Darkening of urine (port wine urine) may be described • Assays of urinary ad plasma porphyrins
Cyclic vomiting	• Sleep onset clustering of emetic episodes with or without photophobia/phonophobia, abdominal pain, diarrhea, headache but no visual symptoms • Childhood condition (3–9 years onset) 33% develop migraine by adolescence • A diagnosis of exclusion

5-HIAA, 5-Hydroxyindoleacetic acid; MRI, magnetic resonance imaging; CT, computed tomography.

multifocal spikes with occipital predominance in 70% of cases.[85,86]

The differentials are broad, yet metabolic and endocrine paroxysmal events seem to constitute the most essential list to exclude (Table 4.11).[87]

INVESTIGATIONS

In a patient with new onset seizures, investigations aim to treat and correct reversible causes of seizures, e.g., hypoglycemia or meningitis, in addition to reaching a confident pathological diagnosis. Different guidelines use different protocols in investigating patients with new onset seizures.[88]

Biochemistry and Hematology

In all patients, a random venous or capillary blood sugar is useful during a seizure as hypoglycemia is a common cause of seizure in patients with diabetes or metabolic/systemic disorders.[89] Other essential first line biochemical and hematological tests include electrolytes, complete blood picture, and differential, renal and liver function tests.

Other tests are ordered accordingly, depending on the presence of background and presenting neurological and systemic findings. Tables 4.12 and 4.13 provide, respectively, list biochemical and hematological tests used in specialized centers for a small number of highly selected patients with new onset seizures; these tests are

TABLE 4.12: Biochemical investigations ordered in patients with new onset seizures[88]

Investigation	Indication	Presentation/context
Random blood sugar	Hypoglycemia (of any cause)	Seizures with or without encephalopathy
Serum electrolytes	Various disorders	Seizures with or without encephalopathy or systemic disturbance
Serum ethanol level	Alcoholic intoxication	Seizures, disturbed level of consciousness, alcoholic fetor
Serum toxicology screen	Drug, toxin	Unexplained seizures in the setting of encephalopathy, systemic and autonomic disturbance especially in teenage and young people
Serum magnesium	Hypomagnesemia	Neonatal seizures, resistant hypocalcemic seizures
Serum calcium	Hypocalcemia, hypoparathyroidism, pseudohypoparathyroidism, DiGeorge syndrome	Neonatal seizures, jitteriness, dysmorphic features, skeletal abnormalities
Serum lactate	• Mitochondrial diseases • Fructose 1,6 diphosphatase deficiency • Glycogen storage disease type 1 • Multiple carboxylase deficiency	• Seizures and encephalopathy, learning disability, multisystemic involvement (hearing, vision, liver, muscles) • Neonatal seizures with variable combinations of encephalopathy, hypoglycemia, metabolic acidosis
Liver function test	• Hepatic failure of various causes • POLG-related mitochondrial diseased	Seizures, encephalopathy, myoclonus, stigmata of chronic liver disease, or fulminant hepatic failure
Renal function test	Renal failure	Seizures in the setting of encephalopathy, myoclonus, earthy color, uremic bone disease
Thyroid function test	Hypothyroidism, thyroid storm	Various signs and symptoms of corresponding abnormality
Less commonly ordered tests		
Serum copper, ceruloplasmin	• Menkes disease • Wilson disease	Hair change, movement disorders, neuropsychiatric features
RBC folate	Folate deficiency	Megaloblastic anemia and seizures
Serum B12, methylmalonic acid, homocysteine	B12 deficiency	Seizures + megaloblastic anemia, dementia, peripheral neuropathy, subacute combined degeneration of the cord
Homocysteine	Homocystinuria, B12, folate metabolic disorders, molybdenum cofactor, and sulfatide oxidase deficiency	Seizures with myriad presentations depending on the specific condition
Alpha-aminoadipic semialdehyde (α-AASA)	Pyridoxine-dependent epilepsy	Refractory neonatal seizures, response to pyridoxine IV
Acylcarnitines and carnitine levels	• Fatty acid oxidation disorders • Organic aciduria • Mitochondrial diseases	Seizures and encephalopathy
Amino acids	Various indications (e.g., phenylketonuria, nonketotic hyperglycinemia, homocysteinemia)	• Seizures with or without encephalopathy • Different signs and symptoms depending on the specific abnormality
Ammonia	Urea acid cycle disorders • Argininosuccinic acidemia • Carbamoyl phosphate synthetase deficiency • Citrullinemia • Ornithine transcarbamylase deficiency • Amino acid disorders (such as methylmalonic acidemia) • Fatty acid oxidation disorders • Organic acid disorders	Seizures in the setting of acute metabolic encephalopathy that could be precipitated by high protein load, sodium valproate, fasting, and infection

Continued

Continued

Investigation	Indication	Presentation/context
White cell enzymes activity	• Lysosomal storage disease • Mucopolysaccharidosis • Mucolipidosis • Gangliosidosis • Leucodystrophies • Neuronal ceroid lipofuscinosis (NCL1 and NCL2) • Glycoprotein storage disorders	Myriad of presentations (systemic and neurological) in which acute seizures is a rarity except in NCL (one of the progressive myoclonic epilepsies)
Uric acid	Purine metabolism defects (Lesch–Nyhan syndrome)	Learning disability, self-mutilation, seizures, movement disorders
Creatinine	Creatine deficiency syndromes (GAMT, AGAT, and transporter deficiency)	Seizures, learning disability
Biotinidase assay	Biotinidase deficiency	Seizures, myelopathy, brain stem syndromes

RBC, red blood cell; POLG, polymerase gamma; GAMT, guanidinoacetate N-methyltransferase; AGAT, L-arginine:glycine amidinotransferase.

TABLE 4.13: Hematological investigations ordered in patients with new onset seizures[88]

Test	Indication	Presentation/ context
Complete blood picture and differential	Various dyscrasias	Seizures with systemic/CNS signs/symptoms of inflammation, infection, neoplasia
Blood culture	CNS/systemic infection	Seizures with systemic/CNS infection including fever, shock state, neck stiffness, photophobia, cerebrospinal fluid leak prior to seizures
Blood film	Acanthocytosis	Seizures, movement disorders (perioral dyskinesia), peripheral neuropathy
	Macrocytosis/megaloblastic RBCs-B12 and folate deficiency	Myelitis, dementia, peripheral neuropathy, seizures (rare)
	Sickle cells	Seizures, stroke in young, painful crisis
	Blast cells	Leukemia, lymphoma
	Vacuolated lymphocytes in Neuronal ceroid lipofuscinosis	Progressive myoclonus, seizures, mental retardation
Clotting profile	Bleeding tendency	Hemorrhage-induced seizures

RBC, red blood cell; CNS, central nervous system.

outlined alongside the presentation or associated features that justify ordering them. It should be noted that most of these investigations are indicated for rare disorders and are not routinely performed.

Autoimmune Screen

The field of autoimmune epilepsy has been rapidly expanding for the past decade and has contributed to reduction of the cryptogenic category of seizures.[90,91] An autoimmune screen is warranted in patients with acute seizures or status epilepticus where there is either a distant malignancy with no detectable metastasis, signs of malignancy even if the latter is cryptic, and in typical limbic encephalitis with temporal lobe seizures and cognitive and emotional disturbance. It should be

noted that the sensitivity of cerebrospinal fluid (CSF) examination for these antibodies is higher than that of serum (Dalmau, 2013, conference lecture). The range of possible tests is outlined in Table 4.14.

Urine Tests

These are indicated for cases with suspected drug/toxin induced seizures and in suspected metabolic etiology, especially in childhood.

Cerebrospinal Fluid Tests

Lumbar puncture is not routinely indicated in patients with new onset seizures. Cerebrospinal fluid analysis is warranted when the clinical condition and/or preliminary

TABLE 4.14: Antibodies screening (blood, cerebrospinal fluid) in patients with suspected autoimmune seizures[88]

Antibody	Indication	Presentation/context
Antibodies associated with intracellular antigens	LE	Seizures, subacute cognitive decline, behavioral disturbance
Anti-Hu	Paraneoplastic LE (SCLC)	Seizures, sensory polyneuropathy, cerebellar syndrome, autonomic failure
Anti-Ma2	Paraneoplastic LE (testicular cancer)	Seizures, brain stem syndromes, hypothalamic disorders
Anti-CRMP-5/CV2	Paraneoplastic LE (SCLC, thymoma)	Various syndromes: Limbic encephalitis, cerebellar syndrome, radiculo/neuropathy, ophthalmological manifestations
Antiamphiphysin	Idiopathic or paraneoplastic LE (breast, SCLC)	Stiff person syndrome, myelopathy, or cerebellar syndrome
Anti-GAD	Idiopathic LE	
Antiadenylate kinase-5	LE (no tumor detected)	
Antibodies associated with extracellular antigens	LE	Seizures, subacute cognitive decline, behavioral disturbance
Antivoltage-gated potassium channel (VGKC): • LGI1 • CASPR2 • Contactin-2	LE	• Seizures, cognitive decline, neuropsychiatric disturbance, REM sleep behavior disorder, hyponatremia • Faciobrachial dystonic seizures (anti-LGI1) Morvan syndrome (neuromyotonia, peripheral nerve hyperexcitability) (CASPR2)
Anti-NMDA receptor	Paraneoplastic LE (ovarian teratoma)	Seizures, psychiatric and autonomic instability, movement disorders, disturbed level of consciousness
Anti-AMPA (GluR1/GluR2) receptor	Paraneoplastic LE (thymus, breast, SCLC)	Rapidly progressive encephalitis with acute psychosis
Anti-AMPA (GluR3)	Rasmussen's encephalitis	Refractory seizures, hemiatrophy on MRI
Anti-GABA$_B$ receptor	LE (50% paraneoplastic to SCLC)	Focal seizures with secondary generalization
Antiglycine receptor	LE	PERM syndrome
Antigliadin, antireticulin, antiendomysial	Coeliac disease	Malabsorption, bone disease, movement disorders, seizures, cerebellar syndrome
ANA, anti-dsDNA, anti-Smith	Cerebral lupus	Skin, renal, hematological, psychiatric, and musculoskeletal manifestations
Anticardiolipin, lupus anticoagulant	Antiphospholipid syndrome	Recurrent arterial and venous thrombosis, history of recurrent abortions, thrombocytopenia
Antithyroid peroxidase	Hashimoto's encephalopathy	Abnormal thyroid function tests in a setting of seizures, subacute cognitive decline, ataxia, headache, tremor, myoclonus
Oligoclonal (unmatched) bands in CSF	Autoimmunity, infection, parainfectious process	Various, according to etiology

CSF, cerebrospinal fluid; LE, limbic encephalitis; SCLC, small cell lung cancer; PERM, progressive encephalomyelitis with rigidity and myoclonus.

investigation or imaging indicate plausible infectious, inflammatory or autoimmune etiology of the seizures.

Electrodiagnostics

Electroencephalography and polygraphic recordings are of paramount significance in the work up of patients presenting with new onset seizures.[92,93] EEG is an essential tool in investigating paroxysmal disorders, in general, and seizures, in particular. It reflects cortical electrical discharges as detected via scalp electrodes. It can be performed as an outpatient interictal recording, an inpatient video-EEG (vEEG) ictal monitoring, or ambulatory EEG recording. Other forms of recordings, including more invasive techniques such as depth electrodes or subdural grid electrodes, are employed mainly for presurgical localization in patients with established refractory epilepsy.

Electroencephalography is mostly recorded between the attacks, i.e. interictal EEG. An abnormal interictal EEG does not diagnose epilepsy by its own means but simply implies that the patient has high propensity to seizures. An abnormal interictal EEG, therefore, supports the clinical diagnosis of epilepsy. It also may aid in classifying epilepsy syndromes, and can be helpful in detecting triggering factors responsible for seizures such as hyperventilation or photosensitivity. In addition, in patients who present with a first seizure, the presence of epileptiform discharges are associated with two to three fold increase in seizure recurrence (58% risk of recurrence).

A single interictal EEG has a sensitivity of around 50–55% in detecting epileptiform activities. Factors that affect the sensitivity of interictal EEG are outlined in Box 4.2.

The specificity and positive predictive value of EEG, however, are >96%. For common epileptic patterns seen in practice, see Table 4.15.

Activation procedures can help increase the diagnostic yield of EEG by lowering the seizure threshold in differing epileptogenic circuits; these include intermittent photic stimulation, sleep, sleep deprivation, and hyperventilation. Intermittent photic stimulation activates epileptiform discharges in patients with IGE, especially childhood and juvenile absence and myoclonic

> **Box 4.2: Factors affecting sensitivity of interictal EEG**
> - Prolonged recording: Shown to increase sensitivity by 20%
> - Inclusion of sleep recording: Sensitivity rises to 80–85% when EEG combines sleep and waking recordings
> - Repeated recordings: Sensitivity rises up to 92% when four interictal recordings are performed
> - Age: Children are more likely than adults to have an abnormal interictal EEG
> - Type of epilepsy syndrome and seizure types: Untreated IGE such as typical childhood absences will almost always have an abnormal EEG
> - Epileptogenic location: Neocortical temporal lobe seizures are more likely to produce interictal discharges than mesial temporal or frontal lobe seizures
> - Timing of recording: Interictal EEG is believed to be most sensitive in the first 24 hours of a seizure (51 vs. 34% subsequently)
> - Presence of precipitating context/factors; e.g., relation to menstrual cycle in catamenial epilepsy or to flashing lights in photosensitive epilepsy

TABLE 4.15: The most common epileptic patterns that are encountered in clinical practice

Pattern	Definition/notes
Focal spikes/sharp waves	Usually indicate an epileptogenic focus. Spikes: <70 ms; sharp waves: 80–500 ms, single or polyspikes, focal or multifocal, anterior, or posterior predominant
Generalized spikes/spike-wave complexes	Symmetrical distribution and amplitude bilaterally, anterior posterior predominance • 2–2.5 Hz if seen in children with developmental delay, neurological impairment, and lapses of consciousness and tone, in association with abnormal background rhythm usually highly suggestive of atypical absences • 3 Hz is characteristic of typical absence seizures, with interictal occipital delta • 4–6 Hz with prominent photosensitivity is usually seen in juvenile myoclonic epilepsy
Slow spike-wave complexes	• Usually encountered in the setting of epileptic encephalopathies, such as Lennox–Gastaut syndrome, where background is usually slow and the complexes demonstrate 1.5–2.5 Hz frequency
Rhythmical temporal delta waves	• Highly specific for temporal lobe epilepsy
Others (less common and more specific patterns)	• Hypsarrhythmia: typically seen in West syndrome • Burst suppression: in infants with spasms indicates Ohtahara syndrome • Continuous spike-wave during slow sleep or electrical status epilepticus during slow sleep: when seen in children with acquired aphasia is highly specific for Landau–Kleffner syndrome • Generalized spike-wave photosensitivity: when seen in infants with febrile seizures, myoclonic jerks, and atypical absences are highly specific for Dravet syndrome • A combination of photosensitivity, generalized spike-wave, progressive background slowing+/− giant somatosensory-evoked potential and facilitated motor evoked potential in patients with progressive myoclonus, seizures, ataxia with or without cognitive decline is characteristic of progressive myoclonic epilepsy

epilepsy. The same applies to sleep deprivation which is shown to increase sensitivity of outpatient EEG by 30–70% and can convert a negative 1st EEG into an abnormal one in 52% of cases. Hyperventilation seems to be most useful in patients with absence seizures where untreated patients have reproducible, EEG, and clinical, seizures with up to 3 minutes of hyperventilation in around 90% of cases.

Ictal EEG, however, is the next step if repeated interictal EEGs (wakefulness, sleep, and with activation procedures) are negative or inconclusive, which is a usual scenario. Ictal EEG, in most of the centers, is combined with video monitoring of the ictal manifestations; this allows precise studying of electroclinical correlation. Ictal EEG, thus, is helpful in determining whether a paroxysmal event is epileptic or not, and if epileptic, classifying it to generalized or focal. Also, ictal EEG can help quantify the seizure activity and detect minor seizures manifesting as disturbed cognitive status or subjective experience, for instance.

It should also be remembered that EEG is also supporting/excluding the diagnosis of several pathologies, e.g., background triphasic waves in Creutzfeldt-Jacob disease or subacute sclerosis panencephalitis, or when combined with other electrodiagnostics, movement disorders such as dystonia and nonepileptic myoclonus.

However, there are some issues regarding EEG that need to be considered by any healthcare professional who requests an EEG study for a paroxysmal disorder:

- A normal EEG study does not exclude a clinical diagnosis of epilepsy and therefore, more prolonged and combined recordings may be required (see the paragraphs on sensitivity above)
- Similarly, not every abnormal EEG means that the related event is epileptic.[94] These abnormal rhythms fall into two major categories
  - Epileptiform discharges that are not caused by epilepsy:
    - Age-related or normal EEG variants, e.g., wicket spikes, and temporal theta rhythms.
    - Epileptiform discharges caused by drugs and metabolic encephalopathies.
  - Nonepileptiform abnormal EEG patterns may lead to erroneous diagnosis of epilepsy if the overall picture is overlooked. The most common examples include diffuse/focal slow waves, voltage asymmetry or frontal intermittent rhythmic delta activity. These can be seen in acute brain injury, toxic metabolic encephalopathies or, more commonly, in conditions commonly mistaken for

epilepsy, such as syncope or migraine. It is worth mentioning though, that these abnormalities may be encountered in the postictal state of epileptic seizures.

Hence, experts often warn against ordering EEGs in patients with presumptive diagnosis of syncopal attacks, migraine or psychogenic nonepileptic attacks because of the grave consequences of false positive results.[95]

Polygraphy refers to the combined recording of EEG and other parameters including electromyography, autonomic functions (heart rate, blood pressure, etc.), and speech to provide overall view of whether or not topographically various events are associated or causally related.

Combined EEG/EMG recording is essential in diagnosis and classification of myoclonic jerks; this combination can show the relationship between cortical spike/sharp wave and the muscle contraction detected by the EMG. When EEG is negative, a usual scenario due to small epileptogenic zone, back averaging is used to detect a possible EEG abnormality.[96-98] Polygraphy based criteria have been set to differentiate epileptic versus nonepileptic cortical myoclonus. Further details can be found in reviews and textbooks and are beyond the scope of this summarized chapter.

Neuroimaging

The aim of neuroimaging is not to diagnose epilepsy but rather to establish an etiology for the seizures/epilepsy, notwithstanding, the detection of an epileptogenic lesion, e.g., a glioma, in the context a paroxysmal event may highly support a diagnosis of epilepsy.[99] In several circumstances, neuroimaging is indicated on emergent basis in patients with new onset seizures.[100]
These indications include:

- Head trauma
- History of cancer
- History of anticoagulants use
- History or suspicion of AIDS or immune-compromised state
- Persistent headache
- Fever
- Neurological deficit
- Persistent altered mental status (+/– intoxication)
- Focal seizures in patients older than 40 years (probable indication).

In the emergency setting, the most commonly encountered imaging diagnoses include stroke, intracranial hemorrhage, tumors, infection, arteriovenous malformation, subdural hematoma, calcifications, atrophy, and cortical developmental malformations.[100] In contrast, about 10% of patients with a new-onset unprovoked seizures will have abnormalities on neuroimaging that might explain their seizures, although this depends on the imaging methods employed.[3] In addition, neuroimaging might provide a rough estimate of the seizure prognosis. For instance, in a patient with seizures and normal MRI, the chance of being controlled with antiepileptic drugs is much higher (50%) than if hippocampal sclerosis were identified (11%).[101]

Neuroimaging is of paramount role in patients with refractory epilepsy in whom surgical treatment is planned, where EEG and anatomical and functional imaging is the cornerstone in assessment and decision making (see chapter 5 for refractory epilepsy).

MRI is the imaging modality of choice in evaluating patients with seizure disorders; nonetheless, in large number of acute management facilities, readily accessible MRI facilities are not available, also, the circumstances of the patient may not permit the prolonged MRI examination. Therefore, CT is a convenient alternative in the acute setting. Neuroimaging is indicated in all patients with seizures unless these have had a definitive diagnosis of IGE or benign childhood epilepsy with centrotemporal spikes.[102] The ILAE has proposed the selected indications for MRI examination in patients with epileptic disorders.[102]

Indications of neuroimaging in patients with epilepsy
- Focal or multifocal onset of seizures at ANY age
- Onset of unclassified or apparently generalized seizures in the first year of life or in adulthood
- Examination reveals fixed neurological deficit or the presence of abnormal background developmental or neurological status
- Drug-resistant seizures
- Loss of control of seizures using antiepileptic drugs, indicating progressive disease.

The spectrum of abnormalities on MRI in people with new-onset unprovoked seizures include hemorrhage, hematoma, ischemia, vascular anomalies, encephalitis, abscess, tumors, cortical dysplasia, malformation of cortical development, hippocampal sclerosis, tubers, hemiatrophy in Rasmussen's encephalitis, among myriad pathologies. The current protocols[102,103] include detailed description of the types of sequences required for suspected pathologies; these are outlined in Box 4.3.

Other imaging studies, including functional imaging, are less essential in acute or newly diagnosed cases of seizures as their main indications are in functional mapping and presurgical evaluation.[102]

Box 4.3: Neuroimaging in new onset seizures

- Use MRI as the standard: FLAIR for screening, T2W for confirmation, and T1W 3D for anatomical reference and quantification. In infants <6 months, use T1W only, from 6 to 18 months, use T1W and T2W, and FLAIR from 18–24 months onward
- Use CT
  - In acute settings when MRI is not available
  - When MRI is not suitable for the patient (e.g., pacemaker, or cochlear implant or patient on ventilator)
  - When the cause of seizure is suspected calcification, e.g., cysticercosis, where CT scan is of high sensitivity
- Use axial sequences for suspected extratemporal, especially frontal lobe, epileptogenic zone
- Use coronal sequence for suspected temporal lobe epileptogenic zone
- Slice thickness should be as minimal as possible, ≤5 mm
- Gadolinium enhancement is used only when native images provide no definitive results; best utilized for visualization of tumors, vascular anomalies, and normal variants
- special indications
  - Calcification and hemosiderin deposition: T2*-gradient ECHO
  - Focal cortical dysplasia:
    - T2W sequence with slice thickness <1.5 mm
    - Coronal/sagittal T1W 3D volume acquisition
    - 3D T2W or FLAIR
    - Phase array surface coils

REFERENCES

1. Fisher RS, Boas WvE, Blume W, et al. Epileptic seizures and epilepsy: definitions proposed by the International League Against Epilepsy (ILAE) and the International Bureau for Epilepsy (IBE). Epilepsia. 2005;46(4):470-2.
2. Hauser WA, Beghi E. First seizure definitions and worldwide incidence and mortality. Epilepsia. 2008;49:8-12.
3. Wiebe S, Tellez-Zenteno JF, Shapiro M. An evidence-based approach to the first seizure. Epilepsia. 2008;49 (Supp 1):50-57. Epub 2008/02/22.
4. Blume WT, Lüders HO, Mizrahi E, et al. Glossary of descriptive terminology for ictal semiology: report of the ILAE task force on classification and terminology. Epilepsia. 2001;42(9):1212-8.
5. Berg AT, Berkovic SF, Brodie MJ, et al. Revised terminology and concepts for organization of seizures and epilepsies: report of the ILAE Commission on Classification and Terminology, 2005-2009. Epilepsia. 2010;51(4):676-85. Epub 2010/03/04.
6. Noachtar S, Arnold S. Clonic seizures. In: Luders H, Noachtar S (Eds). Epileptic Seizures: Pathophysiological and Clinical Semiology. Philadelphia: Churchill Livingstone; 2000. pp. 412-24.
7. Critchley M, Crithley EA. John Hughlings Jackson: Father of English Neurology. New York: Oxford University Press; 1998.
8. Werhahn KJ, Noachtar S, Arnold S, et al. Tonic seizures: their significance for lateralization and frequency in different focal epileptic syndromes. Epilepsia. 2000;41(9):1153-61. Epub 2000/09/22.
9. Panayiotopoulos CP. A Clinical Guide to Epileptic Syndromes and Their Treatment, 2nd edition. London: Springer Healthcare Ltd; 2010.

10. Hallett M. Myoclonus: relation to epilepsy. Epilepsia. 1985;26:S67-S77.

11. Alexopoulos AV, Jones SE. Focal motor seizures, epilpepsia partialis continua and supllemetary sensorimotor seizures. In: Wyllie E (Ed). Wyllie's Treatment of Epilepsy, Principles and Practice, 5th edition. Philadelphia: Lippincott Wlliams & Willkins; 2011.

12. McLachlan RS. The significance of head and eye turning in seizures. Neurology. 1987;37(10):1617-9. Epub 1987/10/01.

13. Kanner AM, Morris HH, Luders H, et al. Supplementary motor seizures mimicking pseudoseizures: some clinical differences. Neurology. 1990;40(9):1404-7. Epub 1990/09/01.

14. Engel J, Pedley TA, Aicardi J. (Eds). Epilepsy: A Comprehensive Textbook, 2nd edition. Philadelphia: Lippincott Williams & Wilkins; 2008.

15. Arroyo S, Lesser RP, Gordon B, et al. Mirth, laughter and gelastic seizures. Brain. 1993;116 (Pt 4):757-80. Epub 1993/08/01.

16. Freeman JL, Eeg-Olofsson O. Gelastic seizures. In: Engel J, Pedley TA (Eds). Epilepsy: A Comprehensive Textbook, 2nd Edition. Philadelphia: Lippincott Williams & Wilkins; 2008.

17. Chee MW, Kotagal P, Van Ness PC, et al. Lateralizing signs in intractable partial epilepsy: blinded multiple-observer analysis. Neurology. 1993;43(12):2519-25. Epub 1993/12/01.

18. Kellinghaus C, Kotagal P. Lateralizing value of Todd's palsy in patients with epilepsy. Neurology. 2004;62(2):289-91. Epub 2004/01/28.

19. Gallmetzer P, Leutmezer F, Serles W, et al. Postictal paresis in focal epilepsies—incidence, duration, and causes: a video-EEG monitoring study. Neurology. 2004;62(12):2160-4. Epub 2004/06/24.

20. Blakeley J, Jankovic J. Secondary paroxysmal dyskinesias. Mov Disord. 2002;17(4):726-34.

21. Perrig S, Jallon P. Is the first seizure truly epileptic? Epilepsia. 2008;49:2-7.

22. McKeon A, Vaughan C, Delanty N. Seizure versus syncope. Lancet Neurol. 2006;5(2):171-80. Epub 2006/01/24.

23. Brenner RP. Electroencephalography in syncope. J Clin Neurophysiol. 1997;14(3):197-209. Epub 1997/05/01.

24. Lempert T, Bauer M, Schmidt D. Syncope: a videometric analysis of 56 episodes of transient cerebral hypoxia. Ann Neurol. 1994;36(2):233-7. Epub 1994/08/01.

25. Kristina M, Markus R, Appleton R. Differential diagnosis of epilepsy. In: Simon S, Renzo G, Mark C, Lhatoo S (Eds). Oxford Textbook of Epilepsy and Epileptic Seizures, 1st edition. Oxford: Oxford University Press; 2013.

26. Kotsopoulos IA, de Krom MC, Kessels FG, et al. The diagnosis of epileptic and non-epileptic seizures. Epilepsy Res. 2003;57(1):59-67. Epub 2004/01/07.

27. Jain SK, Ettinger AB. Psychogenic nonepileptic events imitating epileptic seizures. In: Panayiotopoulos CP (Ed). Atlas of Epilepsies. London: Springer-Verlag; 2010.

28. Malow BA. Paroxysmal events in sleep. J Clin Neurophysiol. 2002;19(6):522-34. Epub 2002/12/19.

29. Jobst BC. Focal hyperkinetic seizures. In: Panayiotopoulos CP (Ed). Atlas of Epilepsies. London: Springer-Verlag London Limited; 2010.

30. Holthausen H, Hoppe M. Hypermotor seizures. In: Luders HO, Noachtar S (Eds). Epileptic Seizures: Pathophysiology and Clinical Semiology. Philadelphia: Livingston Churchill; 2000. pp. 439-48.

31. Engel J Jr. A proposed diagnostic scheme for people with epileptic seizures and with epilepsy: report of the ILAE task force on classification and terminology. Epilepsia. 2001;42(6):796-803. Epub 2001/06/26.

32. Panayiotopoulos CP. Epileptic encephalopathies in infancy and early childhood. In: Panayiotopoulos CP (Ed). The Epilepsies, Seizures, Syndromes and Management. Chipping Norton: Bladon Medical Publishing; 2005. pp. 137-206.

33. Caraballo RH, Capovilla G, Vigevano F, et al. The spectrum of benign myoclonus of early infancy: Clinical and neurophysiologic features in 102 patients. Epilepsia. 2009;50(5):1176-83. Epub 2009/01/30.

34. Luders H, Acharya J, Baumgartner C, et al. Semiological seizure classification. Epilepsia. 1998;39(9):1006-13. Epub 1998/09/17.

35. Duncan JS. Typical absences and related epileptic syndromes. Duncan JS, Panayiotopoulos CP (Eds). London: Churchill Livingstone International; 1995.

36. Thomas P, Beaumanoir A, Genton P, et al. 'De novo' absence status of late onset: report of 11 cases. Neurology. 1992;42(1):104-10. Epub 1992/01/01.

37. Lennox WG, Lennxo MA. Epilpesy and Related Disorders. Boston: Little Brown and Company; 1960.

38. Penry JK, Porter RJ, Dreifuss RE. Simultaneous recording of absence seizures with video tape and electroencephalography. A study of 374 seizures in 48 patients. Brain. 1975;98 (3):427-40. Epub 1975/09/01.

39. Wyllie E. Wyllie's Treatment of Epilepsy. 5th edition. Wyllie E, Cascino G, Gidal B, Goodkin H (Eds). Philadelphia: Wolters Kluwer- Lippincott Williams & Wilkins; 2011.

40. Browne TR, Dreifuss FE, Penry JK. Clinical and EEG estimates of absence seizure frequency. Arch Neurol. 1983;40:469-72.

41. Harding GFA, Jeavons PM. Photosensitive Epilepsy, 2nd edition. London: MacKeith Press; 1994.

42. Dalby MA. Epilepsy and 3 per second spike and wave rhythms. A clinical, electroencephalographic and prognostic analysis of 346 patients. Acta Neurol Scand. 1969:Suppl 40:3+. Epub 1969/01/01.

43. Kotagal P, Lüders HO, Williams G, et al. Psychomotor seizures of temporal lobe onset: analysis of symptom clusters and sequences. Epilepsy Res. 1995;20(1):49-67.

44. King MA, Newton MR, Jackson GD, et al. Epileptology of the first-seizure presentation: a clinical, electroencephalographic, and magnetic resonance imaging study of 300 consecutive patients. Lancet. 1998; 352(9133):1007-11.

45. Duncan J. The current status of neuroimaging for epilepsy. Curr Opin Neurol. 2009;22(2):179-84. Epub 2009/03/21.

46. Rosenow F, Wyllie E, Kotagal P, et al. Staring spells in children: descriptive features distinguishing epileptic and nonepileptic events. J Pediatr. 1998;133(5):660-3.

47. Carmant L, Kramer U, Holmes GL, et al. Differential diagnosis of staring spells in children: a video-eeg study. Pediatr Neurol. 1996;14(3):199-202.

48. Ness PCV, Lesser RP, Duchowny MS. Neocortical sensory seizures. In: Engel J, Pedley TA (Eds). Epilepsy: A Comprehensive Textbook, 2nd Edition. Philadelphia: Lippincott Williams & Wilkins; 2008.

49. So NK. Epileptic auras. In: Wyllie E (Ed). Wyllie's Treatment of Epilepsy Principles and Practice, 5th edition. Philadelphia: Wolters Kluwer/Lippincott Williams & Wilkins; 2011.

50. Stern JM. Focal vertiginous seizures. In: Panayiotopoulos CP (Ed). Atlas of Epilepsies. London: Springer-Verlag Limited; 2010.

51. Foldvary N, Acharya Y, Lueders HO. Auditory auras. In: Lueders HO, Nochatar S (Eds). Epilepsy Seizures: Pathophysiology and Clinical semiology. Philadelphia: Churchill Livingstone; 2000. pp. 304-12.

52. Jobst B, Williamson P. Anatomical–clinical localization of ictal behavior. In: Kaplan PW, Fisher RS (Eds). Imitators of Epilepsy. New York: Demos Medical Publishing, Inc; 2005.

53. Panayiotopoulos CP. Visual phenomena and headache in occipital epilepsy: a review, a systematic study and differentiation from migraine. Epileptic Disord. 1999;1(4):205-16.

54. Daroff RB, Fenichel GM, Jankovic J, et al. Bradley's Neurology in Clinical Practice. 2nd edition. Saunders; 2012.

55. Mothersill IW, Hilfiker P, Kramer G. Twenty years of ictal EEG-EMG. Epilepsia. 2000;41(Suppl 3):S19-23. Epub 2000/09/23.

56. Lipinski CG. Epilepsies with astatic seizures of late onset. Epilepsia. 1977;18(1):13-20. Epub 1977/03/01.

57. Aicardi J. Lennox-Gastaut syndrome. In: Wallace S (Ed). Epilepsy in Children. London: Chapman & Hall; 1996. pp. 249-61.

58. Guerrini R. Epilepsy in children. Lancet. 2006 Feb 11;367(9509):499-524.

59. Gastaut H, Broughton R. Epileptic Seizures: Clinical and Electro-encephalographic Features, Diagnosis and Treatment. Springfield: Charles C. Thomas; 1972.

60. Doose H. Myoclonic-astatic epilepsy. Epilepsy Res Suppl. 1992;6:163-8. Epub 1992/01/01.
61. Oguni H, Fukuyama Y, Tanaka T, et al. Myoclonic-astatic epilepsy of early childhood—clinical and EEG analysis of myoclonic-astatic seizures, and discussions on the nosology of the syndrome. Brain Dev. 2001;23(7):757-64. Epub 2001/11/10.
62. Koutroumanidis M, Ferrie CD, Valeta T, et al. Syncope-like epileptic seizures in Panayiotopoulos syndrome. Neurology. 2012;79(5):463-7. Epub 2012/07/21.
63. Brust JC, Plank CR, Healton EB, et al. The pathology of drop attacks: a case report. Neurology. 1979;29(6):786-90. Epub 1979/06/01.
64. Kang SY, Kim JS. Anterior cerebral artery infarction: stroke mechanism and clinical-imaging study in 100 patients. Neurology. 2008;70(24 Pt 2):2386-93. Epub 2008/06/11.
65. Gerstner E, Liberato B, Wright CB. Bi-hemispheric anterior cerebral artery with drop attacks and limb shaking TIAs. Neurology. 2005;65(1):174. Epub 2005/07/13.
66. Tumarkin A. The otolithic catastrophe: a new syndrome. Br Med J. 1936;2(3942):175-7. Epub 1936/07/25.
67. Perez-Fernandez N, Montes-Jovellar L, Cervera-Paz J, et al. Auditory and vestibular assessment of patients with Meniere's disease who suffer Tumarkin attacks. Audiol Neurootol. 2010;15(6):399-406. Epub 2010/04/15.
68. Ishiyama G, Ishiyama A, Baloh RW. Drop attacks and vertigo secondary to a non-meniere otologic cause. Arch Neurol. 2003;60(1):71-75. Epub 2003/01/21.
69. Criscuolo GR, Symon L. Intraventricular meningioma. A review of 10 cases of the National Hospital, Queen Square (1974-1985) with reference to the literature. Acta Neurochir. 1986;83(3-4):83-91. Epub 1986/01/01.
70. Kumar V, Behari S, Kumar Singh R, et al. Pediatric colloid cysts of the third ventricle: management considerations. Acta Neurochir. 2010;152(3):451-61. Epub 2009/10/27.
71. Pollack IF, Schor NF, Martinez AJ, et al. Bobble-head doll syndrome and drop attacks in a child with a cystic choroid plexus papilloma of the third ventricle. Case report. J Neurosurg. 1995;83(4):729-32. Epub 1995/10/01.
72. Lee MS, Choi YC, Heo JH, et al. "Drop attacks" with stiffening of the right leg associated with posterior fossa arachnoid cyst. Mov Disord. 1994;9(3):377-8. Epub 1994/05/01.
73. Bardella L, Maleci A, Di Lorenzo N. [Drop attack as the only symptom of type 1 Chiari malformation. Illustration by a case]. Rivista di patologia nervosa e mentale. 1984;105(5):217-222. Epub 1984/09/01. "Drop attack" unico sintomo di malformazione di Chiari I. Illustrazione di un caso].
74. Bassetti C, Aldrich MS. Narcolepsy, idiopathic hypersomnia, and periodic hypersomnias. In: Culebras A (Ed). Sleep Disorders and Neurological Disease. New York: Basel: Marcel Dekker; 2000. pp. 323-54.
75. Gelardi JM, Brown JW. Hereditary cataplexy. J Neurol Neurosurg Psychiatry. 1967;30(5):455-7. Epub 1967/10/01.
76. Vanier MT. Niemann-Pick disease type C. Orphanet J Rare Dis. 2010;5:16. Epub 2010/06/08.
77. Nelson GB, Hahn JS. Stimulus-induced drop episodes in Coffin-Lowry syndrome. Pediatrics. 2003;111(3):e197-202. Epub 2003/03/04.
78. Mothersill I, Grunwald T, Kr̈amer G. Sudden falls. In: Schmitz, Tettenborn, Schomer (Eds). The Paroxysmal Disorders. New York: Cambridge University Press; 2010.
79. Tijssen MAJ, Vergouwe MN, van Dijk JG, et al. Major and minor form of hereditary hyperekplexia. Mov Disord. 2002;17(4):826-30.
80. Engel J, Williamson PD. Limbic seizures. In: Engel J, Pedley TA (Eds). Epilepsy: A Comprehensive Textbook, 2nd edition. Philadelphia: Lippincott Williams & Wilkins; 2008.
81. Duncan JS, Fish DR, Shorvon SD. Diagnosis: Is It Epilepsy? In Clinical Epilepsy (in Advances in Neurology series). Churchill Livingstone, Edinburgh, 1995.
82. Pellock J. Other nonepileptic paroxysmal disorders. In: Wyllie E (Ed). Wyllie's treatment of epilepsy, 5th edition. Philadelphia: Wolters Kluwer, Lippincott, Williams & Wilkins; 2011.
83. Kanner AM, Ettinger A. Anxiety disorders in epilepsy. In: Engel J, Pedley T (Eds). Epilepsy: A Comprehensive Textbook, 2nd edition. Baltimore: Lippincott, Williams & Wilkins; 2008.
84. Ferrie CD, Caraballo R, Covanis A, et al. Autonomic status epilepticus in Panayiotopoulos syndrome and other childhood and adult epilepsies: a consensus view. Epilepsia. 2007;48(6):1165-1172. Epub 2007/04/20.
85. Rossetti AO, Kaplan PW. Seizure semiology: an overview of the 'inverse problem'. Eur Neurol. 2010;63(1):3-10. Epub 2009/11/20.
86. Koutroumanidis M. Panayiotopoulos syndrome: an important electro-clinical example of benign childhood system epilepsy. Epilepsia. 2007;48(6):1044-53.
87. Kaplan PW, Basaria S. Metabolic and endocrine disorders resembling seizures. In: Engel J, Pedley T (Eds). Epilepsy: A Comprehensive Textbook, 2nd edition. Philadelphia: Lippincott Williams & Wilkins; 2008.
88. Shorvon S. The biochemical, haematological, histological, immunological, and genetic investigation of epilepsy. In: Shorvon S, Renzo Guerrini, Cook M, Lhatoo S (Eds). Oxford Textbook of Epilepsy and Epileptic Seizures. Oxford: Oxford University Press; 2013.
89. Turnbull TL, Vanden Hoek TL, Howes DS, et al. Utility of laboratory studies in the emergency department patient with a new-onset seizure. Ann Emerg Med. 1990;19(4):373-7. Epub 1990/04/01.
90. Lancaster E, Dalmau J. Neuronal autoantigens—pathogenesis, associated disorders and antibody testing. Nat Rev Neurol. 2012;8(7):380-90. Epub 2012/06/20.
91. Lunn M. Inflammatory and immunological diseases of the nervous system. In: Shorvon S, Andermann F, Guerrini R (Eds). The Causes of Epilepsy. New York: Cambridge University Press; 2011.
92. Aminoff MJ. Electroencephalography: general principles and clinical applications. In: Aminoff MJ (Ed). Electrodiagnostics in Clinical Neurology, 6th edition. Philadelphia: Saunders; 2012.
93. Binnie CD, Prior PF. Electroencephalography. J Neurol Neurosurg Psychiatry. 1994;57(11):1308-19. Epub 1994/11/01.
94. Benbadis SR, Lin K. Errors in EEG interpretation and misdiagnosis of epilepsy. Which EEG patterns are overread? Eur Neurol. 2008;59(5):267-71. Epub 2008/02/12.
95. Panayiotopoulos CP. EEG in the diagnosis and management of epilepsies. In: Panayiotopoulos CP (Ed). A Clinical Guide to Epileptic Syndromes and Their Management, 2nd edition. London: Springer; 2010.
96. Obeso JA, Rothwell JC, Marsden CD. The spectrum of cortical myoclonus. From focal reflex jerks to spontaneous motor epilepsy. Brain. 1985;108(Pt 1):193-224. Epub 1985/03/01.
97. Skidmore CT. Focal myoclonic seizures. In: Panayiotopoulos CP (Ed). Atlas of Epilepsies. London: Springer-Verlag Limited; 2010. pp. 435-6.
98. Pohlmann-Eden B, Newton M. First seizure: EEG and neuroimaging following an epileptic seizure. Epilepsia. 2008;49:19-25.
99. Manford M. Assessment and investigation of possible epileptic seizures. J Neurol Neurosurg Psychiatry. 2001;70(supp 2):ii3-ii8.
100. Greenberg MK, Barsan WG, Starkman S. Neuroimaging in the emergency patient presenting with seizure. Neurology. 1996;47(1):26-32.
101. Semah F, Picot MC, Adam C, et al. Is the underlying cause of epilepsy a major prognostic factor for recurrence? Neurology. 1998;51(5):1256-62. Epub 1998/11/18.
102. Recommendations for neuroimaging of patients with epilepsy. Commission on Neuroimaging of the International League Against Epilepsy. Epilepsia. 1997;38(11):1255-6. Epub 1998/05/14.
103. Woermann FG, Vollmar C. Clinical MRI in children and adults with focal epilepsy: a critical review. Epilepsy Behav. 2009;15(1):40-49.

Chapter 5

Approach to Intractable Epilepsy

Gagandeep Singh

INTRODUCTION

Epilepsy affects 50 million people worldwide.[1] The prognosis for seizure control for majority of the people with newly diagnosed epilepsy is excellent. Even in the early nineteenth century when treatment of epilepsy comprised largely of bromides alone, remission was documented in nearly half of the newly diagnosed cases. With modern antiepileptic drugs (AEDs), approximately 60% of those given a diagnosis of epilepsy in specialist care go in to a period of sustained remission.[2] The remaining 40% continue to have seizures. The term chronic active epilepsy refers to epilepsy in which seizures continue to occur five or more years after initiation of therapy. In a proportion of those with chronic active epilepsy, seizures remain uncontrolled despite adequate AED therapy. People with epilepsy in this category are loosely referred to have intractable epilepsy; they constitute about 20% of all cases with newly diagnosed epilepsy, followed up over a period of time. Till very recently, no uniform definition for intractable epilepsy existed. Various experts defined intractable epilepsy differently. For instance, Gilman et al. used the criteria of resistance to first-line AED therapy (comprising of phenobarbital, phenytoin, carbamazepine, and valproate) at maximally tolerated serum concentrations (hence, doses of the AED) both as a single agent (monotherapy) and in at least one combination (polytherapy) and to one second-line (adjunctive) therapy.[3] A commonly accepted principle evolved and used by many neurologists is the rule of twos, which connotes the occurrence of at least two seizures every month, despite treatment with maximally tolerated doses of two appropriate AEDs for a period of two years. The International League Against Epilepsy (ILAE) has recently proposed criteria for characterization of epilepsy as intractable.[4] Although somewhat complicated, these criteria need to be applied both in clinical practice, and research in order to ensure uniformity between clinicians working in different centers as well as among researchers.

The response to treatment in newly diagnosed epilepsy is excellent. However, this does not mean that the prognosis is invariably poor for those with chronic and intractable epilepsy. A range of newer AEDs (Table 5.1A), a new therapy (vagus nerve stimulation), and a range of surgical options (Table 5.1B) (including radiosurgery, which is currently under evaluation in a multicenter international trial), are now available for people with intractable epilepsy. Although the results of treatment changes (i.e., the use of alternative AEDs) in people with epilepsy who fail an appropriately chosen first-line AED are generally not good (only about 10% of such people achieve seizure freedom), the response to carefully considered surgery is excellent with up to 70–80% of appropriately chosen people attaining seizure remission.[2] Indeed, since the response to alternative medical treatment is poor, the emphasis now is to identify candidates with intractable epilepsy who are likely to benefit from epilepsy surgery. A carefully planned randomized trial clearly established that early surgery in people with intractable mesial temporal lobe epilepsy offers significantly between seizure control and quality of life in comparison to best medical treatment.[5] Hence, a systematic approach to people with intractable epilepsy in order to establish their surgical candidacy as well as

TABLE 5.1A: Newer AEDs and therapies for the treatment of epilepsy

Generation	Drugs
Second-generation AEDs	• Lamotrigine* • Topiramate* • Gabapentin* • Levetiracetam* • Zonisamide* • Vigabatrin • Felbamate • Pregabalin* • Tiagabine
Third-generation AEDs	• Retigabine • Eslicarbazepine* • Lacosamide*
AEDs in development	• Brivaracetam • Carisbamate • Ganaxolone • Remacemide • Rufinamide • Sulfinamide • Talampanel • Stiripentol
Therapy	Vagus nerve stimulation

*Drugs that are available in India.
AED, antiepileptic drug.

TABLE 5.1B: Surgical options in the management of intractable epilepsy

Type of surgery	Procedure
Resective	• Anteromesial temporal lobe resection • Selective amygdalohippocampectomy • Lesionectomy
Disconnective	• Corpus callosotomy • Functional hemispherectomy • Multiple subpial transection

to consider alternative treatment with AEDs that have not been used is desirable. The approach to evaluation of patients with intractable epilepsy forms the basis of this chapter.

PSEUDOINTRACTABLE EPILEPSY

A key step in the evaluation of "difficult to control" epilepsy is to rule out situations in which the patient appears to continue to have seizures but the epilepsy is not truly intractable. Three such situations exist and are described below.

The Diagnosis is Not Epilepsy

Up to 20–30% of referrals to video-EEG telemetry units for evaluation of apparently intractable epilepsy actually are given the label of nonepileptic seizures (also referred to as psychogenic seizures) following evaluation. Hence, in these patients the reason for failure to control epilepsy is not resistance to AEDs, but that the underlying condition which closely simulates epilepsy, is actually not epilepsy but a conglomeration of nonepileptic conditions such as psychogenic seizures, syncope, and breath-holding spells, which would not be expected to respond to treatment with AEDs. For many of these patients, it is relieving when the workup with video-EEG telemetry ends up with withdrawal or reduction in AEDs, reassurance that the condition is benign and appropriate psychiatric and psychosocial interventions.

The Diagnosis is Epilepsy

The diagnosis is epilepsy but the choice of AED or its dose is inappropriate. A well-known example (Case study 5.1) is the case of juvenile myoclonic epilepsy. In general, an essential step in the approach to epilepsy is classification and assignment of an epilepsy syndrome, which in turn dictates the choice of AED. If the syndrome is inappropriately classified, the choice of AED is often incorrect. It is not uncommon to see a case of juvenile myoclonic epilepsy, in which the occurrence of myoclonic jerks is neither reported by the patient nor enquired in a penetrating manner by the treating physician and hence missed. This particular epilepsy syndrome is well treated with valproate but due to misdiagnosis, it is not uncommon that treatment with an AED such as carbamazepine is instituted, which in turn leads to exacerbation of myoclonus. Later, once the syndrome is appropriately identified and treatment changed from carbamazepine to an alternative AED (e.g., valproate), the seizures (particularly myoclonus) respond well to the treatment change. Likewise, incorrect doses (usually suboptimal doses) of AEDs might be responsible for inadequately controlled seizures and in such cases, the institution of appropriate dosages guided by the clinical response and, in many cases, serum levels of AEDs might lead to control of pseudointractable epilepsy.

A 19-year-old gentleman came to the clinic with the history of recurrent generalized tonic–clonic seizures over the past 4 years. For the first 2 years, he had only two generalized tonic–clonic seizures, both in the early morning following late nights for studying for his examinations. An EEG examination and MRI of the brain were essentially normal. He was then started on AED treatment with carbamazepine. His seizures continued thereafter at a regular frequency of 3–4 seizures/year, often precipitated by overnight sleep deprivation due to a variety of reasons and rarely by alcohol ingestion.

During the clinic interview, the history of early morning myoclonic jerks was probed and he admitted after some thought that he did have some clumsiness in the early mornings in the form of holding objects with his hands. A longer duration EEG (Fig. 5.1) revealed generalized bursts of polyspike-wave discharges. A diagnosis of juvenile myoclonic epilepsy was made, treatment switched from carbamazepine to valproate. The patient is seizure-free for 2 years now.

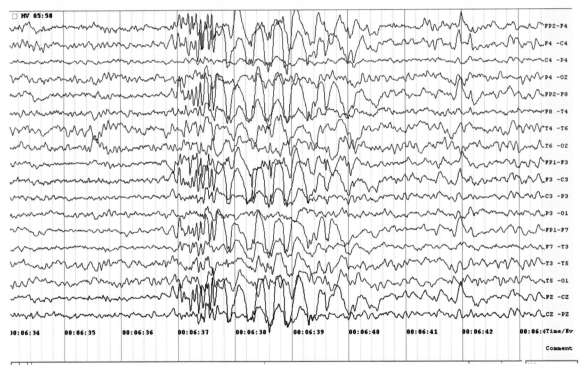

Fig. 5.1: EEG of a patient with juvenile myoclonic epilepsy (JME) showing generalized poly-spike wave discharges.

Poor Compliance

In some instances, although the diagnosis of epilepsy and the choice and dose of AED might be appropriate, the patient is poorly adherent to the dosage schedule of the AED/s. This might be an issue in adolescents, those with chronic epilepsy and those requiring multiple doses of several AEDs (polytherapy).

DEFINITION OF INTRACTABLE EPILEPSY

Chronic epilepsy in which seizures continue to occur despite appropriate AED treatment has been variously referred to in medical literature as medically intractable epilepsy, medically refractory epilepsy, and pharmaco (or drug)-resistant epilepsy. Till recently, there has been no uniformly accepted definition of intractable epilepsy. Definitions or criteria used have varied according to the setting in which they have been applied, e.g., epidemiological, presurgical evaluation, and clinical drug trials of newer AEDs. Lately, the ILAE proposed an algorithmical approach to the diagnosis of drug-resistant epilepsy.[2] A first step in the process is to decide whether seizures are controlled completely or whether the AED treatment instituted has failed (Fig. 5.1). The next step is to decide the appropriateness of AED treatment

Dayanand Medical College and Hospital, Ludhiana
Department of Neurology
Antiepileptic Drug Chart

Patient name: Age/Sex:

Drug	Start date	Stop date	Maintenance dose	Maximum dose	Adverse effects	Level of seizure control

Fig. 5.2: An example of historical record of antiepileptic drug use.

regimen/s (all AEDs used by the patient so far) used, and in this step it needs to be ascertained if the choice, dose prescribed, duration of treatment, and intake of drug are appropriate for the epilepsy syndrome. We recommend that a detailed drug history in the past be obtained from the patient and through review of past medical records. The duration of use of each AED, the maximal dose used, the side effects recorded, and the degree of seizure control with AEDs used are recorded and critically analyzed using drug charts (Fig. 5.2). This chart helps in critically analyzing, which of the AEDs used so far have been used appropriately or vice versa. Examples of inappropriately used AED regimens include the use of ethosuccimide in a patient with intractable temporal lobe epilepsy, or phenytoin in a dose of 100 mg/day in a gentleman weighing 90 kg. Once appropriateness of intervention with AEDs has been established, then drug-resistant epilepsy can be defined as failure of adequate trials of two tolerated and appropriately chosen and used AED schedules (whether as monotherapies or in combination) to achieve sustained seizure freedom. A final step is to determine what constitutes seizure freedom. The ILAE defines seizure freedom as a seizure-free duration that is at least three times the longest interseizure interval prior to starting a new intervention. This seizure-free duration

would need to be observed. If the seizure-free duration is too short, e.g., in days or weeks, then a minimum seizure-free period of 12 months is required in order to label the patient as seizure-free. If, on the other hand, the patient has one or more seizures within the stipulated time period, he or she would be deemed to have failed treatment. This stepwise protocol for the ascertainment of medically intractable epilepsy is relevant and should be followed in all referral centers for care of intractable epilepsy.

From Medically Intractable Epilepsy to Surgically Remediable Epilepsy: The Steps Involved

A seminal randomized trial of early epilepsy surgery versus best medical treatment in medically intractable mesial temporal lobe epilepsy clearly established the superiority of surgical treatment. Seizure-free rates were 58% in the surgically treated group and only 8% in the medically treated group.[5] In general, seizure freedom is reported in 70–80% of surgically treated mesial temporal lobe epilepsy due to mesial temporal sclerosis. The rates of seizure freedom are similar in the case of lesionectomies undertaken for low-grade epileptogenic tumors. In the case of extratemporal epilepsies, the rates of seizure freedom following surgical treatment are less and may vary from 30 to 60%.

As alluded to earlier, about 20–30% of all newly diagnosed epilepsies eventually turn out to be medically intractable. Recent follow-up studies in specialist epilepsy care centers have shown that once two appropriately chosen and given AEDs fail to ensure seizure freedom, the chances that a third AED would be able to offer seizure freedom to the patient are <10%.[2] Hence, the emphasis is on the early identification of medically intractable epilepsy. Since, the results of further medical treatment in patients with established intractable epilepsy are poor, alternative treatments such as surgery, vagus nerve stimulation, dietary therapies (e.g., ketogenic diet in children), and certain experimental therapies need to be considered. Hence, the 20–30% proportion of intractable epilepsy patients constitutes a pool of potential candidates for epilepsy surgery. When subjected to intensive evaluation with a battery of investigations [including video-EEG telemetry, specialized epilepsy-protocol magnetic resonance imaging (MRI), ictal and interictal single photon emission computed tomography (SPECT), neuropsychological evaluation and many a times, long-term invasive EEG monitoring using subdural grid or depth electrodes] in addition to expert clinical judgment, roughly one-fourth of the pool would eventually be declared to be good candidates for surgical treatment. Thus, the actual proportion of people with newly diagnosed epilepsy in whom epilepsy would truly be surgically remediable is 4–5%.

It is essential that all patients with medically intractable epilepsy should be referred to a specialized center for epilepsy that is equipped with expertise and facilities for the presurgical evaluation of epilepsies. The number of centers that offer presurgical evaluations and epilepsy surgery are limited, both in Western affluent countries and, even more so, in low- and middle-income countries. These centers have the necessary equipment (Box 5.1) and a team of experts, including a neurologist with expertise in the presurgical evaluation, a neuroradiologist, a neuropsychologist, a psychiatrist, a nuclear medicine specialist, and a neurosurgeon. The investigative workup for epilepsy surgery is time consuming, labor intensive, and expensive. After necessary investigative workup, the team meets and discusses the suitability of the patient for surgery. The centers for epilepsy vary in the level of expertise and facilities for presurgical evaluation and surgery. Hence, two different levels of epilepsy surgery, and presurgical facilities are available (Table 5.2). In general, the

Box 5.1: Equipment required for presurgical workup
- Video-EEG telemetry (scalp recordings)
- MRI (1.5 or 3 T)
- SPECT
- PET
- Electrocorticography
- Magnetoencephalography

MRI, magnetic resonance imaging; SPECT, single photon emission computed tomography; PET, positron emission tomography.

TABLE 5.2: **Levels of epilepsy surgery**

Level	Investigations	Surgeries
Level 1	Routine interictal EEG, surface video-EEG, MRI (1.5 T) using epilepsy protocols, neuropsychology	Anteromesial temporal lobe resections, standard lesionectomies
Level 2	In addition to above, SPECT (ictal and interictal) SISCOM, PET, MRI applications like functional MRI, ideally 3 T MRI, intracranial EEG	Electrocorticography-guided resections, multilobar resections, functional hemispherectomy, multiple subpial resections, corpus callosotomy, intracranial grid and depth electrode placement, vagus nerve stimulation

EEG, electroencephalogram; MRI, magnetic resonance imaging; SPECT, single photon emission computed tomography; PET, positron emission tomography.

number of epilepsy surgery centers is limited and there is a huge surgical treatment gap in most countries of the world. This treatment gap is the difference between the proportion of patients who require surgical treatment and those who actually are able to get surgical treatment. The reasons for the surgical treatment gap are the limited number of epilepsy surgery centers, cost and expense of presurgical evaluation, and lack of awareness among physicians of the utility of epilepsy surgery.

CONCEPTUAL ISSUES IN PRESURGICAL WORKUP

The basic aim of presurgical workup is to select patients for epilepsy surgery. This involves, firstly, a firm determination that the patient would benefit from surgery, and secondly, that risks associated with surgery are insignificant in comparison to the benefits offered. Few important terms that are relevant to the understanding of presurgical workup are given in Box 5.2.[6] The purpose of epilepsy surgery is to provide complete seizure freedom,

Box 5.2: Relevant terms for the understanding of presurgical workup

Epileptogenic zone: Area of the cerebral cortex that is indispensable for the generation of seizures and the removal of which leads to seizure freedom

Symptomatogenic zone: Area of cerebral cortex that generates the initial seizure manifestations, usually an aura or focal motor manifestations

Seizure onset zone: Area of cerebral cortex from where seizures begin. Generally, it is smaller than the epileptogenic zone, and it may or may not correspond to the symptomatogenic zone

Irritative zone: Area of cerebral cortex that generates interictal spikes defined by using EEG, MEG, or electrocorticographic studies

Functional deficit zone: Area of cortex in relation to the epileptogenic zone that is functionally abnormal, e.g., the motor cortex in a patient who has a hemiparesis, and partial motor seizures involving the contralateral upper limb

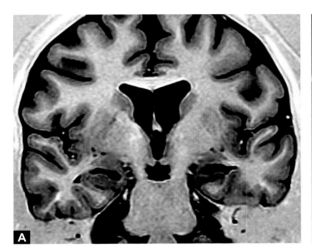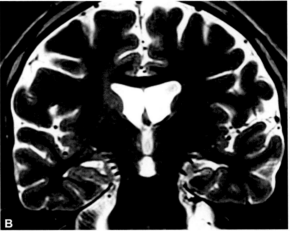

Figs 5.3A and B: **(A)** T1-weighted oblique coronal image showing left-sided hippocampal atrophy; **(B)** T2 oblique coronal image showing hyperintensity of the left hippocampus.

while at the same time ensuring that it does not lead to unacceptable neurological morbidity or deficit/s. These two objectives are usually met by complete resection of the epileptogenic zone and preservation of the eloquent cortex of the brain.

MAGNETIC RESONANCE IMAGING

Magnetic resonance imaging is usually the starting point in the investigation of intractable epilepsy. It is indispensable for identifying and outlining the epileptogenic lesion. The use of special sequences and protocols, which have been adopted in most epilepsy surgery centers, has made MRI exquisitely sensitive for the detection of epileptogenic lesions such as hippocampal sclerosis, cortical dysplasia, tumors, and other lesions such as cavernous hemangioma (Figs 5.3 to 5.5).[7] Epilepsy protocol MRI begins with T1-weighted, T2-weighted, and fluid attenuation inversion recovery (FLAIR) sequences.

Visual inspection, by an experienced neuroradiologist, of oblique coronal 1–2 mm cuts taken perpendicular to the long axis of the hippocampus using T1-weighted, FLAIR, T2-weighted sequences are extremely sensitive and specific for the detection of hippocampal pathology. The T1-weighted sequence detects hippocampal atrophy and abnormalities of the internal architecture of the hippocampus and FLAIR and T2-weighted sequences detect hippocampal hyperintensities suggestive of hippocampal sclerosis. When hippocampal sclerosis is not detectable on visual inspection, hippocampal volumetry using T1-weighted volume acquisition scans and the quantitative measurement of T2 relaxation times can uncover subtle hippocampal abnormalities. At present, hippocampal volumetry and measurement of T2 relaxation times are mainly used for research purposes. T2-weighted and FLAIR sequences frequently reveal focal areas of cortical thickening and blurring of the gray-white matter junction suggestive of cortical dysplasia.

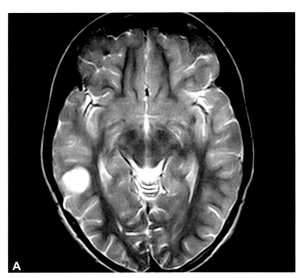 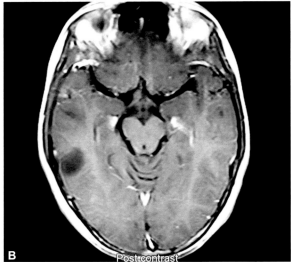

Figs 5.4A and B: **(A)** Axial T2-weighted image showing a dysembroblastic neuroepithelial tumor in the lateral temporal location; **(B)** Axial T1-weighted image showing the hypointense lesion in the same location.

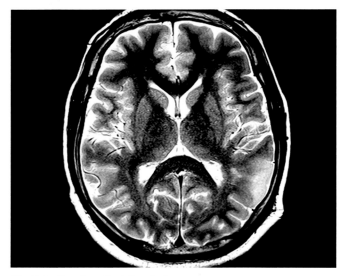

Fig. 5.5: Focal cortical dysplasia

The detection of subtle cortical dysplasia requires an experienced observer. Advanced MRI methods such as three-dimensional volume reconstruction, curvilinear reformatting, and automated segmentation and quantification of the cerebral cortex are being increasingly used for the detection of cortical developmental abnormalities.[8] The gradient echo sequences are useful for the detection of cavernous hemangioma. Finally, the increasing availability of 3T MRI has led to its application in epilepsy, and initial experience has shown that it is superior to 1.5T for the detection of subtle cortical developmental abnormalities.[9]

VIDEO-EEG TELEMETRY

Long-term monitoring with video-EEG telemetry is indispensable in the presurgical evaluation of medically intractable epilepsy. Telemetry is an expensive, time-consuming investigation both from the patient and medical personnel point of view. It involves, long-term EEG monitoring using standard EEG montages (with some additions in some instances) in addition to continuous video monitoring over several days. During this period, AEDs might be carefully and skillfully reduced in order to enhance the chances of occurrence of seizures. Telemetry is usually performed in the epilepsy monitoring unit, which are specialized wards with purpose-trained personnel. Video recording of the seizures allows the opportunity of viewing the semiology of the seizures, which can provide considerable insights into the localization and lateralization of seizures, crucial to the determination of the need for epilepsy surgery. In addition, specially trained medical personnel carry out clinical testing and interaction with the patient, which helps in establishing whether or not consciousness was retained during and after the seizure, and this inturn helps in detecting ictal and post-ictal speech disorders. The purpose behind telemetry is to confirm the diagnosis of epilepsy and its syndromic assignment, to rule out non-epileptic seizures, and to confirm the relationship of the epileptogenic lesion identified on MRI to the seizures (both clinically and electrically). Analysis of seizure semiology is an extremely useful tool in localization and lateralization of the seizure onset (Tables 5.3 to 5.5).[6,10]

TABLE 5.3: Lateralizing ictal and postictal symptoms and signs in patients with temporal lobe or extratemporal epilepsy

Symptoms/signs	Lateralization and localization of epileptogenic zone
Definite symptoms/signs	
Forced head-version (<10 s) before secondary generalization	Contralateral, temporal, extratemporal
Unilateral ictal dystonia	Contralateral, temporal, extratemporal
Ictal speech	Nondominant, temporal
Preserved consciousness during ictal automatisms	Nondominant, temporal
Postictal dysphasia	Dominant, temporal
Postictal nose wiping	Ipsilateral, temporal
Unilateral eye blinking	Ipsilateral, temporal
Figure of four	
Auras	
Somatosensory	• Contralateral, primary somatosensory cortex (areas 1, 2, and 3b) • Ipsilateral (if unilateral), secondary somatosensory areas (parietal operculum/SSII) • Contralateral (mostly), SSMA
Simple visual	Contralateral, primary visual cortex (areas 17, 18, and 19)
Complex visual	Contralateral (if unilateral), temporo-occipital junction and basal temporal cortex
Simple auditory	Contralateral (if unilateral), primary auditory cortex (area 41)
Complex auditory	Contralateral (if unilateral), auditory association cortex (areas 42 and 22)
Vertiginous	Nonlateralizing (often right), temporo-occipital junction
Olfactory	Nonlateralizing, orbitofrontal region, amygdala, and insula
Gustatory	Nonlateralizing, parietal operculum, and basal temporal cortex
Autonomic	Nonlateralizing, insula, amygdala, anterior cingulum, and SSMA
Abdominal	Nonlateralizing, anterior insula, frontal operculum, mesial temporal lobe, and SSMA
Fear	Nonlateralizing, amygdala, hippocampus, and mesial frontal lobe
Déjà vu/jamais vu	Nonlateralizing (often ND), uncus, entorhinal cortex, and temporal neocortex
Multisensorial	Nonlateralizing, mesiobasal limbic cortex, temporal neocortex, TPO junction
Cephalic/whole body	Nonlateralizing, amygdala, entorhinal cortex, and temporal neocortex/SSII, and SSMA
Simple motor	
Myoclonic/negative	Contralateral (if unilateral), primary motor cortex (area 4) and premotor cortex (area 6)/primary somatosensory area
Myoclonus	Contralateral (if unilateral), primary motor cortex and SSMA
Tonic	Nonlateralizing, anterior cingulum, orbitofrontal region, frontopolar region, opercular-insular cortex, and medial intermediate frontal area
Complex motor	
Hypermotor	Nonlateralizing, mesial temporal and anterior cingulum
Automotor	Nonlateralizing, hypothalamus, anteromesial frontal region, and basal temporal area
Gelastic	Nonlateralizing, limbic temporal structures, cingulum, intermediate frontal (area 8), and orbitofrontal areas

Continued

Continued

Symptoms/signs	Lateralization and localization of epileptogenic zone
Dialeptic	
Autonomic	
Tachycardia/Hyperventilation	Nonlateralizing (often right), amygdala, insula, anterior cingulum, and medial prefrontal cortex
Piloerection	Ipsilateral
Mydriasis	Ipsilateral (if unilateral)
Semiologic features	
Automatisms	
Oral automatisms	Temporal lobe, typically hippocampal
Bipedal automatisms	Frontal lobe seizures
Ictal laughter (gelastic)	Hypothalamic, mesial temporal or frontal cingulate origin
Motor abnormalities	
Early nonforced head turn	Ipsilateral to seizure origin
Focal clonic jerking	Contralateral to seizure origin, perirolandic
Asymmetric clonic ending	Ipsilateral to seizure origin
Fencing posture	Contralateral frontal lobe (supplementary motor) seizures
Unilateral ictal paresis	Contralateral to seizure origin
Postictal Todd's paresis	Contralateral to seizure origin
Autonomic features	
Ictus emeticus	Right temporal seizures
Ictal urinary urge	Right temporal seizures
Piloerection (goose bumps)	Left temporal seizures

SSMA, supplementary sensorimotor area.

TABLE 5.4: Differentiating staring due to absence from that of complex partial seizures

Features	Absence	Complex partial
Sleep activation	None	Common
Hyperventilation	Induces the seizures	No activating effect
Seizure frequency	Frequent, many per day	Less frequent
Seizure onset	Abrupt	Slow
Aura	None	Often preceded by a simple partial seizure
Automatism	Rare	Common
Progression	Minimal	Evolution of features
Cyanosis	None	Common
Motor signs	Rare, or minimal	Common
Seizure duration	Brief (usually <30 s)	Minutes
Postictal confusion or sleep	None	Common
Postictal dysphasia	None	Common in seizures origination from the dominant hemisphere

TABLE 5.5: Semiology of frontal versus temporal lobe seizures

Features	Frontal lobe	Temporal lobe
Seizure frequency	Frequent, often daily	Less frequent
Sleep activation	Characteristic	Less common
Seizure onset	Abrupt, explosive	Slower
Progression	Rapid	Slower
Initial motionless staring	Less common	Common
Automatism	Less common	More common and longer
Bipedal automatism	Characteristic	Rare
Complex postures	Early, frequent, and prominent	Late, less frequent, and less prominent
Hyperkinetic motor signs	Common	Rare
Somatosensory symptoms	Common	Rare
Speech	Loud vocalization (grunting, screaming, moaning)	Verbalization speech in non-dominant seizures
Seizure duration	Brief	Longer
Secondary generalization	Common	Less common
Postictal confusion	Less prominent or short	More prominent and longer
Postictal dysphasia	Rare, unless it spreads to the dominant temporal lobe	Common in dominant temporal lobe seizures

For instance, the occurrence of visual aura in one hemifield or a unilateral somatosensory aura correlates with seizure onset in the contralateral hemisphere and hence, has excellent lateralizing value. Indeed a number of symptoms (auras) and ictal and post-ictal signs have now been described which are exquisitely sensitive and specific for the lateralization, particularly, of complex partial seizures of temporal lobe origin (Table 5.3). During telemetry, analysis of the EEG allows definition of the irritative zone and confirmation of the relationship between ictal onset zone and the epileptogenic lesion. This provides extremely useful information for the delineation of the epileptogenic zone.

MAGNETOENCEPHALOGRAPHY

Multiple channel (over 300) magnetoencephalography (MEG) is an expensive investigation, not widely available in most epilepsy centers. However, it is now increasingly recognized that it has potential applications in presurgical evaluation.[11,12] With the combination of increased number of channels available and magnetic source imaging, a specialized technique for data analysis, MEG is superior to scalp EEG for the detection of neocortical spikes, and is particularly useful for the detection of epileptogenic lesions not visualized on MRI, identification of the epileptogenic lesion when several potential lesions are visualized, e.g., multiple tubers in a patient with intractable epilepsy and tuberous sclerosis. Although currently restricted in availability, MEG is likely to play an important role in presurgical evaluation in the future.

Nuclear Imaging (Positron Emission Tomography and Single Photon Emission Tomography)

Positron emission tomography (PET) using 18F-fluoro-deoxyglucose, most commonly, finds application in brain metabolic-functional scanning. It measures the metabolic rate of glucose in various regions of the brain. Interictal PET scan demonstrates reduced glucose metabolism on the side of seizure origin and hence provides useful lateralizing information. This information is particularly useful in MRI-negative cases (e.g., cases of mesial temporal lobe epilepsy, in which MRI does not reveal hippocampal sclerosis, or cases of focal cortical dysplasia, in which MRI might be completely normal).[13] Concordance between the side or lobe showing hypo-metabolism on 18F-fluorodeoxyglucose-PET and the ictal onset zone demonstrated on video-EEG telemetry is a useful indicator in the prediction of the success of epilepsy surgery, especially in MRI-negative cases.

Different applications of PET technology are finding use in presurgical evaluation of intractable epilepsies. 11C-Flumazenil PET measures the relative density of benzodiazepine receptors, which in turn reflect the proportion of gamma-aminobutyric acid (GABA) in various regions of the brain.[14] The transmission of GABA and hence the density of benzodiazepine receptors is reduced in the epileptogenic zone and this is reflected by the regional uptake of the radioactive tracer on PET scan. Another radioactive tracer, 11C-alpha-methyl-L-tryptophan (AMT) has found application in the PET evaluation of tuberous sclerosis.[15] When MRI reveals multiple tubers, AMT-PET provides information on which of the tubers is epileptogenic.

Single photon emission computed tomography has the advantage that it can be used in the lateralization and localization of surgically remediable epilepsies both in the ictal and interictal states. The sensitivity of interictal SPECT is low (about 20-40%); it often demonstrates hypometabolism on the side/lobe of seizure origin.[16] Ictal SPECT is the only nuclear imaging modality that demonstrates the region of seizure origin. The basis of ictal SPECT is an increased blood flow at the focus of seizure origin. The radioactive tracer (either 99 m technetium-hexamethyl propylene amine oxime or 99 mTc-ethylene-dicysteine diethyl ester) is injected intravenously, and is distributed preferentially to the cortical region of seizure onset. The increased uptake of the radioactive tracer at the site of seizure origin represents the area of hypermetabolism and hence, increased blood flow. Ictal SPECT provides reliable lateralization and localization of the epileptogenic zone with a sensitivity of over 90%, provided the tracer is injected within 30 seconds of seizure onset.[17] If, however, injection is undertaken 30 seconds after seizure onset, then the reliability decreases as by this time, the seizure has spread to other cortical regions.

Subtraction ictal SPECT coregistered to MRI is a technique in which the interictal SPECT images are coregistered first subtracted from the ictal SPECT, which accentuates the cortical region of seizure origin.[18] The subtracted image is then coregistered to a structural MRI for better anatomical delineation of the epileptogenic zone. This helps not only in planning the extent of resection but also serves as a guide to the site of implantation of subcortical grid electrodes.

Intracranial EEG

Intracranial EEG recording with video-telemetry is uncommonly indicated particularly for patient selection for level 2 epilepsy surgery. It is undertaken when the relationship of the epileptogenic lesion/s on structural MRI and the seizure onset demonstrated by surface EEG video-telemetry and/or ictal SPECT is unclear

or discordant. Either subdural or depth electrodes are inserted following craniotomy and ictal onset is recorded in the epilepsy monitoring unit. The advantage is that cortical stimulation, in order to map out eloquent functional cortex, can also be undertaken by stimulating the subcortical grid electrodes. The disadvantages of intracranial EEG are that it requires a craniotomy, is expensive, and there is a risk of intracranial infections with long-term recording.

Electrocorticography

For mapping out the epileptogenic zone/s and eloquent cortex better, electrodes might be applied directly to the brain surface during surgery. This records electrical activity from the cortex directly, even though for a short period of time. Since, there are no barriers (skull, cerebrospinal fluid, etc.), between the cortex and the electrodes, the frequency of spikes is higher and their distribution wider than surface EEG. This essentially outlines the irritative zone and guides the extent of cortical resection (tailored resection). Simultaneously, electrical stimulation of the electrocorticography electrodes can be undertaken so as to map out the functional cortex. In surgical practice, the role of electrocorticography is somewhat controversial and experts have deliberated on its advantages and disadvantages vis-à-vis standard resections.

NEUROPSYCHOLOGICAL EVALUATION

Comprehensive neuropsychological evaluation using a battery of tests performed by a clinical neuropsychologist with experience in presurgical evaluation provides useful information, particularly so in two respects.[19] First, certain neuropsychological defects correlate with specific localization of the epileptogenic lesions, e.g., left mesial temporal lobe sclerosis with impaired verbal memory and right mesial temporal sclerosis with nonverbal memory. Second, the degree of preoperative verbal memory impairment is a predictor of postoperative memory decline following left-sided (dominant hemisphere) anteromesial temporal lobe resection (the better the preoperative verbal memory score, the greater the magnitude of decline that is likely following resection of the hippocampus and other mesial temporal structures).

PSYCHIATRIC EVALUATION

There is significant psychiatric comorbidity with epilepsy and this association is all the more apparent in chronic intractable epilepsy. A psychiatrist is an important member of the presurgical evaluation team and psychiatric evaluation forms a core aspect of presurgical evaluation. In general, the presence of significant and severe concomitant psychiatric disorders such as psychosis (except ictal psychosis) or mood disorders and mental retardation that might preclude effective psychosocial rehabilitation of the individual following seizure control with epilepsy surgery constitute a contraindication to epilepsy surgery.

WADA'S TEST AND FUNCTIONAL MRI

The Wada's test was frequently performed during presurgical workup till about a decade ago.[20] It was undertaken for language and memory lateralization and for predicting the extent of postoperative memory decline following anteromesial temporal lobe resections. The test is no longer undertaken, largely because of its invasiveness. To quite an extent, it has been replaced by functional MRI. Various paradigms for functional MRI have been developed and validated and these are useful in three contexts: (i) localization of motor cortex prior to surgery for tumors or dysplastic lesions involving the perirolandic cortex, (ii) lateralization of language function prior to surgery involving the dominant area encompassing the speech regions, and (iii) lateralization of memory function. Of the three, the first two applications have been well developed and are widely used in the clinical setting, while the third is still under development.[21] Another application in development is the EEG spike-triggered functional MRI.[22] The latter involves the use of MRI-compatible EEG equipment including electrodes and recording of EEG for a short period during MRI. The random occurrence of an EEG spike triggers BOLD MRI acquisition, which effectively detects changes in regional or local blood blow associated with the EEG spike. This provides useful anatomical demarcation of the source of spike origin or the irritative zone.

PRESURGICAL MEETING

Epilepsy surgery and presurgical evaluation are essentially a teamwork. The team comprises of a neurologist with special expertise in presurgical workup, a neurosurgeon with expertise in surgical methods involving surgically remediable epilepsy, a neuroradiologist, a neuropsychologist, a psychiatrist, and a nuclear imaging specialist. In epilepsy centers devoted to presurgical workup, the team meets at regular intervals

and discusses and reviews the presurgical workup data in an orderly manner in order to draw a consensus on the surgical, or in cases where further presurgical evaluation is warranted, the presurgical strategies. This approach ensures transparency and minimizes individual bias in treatment approaches. Each center, depending on its level of expertise and technology, has well-defined protocols for presurgical evaluation. These protocols, generally, should be adhered to.

EPILEPSY SURGERY

Once a decision for epilepsy surgery has been arrived at, the patient is counseled regarding the risks and benefits of the surgical approach. The chances of surgical success are clearly informed both verbally and in writing. In general, the chances of complete seizure freedom following standard anteromesial temporal lobe resection for unequivocal unilateral mesial temporal sclerosis are about 70–80%. The chances of seizure freedom following complete excision (lesionectomy) for an epileptogenic tumor (e.g., dysembroplastic neuroepithelial tumor or ganglioglioma) are also about 70–80%. Seizure freedom following surgery for intractable epilepsy due to cortical dysplasia and other developmental malformations is less (40–60%) as microscopic cortical dysplasia is often widespread and extends well beyond the anatomically demonstrated abnormality seen on MRI. Hence, because resections cannot encompass these areas of microscopic dysplasia, seizures might recur following surgery. Likewise, the chances of success following surgery for extratemporal epilepsies are in the tune of 40–60%. Surgery is sometimes undertaken following patient consent on epileptogenic zones that are defined by procedures such as EEG, nuclear imaging, or MEG but in whom the MRI is essentially normal. In these cases, it can be presumed that the MRI is not sufficiently sensitive to demonstrating the epileptogenic lesion (e.g., microscopic dysplasia). The results of seizure freedom following surgery in nonlesional (MRI-normal) cases are understandably less. Certain surgeries, e.g., corpus callosotomy, disconnection surgeries, and multiple subpial transections, are performed in multilobar epilepsies or when the epileptogenic lesion involves eloquent cortex and hence the chances of postoperative neurological deficits are high. These are essentially palliative procedures. During the meeting, the patient is also counseled about the risks involved in epilepsy surgery. The choice of the surgical procedure depends on the level of expertise of the epilepsy surgery team and the experience of the operating neurosurgeon (Table 5.1B).

CONCLUSION

The success of presurgical workup and epilepsy surgery depends on sound clinical principles and good teamwork between competent experts from different areas of clinical medicine. This multidisciplinary approach is essential to the success of surgery. Although at present only a fraction of patients with intractable epilepsy eventually proceed to surgery, research efforts are currently focusing on the strategies to increase the proportion of intractable epilepsies that might benefit from surgery and also to reduce the morbidity associated with surgery.

REFERENCES

1. Brodie MJ, Shorvon SD, Canger R, et al. Commission on European Affairs: appropriate standards of epilepsy care across Europe. ILEA. Epilepsia. 1997;38(11):1245-50. Epub 1998/05/14.
2. Kwan P, Brodie MJ. Early identification of refractory epilepsy. N Engl J Med. 2000; 342(5):314-9. Epub 2000/02/05.
3. Gilman JT, Duchowny M, Jayakar P, et al. Medical intractability in children evaluated for epilepsy surgery. Neurology. 1994;44(7):1341-3. Epub 1994/07/01.
4. Kwan P, Arzimanoglou A, Berg AT, et al. Definition of drug resistant epilepsy: consensus proposal by the ad hoc Task Force of the ILAE Commission on Therapeutic Strategies. Epilepsia. 2010;51(6):1069-77. Epub 2009/11/06.
5. Wiebe S, Blume WT, Girvin JP, et al. Effectiveness, efficiency of surgery for temporal lobe epilepsy study G. A randomized, controlled trial of surgery for temporal-lobe epilepsy. N Engl J Med. 2001;345(5):311-8. Epub 2001/08/04.
6. Rosenow F, Luders H. Presurgical evaluation of epilepsy. Brain: A Journal of Neurology. 2001;124(Pt 9): 1683-700. Epub 2001/08/28.
7. Kuzniecky R. Magnetic resonance and functional magnetic resonance imaging: tools for the study of human epilepsy. Curr Opin Neurol. 1997;10(2):88-91. Epub 1997/04/01.
8. Bastos AC, Comeau RM, Andermann F, et al. Diagnosis of subtle focal dysplastic lesions: curvilinear reformatting from three-dimensional magnetic resonance imaging. Ann Neurol. 1999;46(1):88-94. Epub 1999/07/13.
9. Knake S, Triantafyllou C, Wald LL, et al. 3T phased array MRI improves the presurgical evaluation in focal epilepsies: a prospective study. Neurology. 2005;65(7):1026-31. Epub 2005/10/12.
10. Chee MW, Kotagal P, Van Ness PC, et al. Lateralizing signs in intractable partial epilepsy: blinded multiple-observer analysis. Neurology. 1993;43(12):2519-25. Epub 1993/12/01.
11. RamachandranNair R, Otsubo H, Shroff MM, et al. MEG predicts outcome following surgery for intractable epilepsy in children with normal or nonfocal MRI findings. Epilepsia. 2007;48(1):149-57. Epub 2007/01/24.
12. Fischer MJ, Scheler G, Stefan H. Utilization of magnetoencephalography results to obtain favourable outcomes in epilepsy surgery. Brain: A Journal of Neurology. 2005;128(Pt 1):153-7. Epub 2004/11/26.
13. Theodore WH. When is positron emission tomography really necessary in epilepsy diagnosis? CurrOpin Neurol. 2002;15(2):191-5. Epub 2002/03/30.
14. Ryvlin P, Bouvard S, Le Bars D, et al. Clinical utility of flumazenil-PET versus [18F]fluorodeoxyglucose-PET and MRI in refractory partial epilepsy. A prospective study in 100 patients. Brain: A Journal of Neurology 1998;121(Pt 11):2067-81. Epub 1998/11/25.
15. Fedi M, Reutens DC, Andermann F, et al. alpha-[11C]-methyl-L-tryptophan PET identifies the epileptogenic tuber and correlates with interictal spike frequency. Epilepsy Res. 2003;52(3):203-13. Epub 2003/01/22.
16. Van Paesschen W, Dupont P, Sunaert S, et al. The use of SPECT and PET in routine clinical practice in epilepsy. Curr Opin Neurol. 2007;20(2):194-202. Epub 2007/03/14.
17. Thadani VM, Siegel A, Lewis P, et al. Validation of ictal single photon emission computed tomography with depth encephalography and epilepsy surgery. Neurosurg Rev. 2004;27(1):27-33. Epub 2003/07/08.
18. Ahnlide JA, Rosen I, Linden-Mickelsson Tech P, et al. Does SISCOM contribute to favorable seizure outcome after epilepsy surgery? Epilepsia. 2007;48(3):579-88. Epub 2007/03/10.
19. Jones-Gotman M. Localization of lesions by neuropsychological testing. Epilepsia. 1991;32 (Suppl 5):S41-52. Epub 1991/01/01.
20. Woermann FG, Jokeit H, Luerding R, et al. Language lateralization by Wada test and fMRI in 100 patients with epilepsy. Neurology. 2003;61(5):699-701. Epub 2003/09/10.
21. Rabin ML, Narayan VM, Kimberg DY, et al. Functional MRI predicts post-surgical memory following temporal lobectomy. Brain: A Journal of Neurology. 2004;127(Pt 10):2286-98. Epub 2004/08/27.
22. Krakow K, Woermann FG, Symms MR, et al. EEG-triggered functional MRI of interictal epileptiform activity in patients with partial seizures. Brain: A Journal of Neurology. 1999;122(Pt 9):1679-88. Epub 1999/09/01.

Chapter 6

Psychogenic Nonepileptic Attack Disorder

Parampreet S Kharbanda

INTRODUCTION

Seizures are common and so are nonepileptic seizure mimics that superficially resemble the epileptic seizures. The term nonepileptic seizures encompasses both nonpsychogenic (syncope, paroxysmal movement disorders, cataplexy, complicated migraine, etc.) and psychogenic episodes that mimic seizures. Psychogenic nonepileptic seizures (PNES) are defined as episodes of paroxysmal impairment of self-control associated with a range of motor, sensory, and mental manifestations, which present as experiential or behavioral response to an emotional or social stress. Though majority of PNES are beyond voluntary control, they can occur in malingering and factitious disorders as well.[1,2]

In this chapter, our focus would be on how to approach, evaluate and manage a patient with PNES. Before we go into these details, it is imperative to have some basic knowledge of PNES.

EPIDEMIOLOGY (BOX 6.1)

Psychogenic nonepileptic seizures are not uncommon, with an incidence ranging from 1.4 to 3 per 1,00,000 per year, and a prevalence of 2–33 per 1,00,000. In one study, on patients who presented to the emergency room with a blackout, 57.4% had epilepsy, 22.3% had syncope, and 18% had PNES. It is estimated that 24% of patients with refractory seizures may be suffering from PNES rather than true seizures. Despite such high estimates, it is noteworthy that most of the patients with PNES are diagnosed quite late in their clinical course with a mean diagnostic delay ranging from 7 to 16 years. Seventy-five percent of patients with PNES have received antiepileptic drugs at least in the beginning.[3,4]

Psychogenic nonepileptic seizures are more common in women than men (3:1). The most common factor in women is sexual abuse, and in men it is work-related problems. PNES commonly start in second or third decade of life, though onset before age 4 and after age 70 has also been reported. Prognosis is better in adults and young children.[3,4]

CLINICAL SEMIOLOGY OF PNES[1-6]

The most common semiology of PNES involves excessive movement of the limbs, trunk, and the head. Seizures with atonia, stiffening or tremor are less common. Though PNES can start abruptly, the onset is usually more gradual than true seizures. Shaking is more asynchronous and asymmetrical in PNES. In true seizures, tonic clonic activity decreases gradually during the course of the seizure, but in PNES the jerks vary in terms of amplitude rather than frequency and may become more severe after a period of relative quiescence. Pelvic thrusting, especially forward thrusting, is more common in PNES. The head may shake from side-to-side. The eyes and mouth are usually tightly closed and any effort to open is

---

Box 6.1: PNES: Some interesting facts

- Mean delay in diagnosis of PNES ranges from 7 to 15 years
- Up to 30% of refractory seizures may be attributable to PNES
- 75% of patients with PNES receive antiepileptic drugs

resisted. Pupillary light response is preserved. Ictal crying and verbal communication are common. Purposeful movements during the state of unconsciousness may be seen. While a patient commonly allows the hands to fall freely on the chest or the bed during PNES, the fall of hands on the eyes is usually avoided. While performing this maneuver, appropriate care must be taken to prevent any injury if in case it may be a true seizure. PNES typically last longer than true seizures with seizure duration exceeding two minutes in most cases, while true tonic clonic seizures are brief and usually last for 50–90 seconds.[1-6]

Regarding autonomic symptoms (Box 6.2), urinary and even fecal incontinence may occur in upto 25% of PNES patients. Cyanosis is rare. Sinus tachycardia may occur especially with convulsive PNES. However, it is more gradual in onset and less marked than true seizures. An important clue here is that in PNES, the degree of sinus tachycardia appears to be proportionate to what is expected on the basis of visible seizure manifestations. Increase in body temperature is common during true seizures, but rare in PNES.[4-6]

The feelings of panic and hyperventilation, though can occasionally occur with true seizures, are much more common with PNES. Also, recall of events during the seizure is much more common in PNES as compared to patients with true seizures.

The clinical contexts in which the seizures occur also help in diagnosis of PNES. Ninety-five percent of PNES episodes occur in the setting of recent distressing personal or social events. In fact, it is difficult to diagnose PNES in the absence of a recent stressor. However, one should realize that patients may lack coherence about their self-representation and it may be difficult to obtain a relevant history sometimes depending on patient's personal and social background.[4-6]

UNDERLYING FACTORS IN ETIOLOGY OF PNES

Psychogenic nonepileptic seizures are by definition psychiatric disorders. According to DSM IV, physical symptoms secondary to psychiatric causes can fall into three categories: somatoform disorders, factitious disorders, and malingering. Somatoform disorders imply an unconscious production of physical symptoms due to an underlying psychological disturbance that is not under voluntary control. These are further classified into conversion disorder and somatization disorder. In factitious disorders and malingering, patients try to deceive the doctor purposefully, only difference being that in malingering, gain is clearly obvious while in factitious disorder, it is not so. Practically, most of the patients with PNES fit into somatoform or conversion disorder with only a small minority fitting into malingering or factitious disorder. The job of a neurologist is to decide whether the index patient is suffering from PNES or not. Further management and classification is best done by a psychiatrist.[4]

PREDISPOSING FACTORS

About 90% of the PNES patients report a history of traumatic experiences in the past. The most common traumatic factors have been sexual abuse (24%) and physical abuse (16%) in childhood (Box 6.3).

There is a significant history of familial dysfunction in PNES with positive family history of psychiatric disorder or epilepsy in a significant proportion. There is high incidence of familial conflicts in PNES patients and they often rate their family members to be less supportive or caring.

In addition, PNES patients have high incidence of psychiatric comorbidities such as somatoform, other dissociative, post-traumatic stress, depressive, or anxiety disorders. They do not cope with stresses or even their illness in a proper fashion. They are less likely than true epilepsy patients to endorse stress as the cause of their symptoms. They often report their lives more stressful as compared to patients with true epilepsy and are more likely to use escape or avoidance to deal with problems.

In addition, PNES patients do less well on neuro-psychological tests. Whether this is due to malingering or lack of effort or due to significant cognitive decline is still debatable though current evidence is more in favor of lack of effort.[2,4,6]

Box 6.2: Autonomic symptoms in PNES

- Urinary and even fecal incontinence may occur in up to 25% of PNES patients
- Sinus tachycardia may occur especially with convulsive PNES. However, the degree of sinus tachycardia appears to be proportionate to what is expected on basis of visible seizure manifestations

---

Box 6.3: Predisposing factors

- 90% of PNES patients report traumatic experiences
- Most common factor in women is sexual abuse and in children it is physical abuse
- PNES patients do less well on neuropsychological tests

PRECIPITATING EVENTS OR TRIGGERS FOR SEIZURES[4]

Psychogenic nonepileptic seizures are known to be precipitated by stressful or traumatic life events such as rape, injury, giving birth, loss of job, separation from family or friends, road traffic or other accidents, interpersonal relationship problems, and legal issues. Though, a life event can be identified in relation to PNES in 91% of patients, in 76% the event is significant only in the context of a previous or ongoing conflict or trauma.

In addition to precipitation, seizure events in PNES are more likely to recur in response to a number of much less significant events or stimuli, such as visits to the doctor, visits to homes of distant relatives, or other insignificant stresses. Seizures can frequently be induced by suggestion in PNES patients such as by vibration of a tunic fork or by flashes of light during video electroencephalography (EEG). For the sake of providing correct information to the patient, some experts recommend using stimuli similar to the ones which can precipitate epileptic seizures, like hyperventilation, photic stimulation etc. However, this can be confusing as these stimuli may actually induce an epileptic seizure.

PERPETUATING FACTORS[4]

Social and/or financial gains are commonly found in patients with PNES especially in more chronic cases. They may acquire a sick role and give responsibilities to others. They are significantly more likely to receive medical-related state benefits than similarly disabled seizure patients.

COEXISTENCE OF PNES AND EPILEPSY[2]

The prevalence of epilepsy in patients with PNES is greater than in general population with estimates ranging from 3 to 60%. Usually in these patients, PNES are preceded by true seizures and PNES may cease once, the true seizures are well controlled. They may manifest for the first time after an epilepsy surgery or once seizures are well controlled with drugs. This fact poses further difficulty in evaluating the patients with PNES.

CLINICAL APPROACH TO DIAGNOSIS

Despite commonly seen in epilepsy centers, PNES often pose a challenge for diagnosis and management. The situation is further confounded by the fact that diagnosis of epilepsy, once made is difficult to undo as misdiagnosis of epilepsy has serious consequences and moreover, PNES and epilepsy commonly coexist in the same patient. Thus, despite ability to diagnose PNES with near certainty, the mean delay in accurate diagnosis continues to range from 7 to 10 years.[2,4]

WHEN TO SUSPECT THE DIAGNOSIS?

The diagnosis of PNES is initially suspected based on odd features on history and examination. Of course, this diagnosis should always be suspected in presence of high frequency of seizures that is unaffected by administration of antiepileptic drugs. Traditionally, some of the symptoms that are highly suggestive of true epileptic seizures include postictal confusion, incontinence, occurrence in sleep, postictal stertorous breathing and significant injury, in particular, tongue-bites. However, some of these signs can occur in PNES also. The value of these signs is much more if these are documented rather than reported by the patient. The circumstances in which the seizure occurs is also important in determining the diagnosis. PNES tend to occur more in the presence of an audience and occurrence in the physician's office or waiting room during the examination is suggestive of PNES (Box 6.4).[2,4,6]

The past medical history may be of greater help in differentiating between PNES and true seizures. A history of other physical symptoms or illnesses (chronic pain, fibromyalgia, chronic fatigue, multiple allergies) or surgeries (laparoscopies, appendectomies, hysterectomies, etc.) is strong indicator of events being PNES rather than true seizures. Past history of psychiatric treatment also favor the clinical diagnosis of PNES. The examination especially mental status examination, level of concern, and over dramatization may provide important clues to diagnosis of PNES.

A video recording of the episode by the patient's caregivers may be of great use and all patients in whom diagnosis of seizure is not clear should be encouraged to obtain a home video of the event. This can be done through the mobile phones. Patient's primary caregivers

---

Box 6.4: Initial clues to diagnosis of PNES

- Tongue bite though rare may occur over tip of tongue in PNES
- PNES tend to occur more often in presence of audience such as in doctor's waiting room
- A homemade video by primary caregivers through mobile phones may help in diagnosis of PNES

can be educated to make a detailed video. Other helpful feature to diagnose PNES is inducibility of episodes by suggestion, as mentioned above.[5,6]

Psychogenic nonepileptic seizures patients differ significantly in their interaction from patient with true seizures. By adopting a receptive stance, whereby the physician starts interaction with open questions (such as why have you come to us?), a variety of interactional features can be found which may help in differentiation between PNES and true seizures (Table 6.1). While patients with epilepsy discuss their symptoms voluntarily and in detail, patients with PNES discuss these symptoms only sparingly. The patients with PNES avoid discussing seizure as a topic while patients with true seizures avidly discuss on this. The PNES patients do not have a coherent concept of seizure and there is no active struggle against

TABLE 6.1: Differences between true versus pseudoseizures[5]

Clinical feature	Nonepileptic psychogenic seizures	Epileptic seizures
Onset	Gradual, in wakefulness	Abrupt, may be during sleep
Duration	Often >2 minutes	1–2 minutes
Response to verbal stimulus	Common	Never preserved in GTCS; may be partially preserved in CPS
Trashing, violent movements of entire body; side-to-side head movement and side-to-side body turning; pelvic thrusting	Occasional/common	Occasional/common in frontal lobe seizures; rare in GTCS
Upper and lower body out of phase movements	Occasional/common	Rare in GTCS
Unilateral head turning	Rare/occasional	Common preceding GTCS
Whole body rigidity	Rare/occasional	Always present in tonic phase of GTCS
Fluctuating course, pauses in motor activity	Common	Very rare
Opisthotonic posturing	Occasional	Absent
Vocalization	At the start of throughout the seizure/emotional content, ictal stuttering	Monotonous epileptic cry in GTCS/continuous moans, animal-like noises; uttering in frontal lobe seizures
Eye closure	Common, forceful	Rare/very rare; never forceful
Tongue bite	Very rare, on the tip	Occasional/common; on the sides
Incontinence	Very rare	Common in GTCS
Prolonged unresponsiveness without prominent motor features	Occasional	Very rare
Ictal heart rate	Not significantly increased	Increased in CPS/GTCS
Postictal memory	Common	Very rare
Postictal confusion	Occasional	Common/very common
Postictal breathing pattern	Rapid, shallow, irregular with pause	Stertorous breathing after GTCS; quite, shallow after frontal lobe seizures
Precipitants	Common	Less obvious
Postictal headache	Very rare	Common
Postictal fatigue/lethargy	Occasional	Common
Burn injury	Never	Occasional
Inducibility with suggestion	Common	Absent
Whispering voice/partial motor response	Very common	Absent
Recall of memory items	Very common	Rare
Avoidance response	Common	Rare
Extensor plantar response after seizure	Absent	Common
Ictal weeping	Occasional	Very rare

GTCS, generalized tonic-clonic seizure; CPS, complex partial seizures.
Very common: >70; common: 30–70%; occasional: 10–29%; rare 5–9%; very rare: <5%.

Box 6.5: Historical features suggestive of psychogenic non-epileptic seizures

- Dramatically high frequency of episodes not responsive to antiepileptic drugs
- Fibromyalgia/unexplained chronic pain
- Episodes in waiting room
- Emotional triggers for episodes
- Psychiatric comorbidity
- Florid review of symptoms

Source: Adapted and modified from Benbadis SR. Continuum (Minneap Minn). 2013;19(3):715-29.

seizure-threat, while patients with true epilepsy recognize seizures as independent external agent and have a coherent concept of it.[4–6] The common historical features that may suggest a diagnosis of PNES are summarized in Box 6.5.

HOW TO CONFIRM THE DIAGNOSIS

Routine EEG is not very helpful in confirming the diagnosis because of its low sensitivity. However, PNES should be suspected when repeated EEGs are normal even in the wake of frequent attacks. Ambulatory EEG, which is being used with increasing frequency, is more useful. It is cost-effective and can record the habitual episode. However, as ictal EEG can be interpreted only in context of video-recording of the event, it is imperative that diagnosis of PNES should be confirmed by video EEG.[4–6]

VIDEO EEG

Video EEG is the gold standard for diagnosis of PNES. In experienced hands, it provides a definitive diagnosis in a majority of the patients, and is especially indicated in patients who continue to have frequent seizures despite medications. Most of the patients tend to have the events within the first 2 days of recording. In one study,[3] video EEG captured events in 75% of the patients when EEG recording was combined with hyperventilation, photic stimulation, and a strong suggestion. For diagnosis of PNES, it is imperative that EEG is normal during the clinical event. Further, seizure semiology should not be consistent with frontal lobe seizures or other epileptic seizures, which may not be associated with EEG changes. Both the seizure semiology and the EEG should be analyzed independently, especially so, as EEG may be normal during some partial seizures that are not associated with loss of awareness. Also movement artifacts may make interpretation of ictal EEG difficult.

Another feature that is helpful in differentiation of true seizures from PNES is that PNES do not occur during EEG confirmed sleep. Therefore, the occurrence of a seizure while a patient is sleeping as seen on EEG strongly argues against the diagnosis of PNES.[5]

An analysis of the ictal semiology may reveal behaviors that are suggestive of PNES. It is important to note that none of these behaviors is 100% specific. For example, while preserved consciousness despite bilateral motor movements may be considered as nonepileptic, this phenomenology may be seen with supplementary motor area seizures. Most patients with PNES show more than one semiologic features that are considered more likely in PNES, thereby making the diagnosis easy.

THE PITFALLS OF VIDEO EEG (BOX 6.6)[2,5]

The commonest pitfall of video EEG recording is that EEG changes associated with some types of partial seizures are not picked by routine scalp EEG and so knowledge of semiology of these seizure types is of utmost importance in order to avoid diagnostic errors. The epileptic seizure types not associated with EEG changes include simple partial seizures with purely subjective phenomena (auras), and simple partial seizures that originate from the frontal lobes especially from the supplementary motor area, basofrontal regions, and medial, the frontal cortex. For example, in case of simple partial seizures without loss of awareness and associated with subjective feelings of déjà vu, and a normal EEG, a positive response to one of the inducing maneuvers may help in clarifying the diagnosis. Frontal lobe seizures are usually brief and tonic or hypermotor but not as dramatically flashing as the PNES. If several episodes are recorded, demonstration of stereotypy strongly suggests a presence of true seizures rather than PNES. It may not be possible to interpret ictal EEG because of contamination by movement artifacts such as those associated with tonic stiffening. Again, in such cases, induction may help to clarify the diagnosis.

Box 6.6: Video EEG: Common pitfalls in diagnosis of PNES

- Video EEG that is gold standard for diagnosis of PNES captures events in 75% of patients
- Most PNES patients have more than semiology features that are consistent with diagnosis of PNES
- Highly stereotyped episodes make diagnosis of PNES unlikely
- In case the doubt persists even after video EEG, it is better to treat the patient with antiepileptic drugs
- Syncope, paroxysmal movement disorders, and parasomnias should always be considered in differential diagnosis of PNES

If after all the maneuvers, doubt still persists as to whether we are dealing with true or pseudoseizures, it is better to treat the patient with antiepileptic drugs and see the response. Other nonepileptic disorders must always be ruled out before labeling a patient to be suffering from PNES. These include syncope, paroxysmal movement disorders, and parasomnias.

INDUCTION TECHNIQUES[2,4,5]

Induction or provocative techniques are particularly helpful in diagnosis of PNES. These techniques are based on the principle of suggestibility which is common to all somatoform disorders. Response to induction is a strong diagnostic indicator for diagnosis of PNES (Box 6.7).

The chief advantage of induction is its high specificity and ease to perform. We have found that many patients can be induced to have an attack even in an outdoor patient department by applying a vibrating tuning fork on the forehead. Induction is especially useful when video EEG monitoring does not yield conclusive results for reasons cited earlier. In such a situation, positive response to induction strongly supports a psychogenic origin.

The techniques commonly used for induction should avoid administration of placebo such as normal saline for ethical concerns. On the other hand, simple maneuvers such as photic stimulation, hyperventilation, and verbal suggestion are equally effective in induction and do not involve patient deception. In our practice, we have found that 128 Hz tuning fork applied on the forehead along with verbal suggestion is as effective as photic stimulation in inducing the episode. If possible, a video EEG should be performed in conjunction with provocative techniques. While this is a routine in developed nations, in developing nations where waiting periods for video EEG exceed several months, induction may be carried out during routine EEG, while the clinician is personally observing the episode. There are however few cautions and caveats

to the process of event induction. Hyperventilation and photic stimulation may also induce true seizures in a person with epilepsy, or epilepsy coexisting with PNES. On the other hand, a patient with epilepsy may "oblige" with a PNES under pressure to deliver. However, the clinical features of the two usually are distinctive.

CONFIRMING DIAGNOSIS IN SPECIAL SITUATIONS[1,2]

Previously Abnormal EEG

Quite often a patient enters in your clinic with vague complaints and an EEG report that is reported as abnormal. In these cases, it is important to re-examine the EEG that has been reported as abnormal. Quite often EEG interpretation is found to be wrong.

Psychogenic nonepileptic seizures in patients with epilepsy or other organic brain disease: In cases with a prior history of definite epilepsy or head injury, one would like to diagnose PNES with extreme caution.

Approximately, 9–15% of patients with PNES are reported to have true epilepsy and these present specific management problems. These patients should be managed by both the neurologist and a psychiatrist in coordination.

In patients with organic brain disease such as multiple sclerosis or stroke, it is likely that any paroxysmal event is diagnosed as seizure. But this is not always true. Thirty percent of paroxysmal events in patients with moderate-to-severe brain injury are diagnosed as PNES. The diagnosis of PNES in patients with traumatic head injury is especially important because of legal issues.

Diagnosis of PNES is unlikely to be made in certain special populations such as the elderly and in patients with prior epilepsy surgery. However, these should be considered especially if the clinical situation is suggestive of PNES based on criteria already discussed in this chapter.

THE MANAGEMENT OF PNES[7-9]

A major component of management of PNES is undertaken under the care of psychiatrists, which is not discussed here, but can be referred to in relevant psychiatry texts. From the neurologist's point of view, an important step in management of PNES is the successful communication of diagnosis to the patient and the family. Only when the patient and the caregivers accept the diagnosis, will they adhere to the recommendations

---

Box 6.7: The role of induction technique in diagnosis of PNES

- Induction is highly specific for diagnosis of PNES and is easy to perform
- A vibrating tuning fork applied to forehead along with verbal suggestion is highly effective in induction of events in patients with PNES
- 9–15% of patients with PNES also have true epilepsy
- 30% of seizure-like events in patients with traumatic brain injury are PNES

of the physician. The patients should be clearly informed regarding the diagnosis rather than using vague and deceptive terms. The neurologist should explain to the patient while being compassionate and understand that most of the patients are not feigning. In case of a doubt, it should be clearly communicated, and further lines of treatment explained to the patient in detail. As, often there has been a long delay of 7–10 years before a definitive diagnosis is established, the patient may react with denial or anger. It is important to make the patient understand that it is good for him/her that he or she has been correctly diagnosed now and will receive proper treatment from now on.

The neurologist should further assist in weaning the patient off from antiepileptic drugs. Regarding driving, there is no evidence that driving is risky. However, caution should be exercised while advising regarding driving. Regarding disability, it is better to involve a mental health care professional and give disability from a psychiatry point of view.

PROGNOSIS[7,9]

These seizures stop in 29% of PNES patients at 6-month follow-up, 42% at 1 year, and 50% at 2-year follow-up. However, most long-term studies suggest poor prognosis with recurrence or continuation of seizures. At 11-year follow-up, two-thirds of patients continue to have seizures, while 50% are dependent on social security. Only 16% of the patients had a good outcome (Box 6.8).

The factors associated with good outcome include rapid recognition of PNES, a young age-at-onset or diagnosis, higher level of intelligence, and higher socioeconomic status. Prognosis is unfavorable in patients with more dramatic PNES (tonic clonic seizures, ictal incontinence, tongue bite, or status), a wider range of physical symptoms, greater dissociative tendencies, and more severe personality problems.

Box 6.8: Prognosis of PNES

- Long-term follow-up in PNES shows poor prognosis with recurrence or continuation of seizures in two-thirds of patients
- The factors that are associated with good outcome include rapid recognition of PNES, a young age at onset or diagnosis, higher level of intelligence, and higher socioeconomic class

---

SPECIAL SITUATIONS

PNES in Children[2,7–9]

The PNES may occur in children as young as 5–6 years of age. The occurrence of PNES in children poses some specific issues that differ from adults. Firstly, children are known to suffer from nonepileptic nonpsychogenic conditions like staring spells that can be a manifestation of behavioral inattention but may be misinterpreted as seizures. This diagnosis is easily clarified on EEG. Interictal EEG in children may be confounded by presence of benign focal epileptiform discharges. Another factor that is very important to consider in children is sexual or physical abuse that should be sought in every case of childhood PNES. Other important precipitating factors include school refusal and family discord. The prognosis of PNES is better in children because of short duration and different stressors than in adults.

CONCLUSION

The PNES constitute a significant proportion of patients with refractory epilepsy. These are often misdiagnosed as suggested by a mean lag of 7–10 years before diagnosis. A judicial clinical suspicion and proper use of laboratory studies for confirmation of diagnosis may go a long way in management of these patients.

REFERENCES

1. Benbadis SR. Differential diagnosis of epilepsy. Continuum Lifelong Learn Neurol. 2007;13(4):48-70.
2. Benbadis SR. Nonepileptic Behavior disorders: diagnosis and treatment. Continuum (Minneap Minn). 2013;19(3):715-29.
3. Reuber M, Elger CE. Psychogenic nonepileptic seizures: review and update. Epilepsy Beh. 203;4:205-16.
4. Reuber M. Psychogenic nonepileptic seizures: answers and questions. Epilepsy Beh. 2008;12:622-35.
5. Mostacci B, Bisulli F, Alvisi L, et al. Ictal characteristics of psychogenic nonepileptic seizures: what we have learned from video/EEG recordings—a literature review. Epilepsy Beh. 2011;22:144-53.
6. Widdess-Walsh P, Mostacci B, Tinuper P, et al. Psychogenic nonepileptic seizures. Handbook Clin Neurol. 2012;107:277-95.
7. Dickinson P, Looper KJ. Psychogenic nonepileptic seizures: a current overview. Epilepsia. 2012;53(10):1679-89.
8. LaFrance WC, Reuber M, Goldstein LH. Management of psychogenic nonepileptic seizures. Epilepsia. 2013;54(Suppl 1):53-67.
9. Gillig PM. Psychogenic no epileptic seizures. Innov Clin Neurosci. 2013; 10(11-12):15-8.

7

Approach to Coma

Vivek Lal

INTRODUCTION

The word coma is derived from the Greek word, "koma" meaning deep sleep. In medicine, coma refers to a state of unconsciousness in which a person cannot be awakened, fails to respond normally to painful stimuli, light, or sound, lacks a normal sleep-wake cycle, and does not initiate voluntary action. However, from a practical point of view, the term "coma" encompasses any deterioration in global mental state either in the level of consciousness (coma in broad sense) or in the ability to maintain a coherent and steady stream of consciousness (confusional states). Confusion and coma represent two wide ends of a spectrum of clinical states, representing a failure of certain global or state-dependent brain functions (i.e., systems for maintaining of arousal or global attention). A wide variety of disorders can present with either of the two clinical states. Because many of these disorders pose an immediate threat to life or are associated with significant morbidity unless immediately attended to, the need for urgent evaluation and management of patients presenting with alteration of sensorium cannot be overemphasized. In this chapter, we discuss the general approach to diagnosis and management of patients presenting with alteration in consciousness.[1]

DEFINITION

The term coma has been used in a broad sense to describe any depression in the level of consciousness. However, alteration in the level of consciousness does not represent an all or none phenomenon. Rather, depression in level of consciousness represents a broad range on a continuum of abnormalities ranging from minimal to moderate-to-severe impairment. Thus, coma can be categorized according to the degree of impairment. These categories range from alertness, whereby a person is normal and capable of normal interpersonal relationship, to coma where a person does not show any response. Between these two stages, lie the stages of confusion, lethargy, obtundation, and stupor or semicoma listed in ascending order of severity. It should be noted that though the various stages represent ascending order of severity of alteration in sensorium, they are not exactly quantitative. Rather, they represent a semiquantitative method of assessment. It is imperative that the observer should clearly record the stage in which a patient's sensorium falls. The exact method for recording the level of sensorium is discussed later. The definitions of various terms are given in Box 7.1.

ANATOMIC SUBSTRATE FOR CONSCIOUSNESS AND ALERTNESS

The structures responsible for maintaining wakefulness are loosely grouped aggregations of neurons in the upper brainstem and medial thalamus, the reticular activating system (RAS). Beginning from the experiments of Moruzzi and Magoun in 1949, several clinic-pathological observations have established that excitatory cholinergic inputs emanating from midbrain and rostral pontine reticular formation ascend to thalamus and excite thalamocortical neurons in thalamic intralaminar and midline nuclei that in turn excite widespread regions of the cerebral cortex. In addition, there are several other neuronal systems [basal forebrain nuclei (acetylcholine), brainstem raphe nuclei (serotonin), locus ceruleus (noradrenaline), and substantia nigra–ventral tegmental area complex (dopamine)] to support arousal, which directly project to cortex, bypassing the thalamus. The complex interplay of these various neuronal systems is not fully understood. However, it is clear that arousal depends on integrity of the structures in the central grey of rostral pons and midbrain, basal forebrain, thalamus, hypothalamus and cerebral cortex. The important causes of coma are listed in Box 7.2.[1]

In contrast to arousal which is primarily a function of RAS, attention depends on both the RAS and the cortical systems for directed attention, e.g., posterior parietal lobes (sensory attention), frontal association cortices (motor attention), and cingulate cortices (motivational aspects of attention). Damage to these structures may cause global inattention or confusional state with modality-specific features of neglect. Acute damage to limbic and paralimbic structures (medial temporal lobes, orbitofrontal cortex, and basal forebrain) may also cause confusional state. Thus in practice, acute confusional states may result from either diffuse or focal lesions of the cerebral cortex, thalamocortical connections, or forebrain/subcortical limbic structures.[1]

CLINICAL APPROACH TO A PATIENT WITH COMA

Unfortunately, as comatose patients cannot provide any information and quite often no eyewitness is available, the physician often has to rely on examination of the patient, both for anatomical localization as well as for identification of the underlying cause of coma. In view of emergent situation, both the history and examination should be brief, but nevertheless performed in an organized manner and at the same time, due consideration should be given to the management of the patient. For instance, delay in protecting the airway of a comatose patient for want of history and examination may result in irreparable damage. Thus, management should be tailored as per the patient's needs and there can be no fixed protocol for management of a comatose patient, though following a predefined approach will help a physician. The classic monograph by Plum and Posner remains the most complete text for management of a comatose patient.

HISTORY[1-3]

In some cases (e.g., head injury or drug intake), the cause of coma may be immediately evident from history. On the contrary, in many other cases, historic information is limited for reasons as already discussed. Some time spend on obtaining a brief focused history is worthwhile, as it may provide important clues to the underlying etiology (Box 7.3).

For instance, sudden onset of coma will suggest a brainstem stroke or sudden massive brain hemorrhage, while a history of fever and seizures before onset of confusional state will suggest a central nervous system (CNS) infection. Similarly, in a diabetic patient, who presents with coma, one would suspect hypoglycemia as the likely etiology and performing a random blood sugar estimation followed by infusion of 25% dextrose will take priority over all other steps.

GENERAL PHYSICAL EXAMINATION[1-4]

A quick and focused general physical examination should be carried out in each patient, as it may provide vital clues to the underlying etiology. Temperature, blood pressure, pulse, respiratory rate, and patterns should be recorded quickly. The presence of fever suggests a systemic infection or a CNS infection (meningitis or encephalitis) or it may be consequent to a CNS lesion affecting the hypothalamus or central pontine tegmentum (rare), convulsive activity, a heat-stroke or drug (anticholinergic drugs) intoxication. Conversely, a low body temperature may occur secondary to drugs (barbiturates, sedatives, and phenothiazines), alcohol, hypoglycemia, peripheral circulatory failure, and hypothyroidism. The authors have seen several patients with hypothyroid coma in whom only clue to underlying etiology was hypothermia and bradycardia and this condition should always be considered in differential diagnosis of any patient who presents in a confusional state and is hypothermic. Hypothermia by itself causes coma only if body temperature falls to <31°C. A marked increase of blood pressure is indicative of hypertensive encephalopathy or raised intracranial pressure (ICP) secondary to brain lesion, while a decrease in blood pressure should arouse suspicion of alcohol or sedative drug intoxication, sepsis, internal hemorrhage, hypothyroidism, or addisonian crisis. Other findings on general physical examination also provide useful clues. For example, the presence of altered sensorium in a plethoric patient with central cyanosis will suggest carbon dioxide narcosis, while the presence of generalized lymphadenopathy may point to systemic infection or a metastatic CNS disease. Fundus examination may reveal evidence of raised ICP (papilledema), subarachnoid hemorrhage (subhyaloid hemorrhage), hypertensive encephalopathy (hemorrhages, exudates, papilledema), or infective endocarditis (Roth spots). The presence of cutaneous petechiae should raise suspicion of an underlying thrombotic thrombocytopenic purpura, meningococcemia, or a coagulopathy with resultant intracerebral bleed.

RESPIRATORY PATTERNS AS A USEFUL ADJUNCT TO LOCALIZATION IN COMA[1-5]

Although, respiratory patterns are helpful in localizing the site of the lesion in the neuraxis (Table 7.1 and Fig. 7.1), it is important to note that the same patterns may also result from a variety of metabolic disorders and, therefore, caution along with a thorough evaluation of the metabolic status of the patient must guide the interpretation.

TABLE 7.1: **Different respiratory patterns and their localizing value**

Type of pattern	Clinical description	Localizing value
Posthyper-ventilation apnea	Prolonged apnea (20–30 seconds) following five deep breaths	Poor: Mild bilateral hemispheric disease, metabolic or toxic encephalopathy, cardiac or respiratory disease
Cheyne–Stokes respiration	Brief periods of hyperpnea alternating with even briefer episodes of apnea	Poor: Bilateral cortical lesions, bilateral thalamic lesions, bilateral lesions affecting pathways from cortex to upper pons, severe metabolic or toxic encephalopathy, severe cardiac or respiratory disease
Hyperventilation	Prolonged and rapid hyperpnea	Poor: Metabolic acidosis, cardiac or pulmonary disease, hypoxia, pontine or midbrain lesions
Apneustic breathing	Long pause at end of inspiration	Lateral tegmentum of lower half of pons
Cluster breathing	Clusters of breaths following each other in irregular pattern	Low pontine or high medullary lesions
Ataxic or Biot's breathing	Chaotic breathing with loss of regularity of alternating pace and depth of inspirations and expirations	Damage to dorsomedial medulla

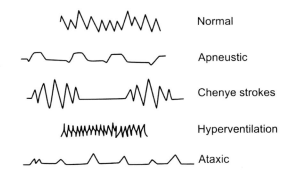

Normal

Apneustic

Chenye strokes

Hyperventilation

Ataxic

Fig. 7.1: Different respiratory patterns in coma.

POSTHYPERVENTILATION APNEA

This condition reflects mild bilateral hemispheric dysfunction. Demonstration of this sign requires active cooperation by the patient. The patient is asked to take five deep breaths that normally decrease the pCO_2 by approximately 10 mmHg and result in brief apnea (<10 seconds) in a healthy individual. In patients with bilateral hemispheric dysfunction, this apnea is prolonged to >20 seconds. The stimulus for rhythmic breathing in hypocapnia arises from the forebrain structures and is abolished in patients with bilateral hemispherical dysfunction, resulting in posthyperventilation apnea.

CHEYNE–STOKES RESPIRATION

This respiratory pattern consists of periods of hyperpnea alternating with brief episodes of apnea. After a period of apnea, the amplitude of respiration increases gradually to a peak and then slowly decreases to apnea. During the hyperpneic phase, the patient becomes more alert, pupils may dilate, eyelids may open, and motor behavior reflects control by higher centers (semipurposeful movements to pain). On the other hand, during the apneic phase, pupils may constrict, eyelids may close, and there may be decorticate posturing. There are many different mechanisms responsible for Cheyne-Stokes respiration (CSR). The respiratory drive becomes critically dependent on pCO_2 due to lack of smoothening effects of the forebrain structures. As the smoothening effect is gone, pCO_2 accumulation leads to hyperpnea that in turn results in drop in pCO_2 levels and apnea followed by repetition of the cycle. Thus, CSR represents a severe form of posthyperventilation apnea. In addition, delay of information transfer regarding pCO_2 levels due to slow circulation time or decrease in alveolar pO_2 and pCO_2

reserves may also result in CSR. In conditions associated with slow circulation times (congestive cardiac failure), a period of hypopnea results in an increase in pCO_2 levels, but this information reaches the respiratory centers slowly due to prolonged circulation time. When this information actually reaches the respiratory centers, there is more than usual rise in pCO_2 resulting in hyperpnea that again is prolonged as slow circulation provides information regarding fall in pCO_2 after a long delay. This results in more than usual fall in pCO_2 resulting in apnea and the cycle is repeated.

The localization value of CSR is limited. It is observed following widespread bilateral cortical lesions, bilateral thalamic damage or with bilateral lesions of descending pathways from cerebral hemispheres to upper pons. In addition, it may be noted with metabolic disturbances (uremia), anoxia, or with heart failure. It may also be seen in some normal elderly people during sleep or in normal individuals residing at high altitudes. In supratentorial mass lesion, CSR may be an indication of an impending transtentorial herniation.

APNEUSTIC BREATHING

This type of breathing is characterized by a prolonged pause at the end of respiration, also called the inspiratory cramp. It has good localizing value, suggesting a lesion of the midcaudal pons usually in the lateral tegmentum.

CLUSTER BREATHING

This type of breathing consists of clusters of breaths following each other in an irregular pattern. It is commonly seen, following low pontine or high medullary lesions.

ATAXIC BREATHING

Also known as the Biot's breathing, this is another respiratory pattern with good localizing value. Here, inspiratory gasps of varying amplitude and length are intermixed with apneic episodes. This pattern follows damage to neurons of reticular formation of medulla and pons, where respiratory rhythms are generated. This respiratory pattern, often seen in agonal patients, heralds complete respiratory failure. The most common etiologies include posterior fossa tumors, cerebellar or pontine hemorrhage, ischemic infarction of medulla, and trauma.

NEUROLOGICAL EXAMINATION[3-7]

The first step in neurological examination is a careful observation of the patient, as it may provide valuable information. For instance, lack of movement on one side of the body may suggest hemiplegia. Intermittent clonic movements of eyelids, fingers, or toes may be the only sign of ongoing seizure activity. Multifocal myoclonus may be an indication of metabolic encephalopathy, e.g., azotemia, anoxia, hyponatremia, drug intoxication (lithium, isoniazid, cyclosporine, haloperidol, etc.), spongiform encephalopathy, or Hashimoto's disease. Similarly, presence of chorea suggests an underlying metabolic disturbance. Decorticate posturing (flexion of elbows and wrist and supination of forearms) suggests bilateral damage above the midbrain, while decerebrate posturing (extension of elbows and wrists with pronation) suggest midbrain or caudal diencephalon damage (Fig. 7.2). A combination of extension of arms with flexion of legs is suggestive of damage in pons. The presence of meningeal signs may suggest an underlying meningitis or subarachnoid hemorrhage as the cause for altered sensorium.

LEVEL OF AROUSAL[4-7]

The patient's level of sensorium should be recorded precisely and clearly. The most commonly used method of recording sensorium is use of the Glasgow Coma Scale (GCS) (Table 7.2). However, though convenient, its use may be limited by the presence of focal deficits especially in stroke. The authors, therefore, recommend a descriptive recording of sensorium rather than just using the GCS. The stimulus required to arouse the patient along with the response of the patient should be noted clearly and documented. This is especially important as any worsening on serial examinations indicates the need for more aggressive therapeutic measures. Consider an example that suggests the need for precise recording (Box 7.4).

Decorticate posturing

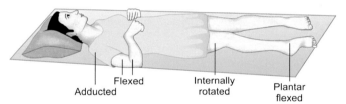

Flexed
Adducted

Internally rotated

Plantar flexed

Decerebrate posturing

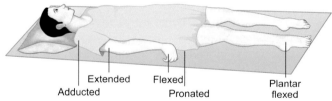

Extended
Adducted

Flexed
Pronated

Plantar flexed

Extension of arms and flexion of legs seen with pontine lesions

Extended Flexed Plantar flexed

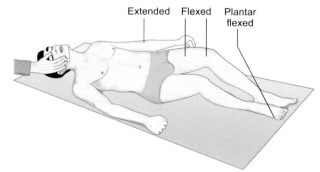

Fig. 7.2: Different posturing seen in patients with coma.

TABLE 7.2: **The Glasgow Coma Scale**

Measure	Characteristic	Score
Eye opening	Spontaneous	4
	To voice	3
	To pain	2
	None	1
Motor response	Obeys	6
	Localizes	5
	Withdraws	4
	Abnormal flexion	3
	Extension	2
	None	1
Verbal response	Oriented	5
	Confused conversation	4
	Inappropriate words	3
	Incomprehensible sounds	2
	None	1

Best possible score -15; least possible score-3.

Box 7.4: The need for precise recording: an example

"The patient was examined at 8 AM in the morning. To obtain a response he needed to be called in a loud voice. When called by his name in a loud voice, he opened his eyes and replied, 'Do not disturb me,' and immediately went back to sleep. He was lethargic at that time." If this patient requires a painful stimulus to obtain the same degree of response after some time interval, it would suggest deterioration in neurological status, though his GCS would still be the same.

The importance of precise and detailed recording of stimulus and response cannot be overemphasized.

EXAMINATION OF THE EYES[4-7]

The eyes provide vital information in evaluation of coma. For instance, conjunctivitis in a patient with fever and altered sensorium should raise suspicion of viral encephalitis. The presence of normal pupil-size and reaction, lids, and extraocular movements suggest that an extended length of the brainstem from midbrain-diencephalic junction to caudal pons is functioning normally. Any lesion along this pathway is likely to affect ocular functions. The fundus examination also provides important clues to etiology of coma. It may reveal papilledema (raised ICP) or subhyaloid hemorrhage (subarachnoid hemorrhage).

PUPILLARY EXAMINATION[4-7]

The pupils should be examined for shape, size, symmetry, and response to light. The pupillary light reflex is of utmost importance as it remains unaffected in metabolic disorders. Abnormalities of the papillary reflex suggest midbrain or third nerve dysfunction. However, there are several exceptions to it. Atropinergic drugs instilled into the eyes, or ingested orally, or given intravenously may dilate the pupils. Such pupils do not react to 1% pilocarpine instilled into the eyes, unlike anoxic pupillary dilation where miosis occurs due to direct action of pilocarpine. Other agents that may result in unreactive pupils include barbiturates, succinylcholine, other anticonvulsants, lidocaine, phenothiazines, methanol, and aminoglycoside antibiotics. Hypothermia and anoxic brain damage may also produce unreactive pupils. From a practical point of view, it is important to note that the pupillary light reaction is often spared in barbiturate intoxication and usually agents other than atropinic drugs cause pupillary dilatation only when taken in massive amount. The common pupillary abnormalities (see Fig. 7.3 and Box 7.5) in coma are summarized in Table 7.3.

Pupillary reactions should be examined by a bright diffuse light and not by an ophthalmoscope. In case of small pupils (<2 mm), light reflex may be difficult to appreciate and a magnifying glass may be helpful. Normally, reactive and round midsized (2.5–5 mm) pupils rule out midbrain damage. Small reactive pupils are commonly seen in sleep and metabolic encephalopathies and reflect bilateral diencephalic function. However,

extreme constriction (pinpoint pupils) is suggestive of pontine tegmental lesions (especially hemorrhage) and reflects sympathetic damage and parasympathetic overactivity. Pin-point pupils with normal reflexive eye movements should alert to the possibility of opiate or cholinergic drug intoxication.

There are many causes of dilated pupils. The common ones include the therapeutic use of atropine or norepinephrine, stimulant drugs (cocaine, phencyclidine, glutethimide, etc.) intoxication or drug withdrawal, and other delirious states. Central herniation with bilateral involvement of the third nerve may result in bilateral unreactive dilated pupils. Pretectal lesions often result in midsized or dilated pupils. Midbrain tegmental lesions may involve the third nerve nucleus with irregular

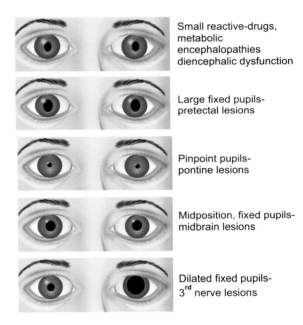

Small reactive-drugs, metabolic encephalopathies diencephalic dysfunction

Large fixed pupils-pretectal lesions

Pinpoint pupils-pontine lesions

Midposition, fixed pupils-midbrain lesions

Dilated fixed pupils-3rd nerve lesions

Fig. 7.3: Pupillary abnormalities in coma.

Box 7.5: Examinations of pupils in coma

- Pupillary light reflexes are extremely resistance to metabolic damage and remain preserved in metabolic encephalopathies until there in brainstem death
- Pinpoint pupils with normal reflex eye movements should point to diagnosis of opiate of cholinergic drug poisoning
- Pupils are fully dilated with third nerve lesion, while mid-dilated in midbrain lesion owing to sparing of sympathetic function with third nerve lesions
- Presence of focal neurological deficits, though rare, does not rule out the possibility of metabolic encephalopathy

TABLE 7.3: Pupillary abnormalities in patients with coma

Condition	Pupillary abnormality
Sleep/metabolic encephalopathy (bilateral diencephalic dysfunction), deep bilateral hemispheric lesions (hydrocephalus or thalamic hemorrhage)	Small pupils that react to light
Pontine tegmental lesions, narcotic or barbiturate overdose	Pinpoint pupils that react to light
Midbrain tectal lesions involving posterior commissure	Midsized of slightly large pupils with absent light reflex; hippus may occur and ciliospinal reflex may be present
Midbrain tegmental lesions involving third nerve nucleus	Irregular (pear shaped) pupils, midsized, often unequal with absent light and ciliospinal responses
Lateral pons, lateral medulla	Ipsilateral Horner's syndrome
Third nerve compression and elongation by a mass lesion	Widely dilated pupil

contraction of iris sphincter resulting in pear-shaped pupils or displacement of pupils to one side (midbrain correctopia). Pupils are midsized and unreactive. By contrast, ciliospinal reflex may be preserved with tectal lesions, though light reflex is absent due to involvement of posterior commissure. Cerebrovascular lesions affecting the oculomotor (pupillomotor) fibers may result in unilateral or bilateral oval pupils. The oval shape is due to paralysis of the pupil sphincter with resultant overactivity of pupil dilators. Compression and elongation of oculomotor nerve secondary to uncal herniation often affects the pupillary function earlier and greater than other the third nerve functions. Unlike a midbrain lesion, the pupil is widely dilated with the third nerve lesions owing to sparing of the sympathetic pathways (Hutchinson pupil). Other abnormalities of the third nerve are unlikely to result in coma unless associated with subarachnoid hemorrhage (posterior communicating artery aneurysm).

EYELIDS[1-7]

In a deeply comatose patient, examination of eyelids is not rewarding. However, in a relatively alert patient, the examination of eyelids may offer important clues to the site of the lesion. A severe unilateral ptosis suggests lesion of nerve fascicle in its intra- or extramedullary

course. Nuclear third nerve lesions are characteristically associated with bilateral ptosis. A partial ptosis associated with a small pupil is suggestive of Horner's syndrome. Bilateral ptosis out-of-proportion to the degree of lethargy is seen with rostral midbrain lesions, as in top of basilar artery infarction. In some cases of pontine infraction, eyelids may remain open due to failure of levator inhibition (eye-open coma).

EYE MOVEMENTS[4-7]

Abnormalities of eye movements suggest lesion at the level of the pons or the midbrain. Eye movement abnormalities in a comatose patient should be assessed systematically. First, look for the primary position of the eyes and the spontaneous movements of the globe by gently lifting the eyelids. The resistance to passive opening of lids, called the lid tone, gradually decreases with increasing depth of coma. In drowsiness, slight divergence of ocular axes is normal. An adducted eye indicates sixth cranial nerve palsy while an abducted eye indicates unilateral third cranial nerve palsy. The clinician should look for any abnormalities of vertical or horizontal gaze as well as for any conjugate or dysconjugate ocular deviations. As voluntary eye movements are often absent in comatose patients, one has to rely on reflexive eye movements (oculocephalic and oculovestibular).

Roving Eye Movements (Ping-Pong Gaze)

This means roving of eyes from one extreme of horizontal gaze to the other and back like a ping-pong ball, each cycle taking 2.5–8 seconds. This finding by itself suggests that the brainstem is intact. The common causes include bilateral cerebral damage (stroke), posterior fossa hemorrhage, basal ganglia infarcts, hydrocephalus, metabolic (hepatic, anoxic), and toxic encephalopathies. The ping-pong gaze is due to lack of cortical inhibition of horizontal gaze centers in the brainstem.

Periodic Alternating Gaze Deviation

In this condition, there is alternating horizontal conjugate eye deviation lasting 1–2 minutes in each direction. It may be seen in metabolic coma such as hepatic encephalopathy.

Repetitive Divergence

In this disorder, the eyes are slightly divergent or in mid-position at rest. Then they slowly deviate out, fully deviate for a brief period, and then return to the midposition. The movements are synchronous in both the eyes. This disorder is very rare and is usually seen in metabolic, especially the hepatic encephalopathies.

Nystagmoid Jerking of Single Eye

These jerks may be horizontal, vertical, or rotatory and suggest pontine damage.

Disconjugate Vertical and Rotatory Movements of the Eyes

Seen with pontine lesions, here one eye rises and intorts while the other one falls and extorts. This needs to be distinguished from sea-saw nystagmus, which, contrary to the common belief, is seldom seen in comatose patients.

Ocular Bobbing

This refers to conjugate, brisk, bilateral downward movement of both eyes followed, after a brief tonic interval, by slow return to midposition. Cold caloric testing may increase ocular bobbing. Ocular bobbing is described as typical when there is associated loss of horizontal eye movement. This form is strongly suggestive of acute pontine injury. On the other hand, atypical ocular bobbing where horizontal eye movements are preserved is not so specific in prediction of site of injury. Ocular bobbing is usually conjugate but may be dysconjugate if there is associated third cranial nerve injury. Ocular bobbing is thought to originate in the mesencephalic and the medullary burst neurons. It is seen with intrinsic pontine lesions (hemorrhage, infarction, tumor, and central pontine myelinolysis), posterior fossa lesions (cerebellar hemorrhage or infarction), toxic and metabolic encephalopathies (anoxic damage, hepatic encephalopathy, organophosphorus intoxication). When present in a patient with coma, it implies a poor prognosis, particularly when associated with absent horizontal eye movements.

Ocular Dipping (Inverse Ocular Bobbing)

This refers to slow downward eye movements followed by fast return to midposition. This has been described with anoxic coma. This reflects diffuse cortical dysfunction as the reflex horizontal eye movements are usually intact.

Reverse Ocular Bobbing

This rare disorder refers to fast upward movement of eyes followed by slow return to midposition. The common causes include, metabolic or toxic encephalopathies, viral encephalitis, and pontine lesions.

Reverse Ocular Dipping (Converse Ocular Bobbing)

This refers to a slow upward movement of eyeballs followed by fast return to midposition. This occurs with metabolic or toxic encephalopathies, viral encephalitis, and pontine lesions.

Vertical Ocular Myoclonus

This rare entity consists of pendular, vertically isolated movements of the eyes seen in severe pontine strokes. Their frequency is 2 Hz and they are commonly associated with palatal tremor.

Saccadic Intrusions without Normal Intersaccadic Interval-Ocular Flutter and Opsoclonus

Both these disorders represent dysfunction of the pontine omnipause neurons resulting in back-to-back saccades without any intersaccadic interval. While the saccades are horizontal in ocular flutter, these are multidirectional in opsoclonus (saccadomania). These disorders are commonly seen with paraneoplastic limbic encephalitis, brainstem encephalitis, toxic or metabolic encephalopathies and in hyperosmolar coma.

Nystagmus

Spontaneous nystagmus is uncommon in coma as the quick or the compensatory phase, which depends on the interaction between the oculovestibular system and the cerebral cortex disappears as the cortical influences are reduced. However, two spontaneous eye movements that resemble nystagmus may be seen in comatose patients. These are retractory nystagmus that consists of irregular jerks of eye backward into the orbit, sometimes occurring spontaneously but usually precipitated by an upward gaze. It results from simultaneous contraction of all six ocular muscles presumable due to dysfunction of cortical mesencephalic inhibitory fibers secondary to mesencephalic lesion. The other is convergence nystagmus that consists of spontaneous slow drifting ocular divergence followed by a quick convergent jerk. It may occur together with retractory nystagmus or in isolation and is result of a lesion in the mesencephalon.

Electrographic Status Epilepticus

This results in brisk, small amplitude, mainly vertical (occasionally horizontal) eye movements.

Abnormalities of Lateral Gaze

Conjugate Gaze

Most lateral conjugate gaze disorders result from destructive lesions, as neither the compressive nor the metabolic lesions affect the supranuclear oculomotor pathways asymmetrically (Table 7.4 and Fig. 7.4). Abnormal conjugate lateral gaze may result from

three conditions. First, a hemispherical lesion results in paresis of gaze to contralateral side resulting in deviation of eyes to the side of the cortical lesion so that the eyes look toward the nonparetic arm and leg. There is no nystagmus. In the second type, an irritative hemispheric lesion (seizure) forcibly deviates the eyes to the contralateral side, but this deviation is transient and is accompanied by nystagmoid jerks. Rarely, a thalamic or basal ganglionic lesion (almost always hemorrhagic) results in forced deviation of eyes to the contralateral side (wrong-way eyes). This may rarely occur with cerebral hemorrhage also. However, in most cases, this forced deviation is replaced within minutes to hours by the more common supranuclear palsy of gaze. The third type of conjugate gaze deviation results from a lesion of the paramedian reticular formation (PPRF), resulting in ipsilateral lateral gaze palsy so that the eyes are deviated to the contralateral side and look toward the paralyzed arm and leg.

TABLE 7.4: **Ocular movement abnormalities in coma**

Spontaneous eye movements	
Type of movement	**Localization**
Roving eye movements (Ping-Pong gaze)	Bilateral cerebral damage; rarely with posterior fossa hemorrhage, basal ganglia infarcts, hydrocephalus, tranylcypromine overdose
Periodic alternating gaze deviation	Metabolic encephalopathy
Repetitive divergence	Metabolic encephalopathy
Nystagmoid jerking of single eye	Mid or lower pontine damage
Ocular bobbing	Intrinsic pontine lesions (tumors, ischemia, demyelination), extra-axial posterior fossa masses (cerebellar hemorrhage or infarction), diffuse encephalitis, Creutzfeldt–Jakob disease, toxic encephalopathies (organophosphorus intoxication)
Typical ocular bobbing	Pontine lesions
Ocular dipping	Diffuse brain dysfunction (anoxic brain damage)
Reverse ocular bobbing	Metabolic encephalopathy, viral encephalitis, pontine hemorrhage, drugs
Reverse ocular dipping	Pontine infarction, metabolic, or viral encephalopathy
Opsoclonus, ocular flutter	Paraneoplastic encephalitis, brainstem encephalitis, metabolic encephalopathy (drugs, hyperosmolar coma)
Refractory nystagmus	Mesencephalic tegmental lesion
Convergence nystagmus	Mesencephalic tegmental lesion
Abnormalities of gaze	
Tonic lateral deviation	Hemispheric lesion (eyes look toward normal side) or pontine lesion (eyes look toward hemiparetic side)
Skew deviation	Brainstem lesion, increased intracranial pressure, hepatic coma
Tonic downward deviation of eyes	Midbrain tectal lesion; metabolic coma
Tonic downward deviation of eyes with convergence	Thalamic hemorrhage
Sustained upgaze	Anoxic coma

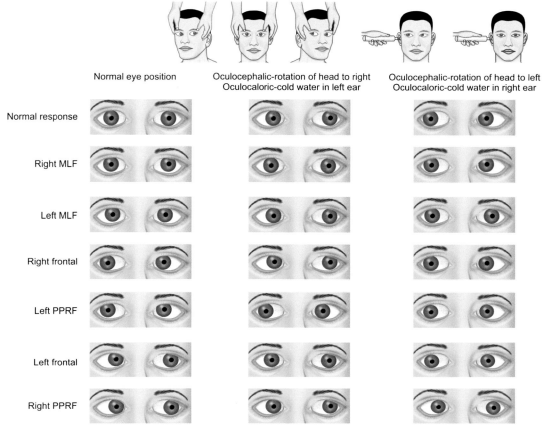

	Normal eye position	Oculocephalic-rotation of head to right Oculocaloric-cold water in left ear	Oculocephalic-rotation of head to left Oculocaloric-cold water in right ear
Normal response			
Right MLF			
Left MLF			
Right frontal			
Left PPRF			
Left frontal			
Right PPRF			

MIF, medical longtitudinal fasciculus; PPRF, paramedian pontine reticular formation.

Fig. 7.4: Some common gaze abnormalities in coma and their response to oculocephalic and oculovestibular maneuvers.

Dysconjugate Gaze

Isolated failure of ocular adduction suggests a lesion of the ipsilateral medial longitudinal fasciculus (MLF), especially if the vertical eye movements and pupils are normal. In comatose patients, MLF involvement is usually bilateral. Rarely, a transient bilateral MLF syndrome may be seen in metabolic coma (barbiturates and amitriptyline intoxication, and hepatic encephalopathy).

Abnormalities of Vertical Gaze

In light coma, upward gaze can be tested by lightly touching the cornea with cotton, when eyeballs tend to roll upward (Bell's phenomenon). Dysconjugate vertical gaze palsy in resting position (skewed deviation) is seen with brainstem lesions, increased ICP and with metabolic encephalopathies (hepatic coma). Persistent downward deviation of the eyes is often noted with midbrain tectal lesion, but may be noted in metabolic encephalopathies also. Tonic downward deviation of eyes with convergence is seen with thalamic hemorrhage due to pressure on dorsal mesencephalon. Sustained upgaze may be observed in anoxic coma and with phenothiazine intoxication. Large midbrain tegmental lesions abolish vertical gaze.

Oculocephalic reflexes (Doll's eye maneuvers) are automatic movements of eyes elicited by moving the head from side-to-side or in the vertical direction. These movements are inhibited by visual fixation that is absent in comatose patients. Signals for oculocephalic movements originate from labyrinths and cervical proprioceptors and require normal activity of the third nerve nucleus, contralateral sixth nerve nucleus, as well of the MLF. A noteworthy point is that induced adduction of globe is less complete than abduction and thus any abnormality noted during this maneuver must be interpreted with caution. Elicitation of normal oculocephalic maneuver means that coma is not due to upper brainstem lesion. On the other hand, an abnormal result on these maneuvers implies damage within the brainstem or profound suppression of brainstem nuclei due to metabolic or toxic encephalopathy (drugs such as phenytoin, barbiturates, tricyclic antidepressants, diazepam, and neuromuscular blocking agents). As discussed earlier, preservation of pupillary functions will distinguish most cases of drug-induced coma from structural brainstem damage.

Oculovestibular Reflexes

Thermal or caloric stimulation of the vestibular apparatus provides a stronger stimulus than oculocephalic reflex and is useful in cases where oculocephalic maneuver is abnormal. Caloric testing is carried out by instilling 50 mL of ice-cold water into the external auditory canal over 30 seconds after elevating the head to 30° and ensuring that the tympanic membrane is intact. Normally, the eyes deviate to the side of the irrigated ear after a brief latency of 30–120 seconds. Vertical movements can be tested by simultaneously irrigating both the ears. This test also checks the integrity of the third and the sixth nerve nuclei, MLF as well as of the brainstem pathways from the labyrinths to the midbrain. If the cerebral hemispheres are functioning (catatonic or hysterical coma), a corrective nystagmus is generated opposite to the side of the tonic deviation. The absence of nystagmus implies damage or profound suppression of both the hemispheres.

OTHER CRANIAL NERVE SIGNS[4,6]

Spontaneous blinking implies an intact seventh cranial nerve function. A normal response to corneal stimulation suggests that both the fourth and the seventh cranial nerves are intact. The presence of the Bell's phenomenon, if present suggests that pathways from the rostral midbrain to the seventh cranial nerve nucleus are intact. The absence of hearing or gag does not have much localizing value in a comatose patient.

Motor and Reflex Signs[4,6]

In a comatose patient, gross assessment of motor functions may provide clues to the site of the lesion. However, this information is not as localizing as in an alert patient. To further complicate the matter, focal deficits such as hemiparesis that are considered as the hallmark of a structural damage to the brain may occasionally be seen with metabolic encephalopathy (particularly, the

hypoglycemic coma). In addition, other motor patterns (decerebrate and decorticate posturing) though originally described secondary to discrete structural lesions in experimental animals are commonly encountered in metabolic coma also. Of course, structural damage to motor pathways can give rise to such patterns that are often asymmetric (Fig. 7.2).

In light coma, useful information may be gathered by just observing the patient. The motor response in these patients varies from lying quietly in bed to thrashing about. Any asymmetry of movement must be noted, as it may be suggestive of motor or sensory deficits. The tone of extremities can be tested by gently elevating the patient's arms or by flexing the legs at the knees. In light coma, patient's arm or leg falls slowly, while a paretic limb falls like a dead weight.

The terms decerebrate and decorticate rigidity refer to experimental studies and do not accurately reflect the clinicopathological correlations. Lower extremity extension and internal rotation with both upper limb flexion and supination (decorticate) or upper limb extension and pronation (decerebrate) are more commonly seen with hemispheric disease rather than the original descriptions in experimental animals. In general, decorticate posturing reflects more superficial, less severe, and more chronic disease at the level of diencephalon or above, while decerebrate posturing is more often seen with brainstem lesion.

In clinical practice, the commonest cause of these posturing especially if symmetric is toxic or metabolic encephalopathy that may be reversible. An abnormal extension of arms with flexion of legs usually suggests damage to the pontine tegmentum. With still lower lesions involving the medulla, all four limbs may be flaccid. Deep tendon reflexes and plantar responses may also suggest a focal lesion, but they are often misleading. Careful observation for subtle movements suggestive of nonconvulsive status, epilepticus should be undertaken in all the patients with coma.

CLINICAL PRESENTATIONS OF DIFFERENT CAUSES OF COMA[1]

Broadly, the causes of coma fall in three categories: (a) toxic metabolic causes, (b) supratentorial structural lesions, and (c) subtentorial structural lesions. Each of these groups has distinctive clinical features and though it may not be possible to determine the precise cause in many cases, an attempt should always be made to classify the cause of coma into one of the three categories, as further management and outcome is entirely specific to each group. The clinical features of each of the broad group are discussed below.

TOXIC METABOLIC ENCEPHALOPATHY[1,6]

In general, the phylogenetically newer brain structures are more prone to metabolic and toxic injury than the older brain structures. As a result, the functions subserved by complex polysynaptic pathways are affected earlier and more severely than the functions subserved by less complex pathways and a fewer neurons. Thus, attention and higher cortical functions are affected earlier and more severely in metabolic insults, whereas the pupillary light reflex remains normal until brainstem death ensues. Usually, the corneal reflexes are suppressed only by the time decerebrate posturing appears, though some eye movements may still be elicited through oculocephalic or oculovestibular stimulation. Although, asymmetric motor or ocular signs argue against the diagnosis of toxic or metabolic encephalopathy, this is not always the case. Hepatic encephalopathy is reported to be associated with downward deviation of the eyes and hypoglycemia with hemiparesis. Also, the focal seizures may occur with metabolic encephalopathies (hyperglycemia, eclampsia, and porphyria).

Toxic metabolic encephalopathies produce certain involuntary movements that are unlikely to occur in patients with focal structural lesions of the brain (Box 7.6). These include asterixis, multifocal myoclonus, generalized myoclonus, tremor, generalized chorea or other dyskinesias, etc. Tremor seen in metabolic encephalopathy is coarse and irregular with a frequency of 8–10 Hz. It is best seen with outstretched hands, but in confused patients, it is best felt by holding the patient's extended fingers. Asterixis is sudden and brief loss of postural tone. It is best demonstrated by holding the patient's hand in dorsiflexion with fingers extended and abducted. It can also be seen in hips by passive flexion and then abduction of hips at 60–90° between the thighs. Though, a classic sign of metabolic encephalopathy, it can occasionally be seen with structural lesions as well. Unilateral asterixis may be seen with contralateral lesions of the mesencephalon, ventrolateral thalamus, primary

Box 7.6: Clues to metabolic encephalopathy
The presence of involuntary movements such as multifocal or generalized myoclonus, generalized chorea and other dyskinesias as well as tremor argue strongly in favor of metabolic encephalopathy

motor cortex, or parietal lobe or with an ipsilateral lesion of the pons or medulla. The damage to corticoreticular pathways or to brainstem reticular formation is the proposed mechanism. Bilateral asterixis may be seen following bilateral mesencephalic or bilateral pontine lesions. Multifocal myoclonus, which means sudden, nonrhythmic, and random twitching of muscles affecting facial and proximal limbs in particular, is usually seen in metabolic encephalopathies especially uremic and hyperglycemic–hyperosmolar encephalopathy, carbon dioxide narcosis, and penicillin intoxication. Generalized myoclonus, which is stimulus-sensitive and affects axial musculature, is characteristic of postanoxic cerebral damage. It may be associated with multifocal myoclonus.

SUPRATENTORIAL STRUCTURAL LESIONS[4]

For supratentorial lesions to cause coma, damage must affect both the cerebral hemispheres (massive brain infarction, bilateral thalamic infarction). The clinical presentation of some of these lesions may resemble metabolic encephalopathy. However, most cerebral infarcts occur more abruptly than metabolic encephalopathies and are associated with asymmetric motor signs even when bilateral. History may be useful in these cases. For instance, a history of sudden severe headache before loss of consciousness may suggest a diagnosis of subarachnoid hemorrhage or pituitary apoplexy or even massive intracerebral bleed.

Unilateral supratentorial lesions (e.g., subdural hematoma, intracerebral hemorrhage, and malignant middle cerebral artery infarctions) can cause coma by affecting the other side through mass effect and midline shift, or by affecting the diencephalic and upper brainstem structures. This is usually associated with either of the two well-defined herniation syndromes (lateral-uncal or central-transtentorial) depending upon the location of the mass and the size of tentorial opening.

LATERAL HERNIATION

This type of herniation occurs when extracerebral or temporal mass lesions push the uncus through the tentorial opening between the ipsilateral aspect of the midbrain and the free edge of tentorium. The herniated tissue presses the third cranial nerve and posterior cerebral artery downward. As a result, ipsilateral pupil dilates and becomes unresponsive to light. This stage is brief and its recognition is of utmost importance as prompt surgical intervention at this time may be

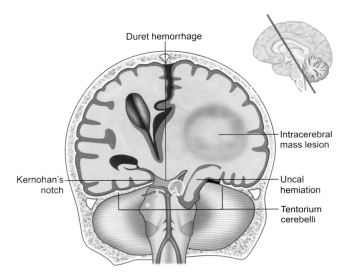

Fig. 7.5: Diagram showing Duret hemorrhage.

lifesaving. Occlusion of posterior cerebral artery results in medial occipital infarct. The herniated uncus pushes the midbrain against the opposite free edge of the tentorium that results in a notch (Kernohan's notch) on the lateral aspect of the midbrain, affecting the cerebral peduncle resulting in hemiparesis on the side of dilated third pupil and on the side of the original cerebral lesion. Furthermore, anteroposterior elongation and downward displacement of the midbrain results in rupture of the paramedian perforating arteries leading to midbrain tegmental hemorrhages (Duret's hemorrhages, Fig. 7.5). The pupil that was large becomes smaller now as the sympathetic pathways become affected, while the other pupil becomes midsized and nonreactive.

Many of the causes of lateral herniation can be treated surgically. However, once herniation with dilated pupil, absent ocular and oculocephalic reflexes or extensor posturing supervenes, prognosis is extremely poor. Survivors are often left with locked-in syndrome or in a persistent vegetative state, though rare cases of recovery have been reported.

Central Herniation

This type of herniation usually occurs secondary to frontal, parietal, or occipital masses. These masses first compress the diencephalon, which then shifts and buckles the midbrain, resulting in flattening of the midbrain and the pons in a rostrocaudal direction. This results in elongation and rupture of the paramedian perforating arteries leading to midbrain tegmental hemorrhages first

followed by pontine tegmental hemorrhages (Duret's hemorrhages, Fig. 7.5). Accordingly, the clinical picture also follows this rostrocaudal progression of brainstem damage.

Early diencephalic stage

This stage is characterized by appearance of somnolence and inattention with frequent deep sighs and yawns. During periods of somnolence, the pupils may become small, but are reactive to light and the eyes may rove from side-to-side. However, the patient is easily arousable and awakens during performance of oculocephalic or oculovestibular reflexes. For this reason, caloric stimulation induces nystagmus in these patients. Gegenhalten and grasp reflexes may be present and plantars are bilaterally extensor.

Late diencephalic stage

At this stage, the patient does not respond to light pain, while heavier stimuli induce decorticate posturing more on the side of previous hemiparesis. CSR is frequent. Pupils are small and reactive. Reflex eye movements produce tonic deviation of the eyes, but no nystagmus. Plantars are bilaterally extensor. A diagnosis and intervention at this stage may result in good recovery, but once the clinical picture evolves into next stage, prognosis is usually poor.

Midbrain-upper pons stage

Breathing becomes quicker and even. Temperature fluctuates and diabetes insipidus may result from stretching of median eminence. Pupils become midsized, unequal, and irregular (pear-shaped and eccentric). Vertical eye movements are absent on reflex eye movement testing. Eyes movements are dysconjugately in both horizontal and vertical planes.

Lower pontine stage

Breathing becomes quicker and shallower. Pupil is the same as in the previous stages, but eye movements disappear. Decerebrate rigidity decreases.

Medullary stage

In this stage, ataxic breathing soon gives way to apnea. Blood pressure drops and pulse becomes irregular.

Although, clinical features of patients with herniation syndrome follows the above pattern, some studies suggest that at least the early depression of alertness may be more related to distortion of brain by horizontal than by vertical displacement of brain tissue. In one

> **Box 7.7: Mass lesions and coma**
>
> - In transtentorial herniation, early surgical intervention is extremely important as once herniation with dilated pupil, absent ocular and oculocephalic reflexes or extensor posturing supervenes, prognosis is extremely poor. Survivors are often left with locked in syndrome or persistent vegetative state
> - A diagnosis and intervention at late diencephalic stage or before may result in good recovery, but once clinical picture evolves into midbrain-upper pons stage, prognosis is usually poor
> - In lobar hemorrhages, hemorrhage of >60 mL, shift of septum pellucidum, effacement of contralateral ambient cistern, and widening of contralateral temporal horn are predictors of subsequent deterioration. With basal ganglionic bleeds, a GCS of <8 or presence of hydrocephalus predicts clinical deterioration

study, horizontal of 0–3 mm of the pineal was associated with alertness, 3–4 mm with drowsiness, 6–8.5 mm with stupor and 8–13 mm with coma. In this study, perimesencephalic cisterns were more often widened than filled by medial temporal lobe.

With regard to lobar hemorrhages, hemorrhage of >60 mL, shift of septum pellucidum, effacement of contralateral ambient cistern, and widening of contralateral temporal horn are predictors of subsequent deterioration. With basal ganglionic bleeds, a GCS of <8 or presence of hydrocephalus predicts clinical deterioration (Box 7.7).

Subtentorial Structural Lesions

Unlike rostrocaudal deterioration secondary to supratentorial mass lesions, where all the structures at a particular brainstem level are affected at the same time, compressive lesions of posterior fossa affect one level more than the other, often asymmetrically, giving rise to unilateral brainstem and cerebellar signs. Compressive lesions of upper brainstem may cause upward transtentorial herniation of the tectum and anterior cerebellar lobule resulting in midbrain dysfunction with coma, hyperventilation, fixed pupils, and vertical ophthalmoplegia. Lower level lesions compress the pons resulting in somnolence, pinpoint reactive pupils, truncal ataxia, and loss of voluntary and reflexive horizontal eye movements while vertical eye movements may still be preserved. Still lower lesions may compress the medulla resulting in apnea and circulatory abnormalities that may precede changes in alertness.

Mass lesions of the posterior fossa may cause downward herniation of tonsil through foramen magnum,

resulting in infarction of tonsil, medulla, and even upper cervical cord. Prognosis is poor in these patients. Another important point to note here is that patients with pre-existing brainstem lesions (multiple sclerosis) may lose all brainstem reflexes transiently on suffering an anoxic or metabolic insult. In these patients, prognostication should be carried out with caution.

DIFFERENTIAL DIAGNOSIS[1,4]

In most of the cases, confusion and coma are related to an underlying medical condition such as overt drug ingestion, hypoxia, stroke, trauma, and liver or kidney failure. It is helpful to classify the clinical presentation of coma into two types: (a) altered sensorium without any lateralizing features or in other words, nonfocal neurological deficits and (b) altered sensorium with lateralizing features or focal neurological deficits. The common causes responsible for both the clinical presentations are listed in Box 7.8.

Further clinical diagnosis can be reached with the help of other clinical features. For example, in the category without lateralizing features, a history of fever, headache, and neck stiffness would suggest meningitis, while a history of fever with seizures would favor a diagnosis of viral encephalitis. The presence of high blood pressure would suggest hypertensive encephalopathy, while unrecordable blood pressure would suggest brain hypoperfusion as the cause of altered sensorium. When in doubt, investigation profile and cerebrospinal fluid analysis can help in settling the diagnosis.

Differentiating Coma due to Toxic Metabolic Causes versus Structural Lesions[2,4]

It is important to differentiate metabolic coma from that due to structural causes as the treatment options and the final outcome vary markedly among these two groups. History may be helpful. For example, any recent change of medications in a diabetic patient would suggest hypoglycemia as the likely cause. A history of opiate addiction in the past would suggest opiate intoxication. Response to empirical treatment given in the emergency room may help settle the issue. A hypoglycemic person wakes up after receiving glucose, while naloxone will help in opiate drug overdose. In general, structural lesions will have some lateralizing features, while metabolic, psychiatric, and toxic coma are characterized by symmetry. The main features of a neurological examination that can help different between metabolic and structural coma are summarized in Table 7.5.

Box 7.8: Differential diagnosis of coma

- Altered sensorium without lateralizing features
  - *Drug intoxications*: Benzodiazepines, barbiturates, opiates, organophosphorus compounds, phenothiazines, butyrophenones, tricyclic antidepressants, stimulant drugs (cocaine, amphetamines, phencyclidine), drugs causing metabolic acidosis (ethanol, methanol, aspirin, ethylene glycol, other hydrocarbons), neuromuscular blocking agents, drug withdrawal syndromes (alcohol, sedative hypnotic), etc.
  - *Metabolic causes*: Anoxia, hypo and hypernatremia, hypercalcemia, hepatic coma, uremia, dialysis disequilibrium syndromes, diabetic ketoacidosis, hyperosmolar coma, hypoglycemia, addisonian crisis, hypo and hyperthyroid states, carbon dioxide narcosis, porphyria, hyperammonemic states
  - *Nutritional deficiencies*: Thiamine deficiency, vitamin B12 deficiency
  - *Septic encephalopathy*: Pneumonia, typhoid, septicemia, etc.
  - Non-convulsive status epilepticus, postseizure states
  - Severe hyper and hypothermia
  - Peripheral circulatory failure or shock of whatever etiology
  - Hypertensive encephalopathy, eclampsia
  - Concussion
  - Acute hydrocephalus
  - Subarachnoid hemorrhage
  - *Meningitis:* pyogenic, tubercular, fungal, carcinomatous or lymphomatous, chemical meningitis, etc.
  - Viral encephalitis
- Altered sensorium with lateralizing features
  - *Intracranial hemorrhage:* Intracerebral hemorrhage, epidural and subdural hemorrhage, trauma
  - *Ischemic stroke:* Malignant middle cerebral artery infarction with midline shift and mass effect, brainstem infarction
  - Brain abscess, subdural empyema
  - Brain tumor with surrounding edema, Gliomatosis cerebri, intravascular lymphoma
  - Cerebral venous sinus thrombosis
  - *Demyelinating disorders*: Acute hemorrhagic leukoencephalitis, acute disseminated encephalomyelitis
  - Cerebral vasculitis, thrombotic thrombocytopenic purpura
  - Metabolic coma with pre-existing deficits
  - Meningitis with arteritis and resultant infarcts

TABLE 7.5: Differentiation of metabolic coma from structural coma

Feature	Toxic metabolic coma	Structural coma
State of consciousness	Fluctuates	Tends to remain static or worsens over time
Deep sighing respiration	Frequent	Infrequent (may occur with pontine lesions)
Papilledema	Rare except for carbon dioxide narcosis, lead intoxication, hypoparathyroidism or malignant hypertension	Common
Pupils	Small, reactive pupils; light reaction is preserved till late (exceptions: drugs with anticholinergic properties, hypothermia, neuromuscular blocking agents, barbiturates)	Light reaction may be affected early depending on the cause
Ocular mobility	May be affected, usually symmetrically	Asymmetric affection of ocular motility
Roving eye movements	Common	Rare
Reflex eye movements	Usually normal (except for phenytoin or barbiturate poisoning)	May be affected
Focal neurological deficits	Usually absent	Usually present
Involuntary movements	Commonly have tremor, generalized chorea, multifocal or generalized myoclonus, asterixis	Rare

Psychogenic Coma[4]

Several features indicate psychogenic coma. The patient may keep his eyes tightly closed and resist eye opening or may stare continuously at one point, interrupted by blinks. Pupils are normal sized and reactive. Oculocephalic reflexes are normal and oculovestibular maneuver elicits nystagmus that requires activity of frontal eye fields. Muscle tone, deep tendon reflexes, and plantar responses are normal.

LABORATORY INVESTIGATIONS[1,2]

The laboratory investigations that are most useful in the evaluation of a comatose patient include a detailed biochemistry profile [blood sugars, renal (blood urea, serum creatinine) and liver function tests (bilirubin, SGOT/SGPT, serum albumin and globulin, serum ammonia) serum electrolytes (sodium, potassium), serum calcium, serum magnesium], hemoglobin, total and differential leucocyte counts, platelet counts, erythrocyte sedimentation rate, C-reactive protein, blood and urine toxicology screen, creatine kinase and creatine kinase MB isoenzyme levels, neuroimaging, electroencephalography (EEG), and cerebrospinal fluid (CSF) analysis.

Any abnormal value on these tests may suggest the underlying etiology. For instance, severe leukocytosis may provide clue to underlying sepsis or pyogenic meningitis as a cause of coma. Blood ammonia should be measured in all the patients, as it may be markedly elevated in hepatic encephalopathy while other liver function tests may be normal. Thyroid function tests may be obtained depending upon the clinical scenario. Serum cortisol levels should be obtained if addisonian crisis is suspected. In the presence of a stressful state like coma, a low or even normal serum cortisol should strongly suggest adrenal insufficiency. If the cause of coma is not obvious, a blood toxicology screen should be obtained and serum osmolality should be measured and osmolar gap should be calculated to detect the presence of unmeasured osmotically active particles.

Neuroimaging[2]

Once the patient is stabilized and appropriate treatment has been given, CT scan of the brain should be carried out with thin (5 mm) section cuts of posterior fossa. Alternatively, magnetic resonance imaging (MRI) of the brain may be performed. Though most of the times a CT scan of the brain would suffice, it may miss acute infarcts.

Therefore, in appropriate clinical settings, an MRI scan of the brain may be required.

Magnetic resonance imaging of the brain may show evidence of a space-occupying lesion with resultant brain edema and evidence of herniation. It may reveal brainstem stroke or bilateral thalamic infarcts testifying basilar artery thrombosis. It may show characteristic changes of central pontine myelinolysis (CPM) secondary to acute correction of hyponatremia or may show bilateral basal ganglionic lesions seen in extrapontine myelinolysis. It may reveal tell-tale signs of anoxic damage to the brain such as bilateral pallidal lesions or diffuse cortical damage. It may help in diagnosis of herpes simplex encephalitis (HSE) by showing characteristic medial temporal, basifrontal and insular lesions or may show evidence of tubercular meningitis. In the presence of an absolutely normal neuroimaging, one should strongly suspect the possibility of a metabolic abnormality as the cause of coma.

Electroencephalography[2]

The major thrust of electroencephalography (EEG) lies in ruling out any ongoing convulsive activity, though it may show other features as well. In hepatic encephalopathy, EEG may show bilaterally synchronous and symmetrical, medium-to-high amplitude triphasic waves with frontal dominance. EEG showing a widespread β-activity is suggestive of drug intoxications. An EEG pattern with ominous prognosis is α-coma that reveals widespread α-activity resembling normal α-rhythm, but with lack of response to environmental stimuli. Normal α-activity on EEG would suggest locked-in syndrome or psychogenic coma. In herpes simplex virus (HSV) encephalitis, EEG may reveal periodic lateralized epileptiform discharges.

Lumbar Puncture[1,2]

In the recent years, lumbar puncture is being used more judiciously. This is because of the widespread availability of neuroimaging. In most cases, a lumbar puncture is carried out after a neuroimaging study has excluded intracerebral hemorrhages, infarctions, or other space-occupying lesions. The examination of CSF is, however, indispensable in ruling out CNS infections and CT-negative subarachnoid hemorrhage.

CONCLUSION

Confusion and coma suggest a failure of brain function with many different etiologies. Coma represents a neurological emergency with significant mortality and morbidity if the underlying cause is not identified and treated urgently. Delay of even a few minutes can make the difference between complete recovery and lifelong dependence. It is extremely important to develop an orderly approach to management of a comatose patient to expedite early diagnosis and recovery. This would require an understanding of the anatomic basis of coma and localizing features of neurological examination, knowledge of various syndromes known to present with coma, a predetermined plan for empirical therapy based on local epidemiological data and a careful consideration of cases where diagnosis is not apparent after neuroimaging, EEG and CSF examination.

REFERENCES

1. Josephson SA, Miller BL. Confusion and Delirium. In: Longo DL, Fauci AS, Kasper DL, Hauser SL, Jameson JL, Loscalezo J (eds). Harrison's principles of internal medicine. 18th edn, McGraw-Hill Companies, New York 2012; pp. 196-201.

2. Feske SK. Coma and confusional states: emergency diagnosis and management. Neurol Clin N Am. 1998;16:237-56.

3. Campbell WW. The Examination in coma. In: Campbell WW (eds). DeJong's the neurological examination. 7th edn. Lippincott Williams and Wilkins, South Asian edition, New Delhi, 2013; pp. 745-62.

4. Brazis PW, Masdeu JC, Biller J. The localization of lesions causing coma. In: Brazis PW, Masdeu JC, Biller J (eds). Localization in Clinical Neurology. 5th edition, Lippincott Williams and Wilkins, South Asian edition, New Delhi, 2007; pp. 557-82.

5. Prasad K, Yadav R, Spillane J. The Unconscious patient. In: Prasad K, Yadav R, Spillane J (eds). Bickerstaff's Neurological Examination in clinical practice. 7th edition, Wiley India. New Delhi, 2013; pp. 245-62.

6. Berger JR. Stupor and Coma. In: Daroff RB, Fenichel GM, Jankovic J, Mazziotta JC (eds).Bradley's neurology in clinical practice. 6th edition, Vol 1, Principles of diagnosis and management, Elsevier publishers, Philadelphia, 2012; pp. 37-55.

7. Ropper AH, Samuels MA. Delirium and other confusional states. In: Ropper AH, Samuels MA (eds). Adams and Victor's principles of neurology. 9th edition, McGraw-Hill Companies, New York 2009; pp. 398-409.

Chapter 8

Delirium and Acute Confusional States

Ellajosyula Ratnavalli

INTRODUCTION

Delirium is characterized by an acute and fluctuating change in attention, cognition, and consciousness usually due to an underlying medical condition. It is a reversible medical emergency and if untreated is associated with a high morbidity and mortality. Delirium is often overlooked or not given due importance.

Delirium is a very common disorder in clinical practice and may be managed by intensivists, emergency physicians, internists, surgeons, oncologists, neurologists, or psychiatrists. It is important to understand the ramifications of the disorder. If psychotic symptoms predominate, the patient may be referred to a psychiatrist who focuses on the treatment of agitation. A neurologist often labels the condition as an "encephalopathy" or a "confusional state" and focuses on investigations and fails to perform a complete cognitive assessment, or does not pay sufficient attention to the risk factors and follow-up (see Box 8.1).

This chapter deals with a comprehensive approach to a patient with delirium. Treatment will not be discussed.

TERMINOLOGY AND DIAGNOSTIC CRITERIA

The term delirium has been used synonymously with acute confusional state, organic brain syndrome, acute brain failure, septic encephalopathy, ICU psychosis (if it occurs in intensive care unit-ICU), and toxic-metabolic encephalopathy.[1] Confusional state appears to be a more general term but delirium is better suited and more specific. "Delirium" should be used when the diagnostic

and statistical manual of mental diseases (DSM-V) criteria are met (Box 8.2).[2] If the criteria are not met, a term "subsyndromal delirium" has been used.[3] Subsyndromal delirium occurs in patients with similar risks to those observed with delirium and is associated with clinical outcomes that are intermediate between normal and delirious patients.

> **Box 8.1: Red flags which should heighten the suspicion of delirium in a hospitalized patient**
>
> - Age >75
> - Sepsis
> - Critical care setting
> - Hypoxia
> - Medications, especially narcotics, anticholinergics
> - Intracranial pathology: stroke, meningitis, epilepsy
> - Substance intoxication (e.g., amphetamines and XTC) or withdrawal (alcohol and benzodiazepines)
> - Pain
> - Head injury
> - Acute or severe medical illness

> **Box 8.2: DSM-V diagnostic criteria for delirium**
>
> - All features should be present
> - Disturbance in attention and awareness
> - Acute onset over hours or days
> - Cognitive impairment
> - No coma and not caused by pre-existing dementia
> - Caused by a medical condition, substance intoxication, substance withdrawal, toxin, or multiple etiologies

PREVALENCE

The overall prevalence of delirium in the community is 1–2% but rises to 14% among those >85 years old.[4-7] Prevalence rate of delirium in hospital admissions is around 18–35%.[5-7] Highest incidence rates are seen in the ICU, postoperative, and palliative care settings.[5,6]

ASSESSMENT OF RISK FACTORS AND CAUSES

Delirium is usually multifactorial and results when a vulnerable patient with several risk factors is exposed to one or more precipitating factors or a noxious insult.[8] In an elderly malnourished patient with a recent fracture, a single dose of sedative may precipitate delirium, while in a young patient, multiple factors such as hyponatremia, sepsis or stroke, and admission to ICU may be necessary. Hence, addressing all the factors in a given patient or individual will be the most effective strategy in the treatment or prevention of delirium.[8]

A predictive model based on four risk factors—vision and cognitive impairment, severe illness and blood urea nitrogen (BUN)/creatinine ratio can identify patients at greatest risk for delirium.[9] In another study, the authors identified five common precipitating factors for delirium: use of physical restraints, bladder catheter, three or more psychoactive medications, malnutrition, and an iatrogenic event.[8]

Prominent risk factors include advanced age and dementia, and previous history of stroke, trauma, hearing, or visual impairment.[5-10] Some of the more common risk factors and causes are outlined in Table 8.1 and Box 8.3. The list is not exhaustive, as practically any acute medical (or neurological) illness can be a precipitating factor or the cause of delirium.[5-12] Drugs, acute infections (particularly urinary tract infections and pneumonia), stroke, and metabolic disturbances (particularly hyponatremia, hypo- and hyperglycemia, renal failure) are common causes of delirium in the elderly.[12]

Drugs are implicated in up to 40% of cases and should always be considered as a cause.[5,11,13,14] Any drug can cause delirium, but some, like antipsychotics, benzodiazepines, dopamine agonists, antibiotics, and nonsteroidal anti-inflammatory drugs, have greater potential. Drugs with high anticholinergic activity like digoxin, nifedipine,

TABLE 8.1: **Risk factors for delirium**

Nonmodifiable	Modifiable
Age >65 years	Hearing and visual impairment
Dementia, mild cognitive impairment	Alcohol misuse
Depression	Medical comorbidities
Past history of delirium	Environmental
History of stroke	Restraints
Medical comorbidities	• Catheter
	• Pain and lack of sleep
	• Special settings

Box 8.3: Common causes of delirium

Systemic infections (cystitis, pneumonia, sepsis)
Neurological
   Acute stroke (right parietal, thalamic)
   Meningoencephalitis
   Epilepsy—nonconvulsive status
   Head injury, subdural hematoma
   Intracerebral hemorrhage
   Hypertensive encephalopathy
   Tumors
Metabolic
   Hyponatremia, hypernatremia
   Hypoglycemia, hyperglycemia
   Hypocalcemia, hypercalcemia
   Hypomagnesemia
Medications
Alcohol withdrawal or intoxication
Drug withdrawal: Benzodiazepine, barbiturates
Substance abuse: cocaine, ecstasy, amphetamines
Toxins: heavy metals, inhalants, insecticides, carbon monoxide
Hypoxia and shock
Hypo- and hyperthermia
Acute myocardial infarction, cardiac failure
Renal, hepatic, or respiratory failure
Nutritional deficiency
   Thiamine
   Niacin
   B12
   Iron
   Folate
Endocrine
   Hypo- and hyperthyroidism
   Cushing's and Addison's
   Hyperparathyroidism
Trauma
Postsurgery
Miscellaneous: porphyria, neoplasms, autoimmune disorders

Common causes are **highlighted.**

Box 8.4: Medications causing delirium

- Central nervous system drugs
  - Benzodiazepines and other sedatives
  - Dopamine agonists
  - Anticonvulsants
  - Tricyclic antidepressants
  - Antipsychotics
  - Lithium
- Corticosteroids
- Analgesics
  - Meperidine
  - Nonsteroidal anti-inflammatory drugs
- Cardiac
  - Furosemide
  - β-Blockers, nifedipine
  - Captopril, digoxin
  - Isosorbide dinitrate
- Warfarin, dipyridamole
- Antihistamines
  - Diphenhydramine
  - Promethazine
- Muscle relaxants
  - Carisoprodol
  - Cyclobenzaprine
  - Methocarbamol
- Antispasmodics
  - Belladonna
  - Hyoscine
- H2 blockers
  - Cimetidine
  - Ranitidine
- Theophylline

Box 8.5: Mnemonic: DELIRIUM(S)

D	Drugs
E	Eyes, ears, and other sensory deficits
L	Low O_2 states (e.g., heart attack, stroke, and pulmonary embolism)
I	Infection
R	Retention (of urine or stool)
I	Ictal state
U	Underhydration/undernutrition
M	Metabolic causes
(S)	Subdural hematoma

Source: Adapted from Saint Louis University Geriatric Evaluation Mnemonics Screening Tools (SLU GEMS).

Box 8.6: Key points

- Old age and dementia are important risk factors for delirium
- Postoperative patients and those admitted to ICU are at an increased risk for developing delirium
- Delirium is multifactorial. Consider multiple precipitating factors in an individual
- Infections, alcohol, or benzodiazepine withdrawal, medications, and metabolic disturbances are common causes of delirium

PATHOPHYSIOLOGY

Historically, delirium has been considered a disorder of consciousness or arousal. Currently, it is regarded as a disorder of cognition with impaired attention and associated global cognitive impairment.[16,17] Considerable advances have been made in our understanding of delirium, but the fundamental pathophysiological basis remains unclear. Delirium is an acute brain failure in response to noxious insults, which unmasks decreased cognitive reserve. There are possibly multiple interacting mechanisms in an individual, which cause disruption of neural networks in the brain leading to cognitive impairment. Changes in neurotransmitters, disruption of blood–brain barrier, inflammation, acute stress response, neuronal injury, hypoxia, and impaired glucose oxidation are some of the mechanisms invoked to explain delirium.[6,17–19] Cholinergic deficiency and dopamine excess or both have frequently been linked to delirium.[19]

TYPES OF DELIRIUM

Three types of delirium have been distinguished.[20–22]

furosemide, H2 blockers, meperidine, and muscle relaxants are also common culprits (Box 8.4).[13,14] Alcohol intoxication or more commonly withdrawal (delirium tremens) and withdrawal from sedative hypnotic drugs and barbiturates are important causes in younger patients with hyperactive delirium. Urinary retention, fecal impaction, restraints, pain, and sleep deprivation can precipitate delirium in an elderly individual.[8,9,15]

Patients undergoing orthopedic, cataract or vascular surgery, cardiopulmonary bypass, or admitted to ICUs as well as those with terminal cancer and acquired immunodeficiency syndrome (AIDS) are particularly vulnerable to developing delirium (see Boxes 8.5 and 8.6).[5,6,9,10]

Hyperactive Delirium

This type of delirium is easy to diagnose as the patient is agitated, restless, and may exhibit disruptive behavior (shouting, abusive), psychosis, and mood lability. Patients are also prone to falls as they get out of bed and pull out intravenous lines or catheters. Delirium tremens or benzodiazepine withdrawal are typical examples but delirium can also occur following anticholinergic and illicit drug usage [cocaine, lysergic acid diethylamide, (LSD)].

Hypoactive Delirium

Hypoactive delirium is seen in metabolic disorders (hyponatremia, hypoglycemia, hepatic, and renal failure) and opiate intoxication, particularly in older patients. It can be missed or more seriously dismissed as a transient and insignificant problem as patients are sluggish, apathetic, confused, and drowsy. Hypoactive delirium is a significant condition, as it considerably prolongs hospital stay.

Mixed Delirium

Features of both hypoactive and hyperactive types are present. The patients may have greater morbidity and mortality.[21] In one study, mixed delirium was the commonest type of delirium (43%), followed by hypoactive (29%), hyperactive (21%), and unclassified (7%) (Box 8.7).[22]

DIAGNOSIS

The diagnosis of delirium is clinical and based on history, behavioral observations, and cognitive assessment.[5,23,24] Examination might help in identifying the cause of delirium. It is important to be methodical and thorough while approaching a patient with delirium. Sometimes delirium might be the only indicator of an underlying disorder (e.g., hypoglycemia and hypoxia) or it can be an atypical presentation of a common disorder (e.g., acute myocardial infarction) in the aged.[6]

Box 8.7: Key points: Hypoactive and hyperactive delirium

- Hypoactive delirium is usually missed or dismissed. Confusion may not be apparent on superficial conversation
- Consider alcohol or benzodiazepine withdrawal or substance abuse in a young individual with hyperactive delirium

---

HISTORY

A meticulous medical and neurological history should be obtained from the patient's family, especially a reliable caregiver living with the patient. This is because the patient may be incoherent and disoriented and unable to give history.[5,6] Details of previous cognitive state and functional abilities are essential in an older individual when distinctions from dementia become important. History of alcohol use or abuse, benzodiazepine and other sedative use, over-the-counter drugs, and herbal remedies is especially important.[11,12,23,25] The treating physician should also ask for a complete list of all the medications the patient is taking, the doses and recent changes if any. History of falls, change in sleep–wake cycle, recent surgery, and past history of delirium should also be elicited. A prodrome of 1–3 days may precede the delirium when the individual may appear anxious, restless, or dull and incontinent and refuse food or medications.

CLINICAL FEATURES[5,6,11,12,25,26]

Essential Features

Onset

Onset is usually acute over a few hours or days and should reflect a sudden change in cognition and behavior from the base line.

Fluctuating Course

Typically, symptoms fluctuate or wax and wane and are usually worse at night.

Altered Consciousness

Clouding of consciousness is a classic sign ranging from attention deficit and distractibility to drowsiness and unconsciousness, all of which fluctuate. Milder degrees are common and easily missed. Paradoxically, a sleepy elderly person may also be startled into aggressive vigilance. The level of consciousness may fluctuate between extremes in the same patient.

Inattention

Impaired attention is one of the hallmarks of delirium (Box 8.8). Patients are distractible, unable to focus, and may not carry out instructions. This can also fluctuate and may worsen toward the evening (sun-downing). A useful bedside test is asking the patient to name days of the week or months of the year backward. Digit span both forward and backward can also be used to assess attention. Normal forward digit span is usually 5–7. Serial subtraction (100–7) is a measure of sustained attention or working memory.

Impaired Cognition

There is impaired abstraction, logic, planning, reason and judgment. Thinking is progressively disturbed and disorganized. Speech is slow or fast and may be incoherent, rambling, circumlocutory and difficult to follow. Paraphasias may be noted on naming, which are usually unrelated to the target word. There can be disturbances in visuospatial abilities and writing.

Disorientation and Memory Impairment

Patients with delirium are disoriented to time and in severe cases, to place, and sometimes to person (Box 8.8). They may insist that they are at home and are unable to recall day, date or month. They may show recent memory impairment, may not remember what they had for breakfast or remember admission details. Remote memory is usually normal. They may appear awake and apparently normal and the physician may be surprised to find that the patient thinks he is at a hotel. It is important to ask specific questions regarding orientation? (Where are you? When did you get admitted? What day is it? etc.).

Supportive Features

Psychomotor Disturbances

Patients can be agitated, overactive, or apathetic. The former is more common in younger patients due to drug intoxication or substance abuse while the latter is more common in older individuals. One state may progress to the other. Groping, picking movements, and sometimes complex stereotyped movements can be observed.

Sleep–Wake Cycle Disturbances

Sleep–wake cycle is almost always disturbed with marked periods of drowsiness during the day and insomnia at night (Box 8.8). Patients are drowsy, lethargic, fall asleep during assessment and may have nighttime insomnia. Nighttime insomnia can lead to wandering. Excessive dreaming with persistence of the experience into wakefulness is also common.

Perceptual Disturbances

Visual hallucinations (insects, animals, shadows, people) or illusions (designs on a bed sheet as ants, bed bugs etc.) predominate. Lilliputian hallucinations are characteristic. Disturbances of body image (body part shrunk or enlarged), depersonalization, and derealization can be seen. Time sense may be distorted—a day may seem like a week. Delusions are often paranoid or persecutory in nature. Perceptual disturbances can occur in up to 40% cases of delirium. Florid changes are seen in delirium tremens, and LSD or cocaine intoxication.

Emotional Disturbances

Apathy is common in older patients but the whole gamut of emotional disturbances like irritability, emotional lability, anger, fear, bewilderment, depression, and euphoria can be seen.

In one study of 100 patients with delirium, inattention and sleep–wake cycle disturbances were the commonest symptoms (73%), followed by impairment in recent memory (64%), psychomotor retardation (37%), agitation (27%), hallucinations (26%), language disturbances (25%), impaired thinking 22%, emotional lability (18%), and delusions (9%) (Box 8.8).[26]

EXAMINATION

Cognitive examination and detailed mental state examination are essential.

Patient's state of consciousness (alert, vigilant, drowsy) should be noted.[5,11,23,24] Attention, orientation, memory, and language (comprehension and speech content) in particular should be assessed. Mood and affect, appearance, motor behavior (restlessness, groping, or picking movements) and eliciting hallucinations and delusions is part of the mental state examination.[25] A mini-mental state examination (MMSE)[27] or the Montreal Cognitive Assessment (MoCA)[28] may be used for formal testing of cognition. Dysgraphia, dysphasia, and dysnomia may be seen.

A complete general, systemic, and neurological examination is necessary in all patients. Raised temperature, tachycardia, and a rash may point toward infection. Smell of alcohol on breath, needle marks, jaundice, and cyanosis on general examination offer clues to the precipitating cause. Signs of autonomic dysfunction like pupillary dilatation, sweating, hypertension, tachycardia may point to intoxication, withdrawal, or substance abuse. Nystagmus, tremor, asterixis, myoclonus, and dysarthria are some of the neurological signs seen in delirium.[5,11,12,25] Focal neurological signs suggest a stroke or a subdural hematoma, meningeal signs point to meningoencephalitis and ophthalmoplegia to Wernicke's encephalopathy. Asterixis is more common in delirium tremens, hepatic encephalopathy, and respiratory failure with hypercarbia.

Sun-downing can be one of the caveats in the diagnosis as patients may be lucid in the morning but the night nurse may report disruptive behavior and confusion.[11] It is important to recognize these subtle indicators and not consider them a part of old age or "psychological reaction to admission". Conversely, an elderly patient sleeping on the doctor's morning rounds may have hypoactive delirium.[5] It is important to rouse the patient and evaluate the mental state. High degree of suspicion and repeated assessments are necessary, as a single evaluation may miss the diagnosis due to the fluctuating nature of delirium. Acute onset of confusion should be regarded as delirium unless proved otherwise, especially if there is no history available (Boxes 8.9 and 8.10, Case study 1).

Box 8.9: Clinical tip

- Check for bladder retention and fecal impaction, which are easily missed and can cause delirium in older patients

---

Box 8.10: Examinaton: Key points

- Delirium is a bedside clinical diagnosis based on history and examination
- Do a complete mental state examination. Test attention and orientation in particular and monitor consciousness and sleep–wake cycle
- A single assessment may miss delirium due to its fluctuating nature. Do repeat assessments
- Minor episodes of confusion, behavioral disturbance, or agitation in elderly should be taken seriously and investigated as appropriate

---

CASE STUDY 1

Mrs S, a 75-year-old woman, resident of a dementia care facility was referred for a change in behavior of 3 days. She had moderate Alzheimer's disease but was interacting with her caregivers and doing some scheduled activities like singing and playing a few games. She was oriented to person and place. Three days before admission, she became lethargic, apathetic, and refused food and medications. Her sleep was disturbed and she was incontinent. She was investigated and found to have hyponatremia and a urinary tract infection.

This is an example of hypoactive delirium common in elderly. Any acute change in a patient with dementia should be investigated rather than dismissed. This patient improved with treatment and did go back to her original level of functioning.

ASSESSMENT TOOLS

Delirium is consistently under-diagnosed especially in the elderly. Studies suggest that up to 30–60% cases may go unrecognized.[7,21] Under-diagnosis may be due to the fluctuating nature of delirium, its overlap with dementia, lack of formal cognitive assessment, missing hypoactive delirium or failure to consider the condition important.

Formal diagnosis can be made using the DSM-V criteria.[2] Confusion assessment method (CAM) is one of the most commonly used tools for screening delirium (Box 8.11).[16] It requires that acute onset and fluctuating course and inattention be present along with disorganized thinking or altered level of consciousness. It takes 5 minutes to administer. The ratings should be completed following cognitive assessment of the patient using the MoCA.[28] In a meta-analysis of 1,071 patients, CAM had a sensitivity of 94% and specificity of 89%.[29] The MMSE is perhaps least useful for identifying a patient with delirium.[24] The severity of delirium can be rated using the Delirium Rating Scale.[30]

Delirium in ICU or critical care setting should be viewed as acute brain dysfunction or failure akin to hepatic, renal, or cardiac failure. It is more difficult to recognize and appreciate, as patients are usually intubated or on ventilatory support. A CAM-ICU is available for detecting ICU delirium[31] (Table 8.2; Figs 8.1 and 8.2). Intensive care delirium screening checklist has also been used to diagnose delirium in the ICU, with a sensitivity of 99% and specificity of 64% (Box 8.12).[32]

A flowchart for approach to a patient with delirium is shown in Fig. 8.3.

Box 8.11: Early screening: CAM

- Improve early detection of delirium using CAM and formal cognitive testing

TABLE 8.2: Confusion Assessment Method for the intensive care unit (CAM-ICU)

Background	• The CAM[16] is a bedside evaluation for diagnosis of delirium • The CAM-ICU[31,32] is an adaptation of CAM for use in ICU patients who are often nonverbal because of intubation and pose communication challenges for the clinicians • It has four features which are determined by the patient, nurse, and family interview • Eight-hourly assessment recommended
CAM-ICU (two-step process)	It is a two-step process • Step 1. Arousal level (RASS) • Step 2. Content of consciousness (CAM-ICU)

Step 1:
Assess the level of sedation: (RASS)[33]
	• Scoring: Based on a 10-point scale
	• Four levels of anxiety or agitation (+1 to +4)
	  ○ One level to denote calm and alert state (0)
	  ○ Five levels of sedation (−1 to −5)
	• Strengths of RASS
	  ○ Two different conditions, sedation, and agitation are evaluated on a single scale
	  ○ Precise, unambiguous definitions for levels of sedation
	  ○ Positive numbers for agitation and negative numbers for sedation offer a logical approach, within a robust 10-level evaluation of consciousness
	  ○ Separates verbal from physical stimulation
	  ○ Relies heavily on duration of eye contact
	  ○ RASS complements the CAM-ICU
	• Psychometric properties
	  ○ RASS has demonstrated excellent inter-rater reliability and criterion, content, and face validity[45]

Step 2: Content of consciousness: CAM-ICU	Feature 1: Acute change or fluctuating course of mental status and Feature 2: Inattention and Feature 3: Altered level of consciousness or Feature 4: Disorganized thinking Psychometric properties Studies have demonstrated: • A high sensitivity of 91–95% • Specificity of 98% • Inter-rater reliability (k = 0.91)[45]
Other specialty versions of CAM-ICU	• The pediatric CAM-ICU (pCAM-ICU) • The Brief-CAM (B-CAM) for the emergency room
Strengths of CAM-ICU	• CAM-ICU serves to detect the onset of delirium as early as possible in order to rectify any modifiable causes • So, it is important to adapt delirium monitoring as standard practice in critically ill patients • CAM-ICU has been found to be reliable and valid in patients with and without dementia[16,31] • CAM-ICU has been found to have the best combination of ease, speed of use, suitability for repetitive use, data acquisition, reliability, and validity
When to discontinue pharmacologic treatment for delirium	• Since, by definition, delirium is a disorder of fluctuations in mental status, a patient is considered free of delirium when CAM-ICU has been negative for 24 hours
Limitations of CAM-ICU	• Although, the CAM-ICU has been validated in mechanically and nonmechanically ventilated critically ill patients, it has not been validated in the non-ICU settings

CAM, Confusion Assessment Method; ICU, intensive care unit; RASS, Richmond Agitation-Sedation Scale.

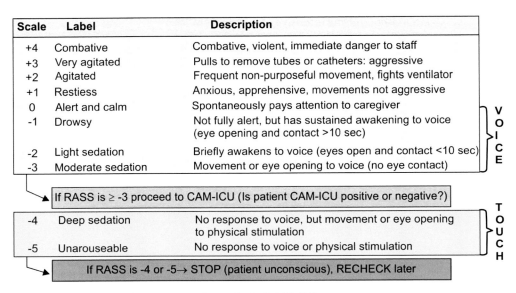

Fig. 8.1: The Richmond Agitation-Sedation Scale (RASS).[44,45]
Courtesy: By courtesy of Curtis N Sessler, Virginia Commonwealth University, Richmond, VA, USA.

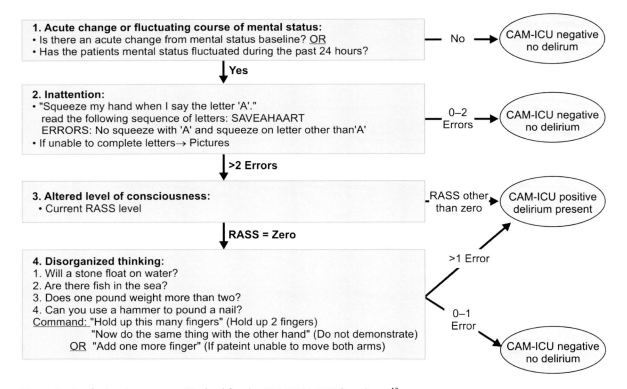

Fig. 8.2: Confusion Assessment Method for the ICU (CAM-ICU) flowsheet.[43]
Courtesy: E Wesley Ely, Vanderbilt University Medical Centre, Nashville, TN, USA.

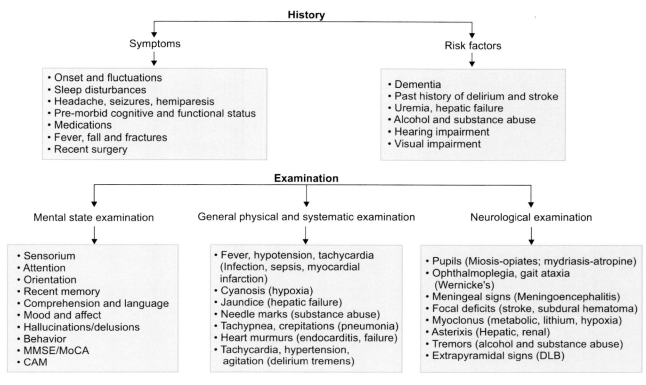

History

Symptoms

- Onset and fluctuations
- Sleep disturbances
- Headache, seizures, hemiparesis
- Pre-morbid cognitive and functional status
- Medications
- Fever, fall and fractures
- Recent surgery

Risk factors

- Dementia
- Past history of delirium and stroke
- Uremia, hepatic failure
- Alcohol and substance abuse
- Hearing impairment
- Visual impairment

Examination

Mental state examination

- Sensorium
- Attention
- Orientation
- Recent memory
- Comprehension and language
- Mood and affect
- Hallucinations/delusions
- Behavior
- MMSE/MoCA
- CAM

General physical and systematic examination

- Fever, hypotension, tachycardia (Infection, sepsis, myocardial infarction)
- Cyanosis (hypoxia)
- Jaundice (hepatic failure)
- Needle marks (substance abuse)
- Tachypnea, crepitations (pneumonia)
- Heart murmurs (endocarditis, failure)
- Tachycardia, hypertension, agitation (delirium tremens)

Neurological examination

- Pupils (Miosis-opiates; mydriasis-atropine)
- Ophthalmoplegia, gait ataxia (Wernicke's)
- Meningeal signs (Meningoencephalitis)
- Focal deficits (stroke, subdural hematoma)
- Myoclonus (metabolic, lithium, hypoxia)
- Asterixis (Hepatic, renal)
- Tremors (alcohol and substance abuse)
- Extrapyramidal signs (DLB)

MMSE, Mini-Mental State Examination; MoCA, Montreal Cognitive Assessment; CAM, Confusion Assessment Method.

Fig. 8.3: Flowchart showing approach to a patient with delirium.

Box 8.12: The intensive care delirium screening checklist

1. Altered consciousness
   - A. Comatose*
   - B. Stuporous*
   - C. Drowsy
   - D. Awake
   - E. Vigilant
2. Inattentive
3. Disorientation
4. Hallucinations or delusions
5. Agitation or retardation
6. Inappropriate speech or mood
7. Sleep–wake cycle disturbance
8. Fluctuation of symptoms

*If consciousness is A or B, delirium cannot be assessed.
Score 1 for each feature, if present. Total score 0–8.
A score of 4 or greater is diagnostic of delirium.

INVESTIGATIONS

Investigations should be done on the basis of patient's history and examination. It is recommended that all patients have a basic workup.[5,6,12,25] Additional investigations may be required depending on the clinical picture. These are outlined in Table 8.3. Delirium is usually multifactorial, so it is better to look at all the possible risk factors and precipitating causes in a given patient. For example, a patient may have hyponatremia, a urinary tract infection and recovering from a fracture surgery.

Electroencephalogram (EEG) can show diffuse slowing to theta or delta with poor organization of background rhythm, which correlates with the severity of delirium.[5,6,33] Electroencephalogram may be useful to detect occult seizures and differentiate delirium from a primary psychiatric disorder. It may show increased fast activity (delirium tremens, sedative overdose) or triphasic waves (hepatic encephalopathy). Routine use is limited

TABLE 8.3: Investigations for delirium

Signs/cause	Investigation
Essential	• Arterial blood gas • Complete blood count • Blood glucose • Serum electrolytes, creatinine • Serum calcium • Liver function tests • Thyroid-stimulating hormone • Electrocardiogram • Urine routine
Infection	• Erythrocyte sedimentation rate • C-reactive protein • Blood culture • Urine culture • X-ray chest
Nutritional	• Serum B12, folate, thiamine • Total protein, A:G ratio • Serum iron and ferritin
Drugs and toxins	• Blood levels • Urine toxicology
Cardiac	• Electrocardiogram • Echocardiography
Focal deficits	• Neuroimaging • Electroencephalography
Meningeal signs	Lumbar puncture
Seizure	Electroencephalography
Others	• Serum magnesium, phosphorous, • Ammonia, autoantibodies • Human immunodeficiency virus antibody

Box 8.13: Key point

• Targeted investigations will yield better results in the workup for delirium

because it is false-negative in 17% and false-positive in 22%.[34]

Neuroimaging should be considered if there are focal signs, signs of raised intracranial tension, head injury, suspected meningoencephalitis, history of a fall or when clinical suspicion of stroke is high. Neuroimaging should also be done when there is no other apparent cause, when history is unavailable or when patient is extremely agitated and cannot be examined. The yield of finding a focal lesion on neuroimaging was <7% if there were no focal signs and 2% in the presence of fever and dementia (Box 8.13).[35]

DIFFERENTIAL DIAGNOSIS

Delirium should be differentiated from dementia, depression, and acute psychosis or schizophrenia.[12,23,25]

A flowchart for the differential diagnosis of delirium is shown in Fig. 8.4.

DELIRIUM AND DEMENTIA

The relationship between delirium and dementia is a complex one. Both are predominantly cognitive disorders and they can frequently coexist. Delirium is an acute confusional state while dementia is chronic (or subacute). Dementia is a risk factor for developing delirium[36] and delirium is very frequent in patients with

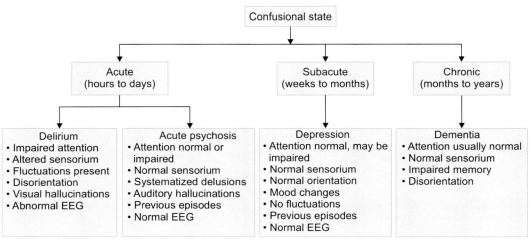

EEG, electroencephalography.

Fig. 8.4: Flowchart showing differential diagnosis of delirium.

dementia, up to 90% patients may develop delirium.[37] Delirium also increases the rate of incident dementia on follow-up (relative risk 5.7)[38] and accelerates the rate of cognitive decline in dementia.[39]

The clinician has to determine whether the patient has delirium, dementia, or delirium superimposed on dementia. It is important to differentiate delirium from dementia (Box 8.14), as the former is treatable and mostly reversible. Acute onset of hours to days differentiates delirium from dementia, which is more subacute or chronic, which develops over months or years. Consciousness is also altered in delirium. Attention is always impaired in delirium, while it is usually preserved in dementia. Most of the other features like disorientation, altered speech, perceptual disturbances etc. are relative and can occur in both. In a study on delirium, dementia, delirium with dementia, and normal controls, inattention and disorganized speech, and thinking were more severe in delirium alone. Forward spatial span was decreased significantly in delirium compared with dementia.[40] Dementia with Lewy bodies has features of dementia and delirium, but usually has a longer history and associated Parkinsonian features.

Depression should be differentiated from hypoactive delirium. Onset is usually subacute (weeks to months) in depression, and the mood symptoms are pervasive without fluctuations.[12,25] Consciousness is normal. Attention is usually normal but occasionally impaired. A high proportion of patients referred to psychiatric services for depression actually have delirium.[25]

Primary psychotic disorders may be difficult to differentiate from delirium. Delirium has psychotic features and if these are prominent, inattention may be masked.[23,25] Electroencephalogram is normal in psychosis. Abnormal EEG showing generalized slowing is suggestive of delirium but a normal EEG cannot rule out delirium. Primary psychotic disorders have predominantly systematized delusions, which are more persistent and consistent.[25] Thought insertion is common in schizophrenia and uncommon in delirium.[23,25] Visual hallucinations strongly suggest delirium, while hallucinations are auditory in schizophrenia.[25]

OUTCOME

Delirium usually lasts for up to a week or two and most patients improve. Some have persistent delirium. In one study, 45% of patients had delirium at one month and in 20% it persisted six months after discharge[41] Persistent delirium in the elderly can be an independent predictor of one year mortality (up to 40%).[42,46] Patients diagnosed with delirium have an overall high morbidity due to a high risk of malnutrition, falls, and pressure sores. Delirium is associated with increased risk of death, dementia, and institutionalization independent of age, sex, comorbid illness, and dementia.[10,38]

CONCLUSION

To conclude, delirium is a preventable disorder common in elderly. It may serve as a model for advancing our understanding of cognitive disorders and dementia and identify vulnerable patients. Further research is necessary to investigate pathogenesis, biomarkers, and effective therapies for delirium.

Acknowledgments

Assistance of Dr Swathy Chandrashekar in the preparation of flow charts and tables is gratefully acknowledged.

REFERENCES

1. Morandi A, Pandharipande P, Trabucchi M, et al. Understanding international differences in terminology for delirium and other types of acute brain dysfunction in critically ill patients. Intensive Care Med. 2008;34: 1907-15.
2. American Psychiatric Association. Task Force on DSM-5, Diagnostic and Statistical Manual of Mental Disorders: DSM-5. 5th edition. Washington, DC: The American Psychiatric Association; 2013.
3. Cole MG, McCusker J, Dendukuri N, et al. The prognostic significance of subsyndromal in delirium in elderly medical inpatients. J Am Geriatr Soc. 2003;51:754-60.
4. Folstein MF, Bassett SS, Romanoski AJ, et al. The epidemiology of delirium in the community: the Eastern Baltimore Mental Health Survey. Int Psychogeriatr. 1991;3:169-76.
5. Inouye SK. Delirium in older persons. N Engl J Med. 2006;354:1157-65.
6. Inouye SK, Westendorp RGJ, Saczynski JS. Delirium in elderly people. Lancet. 2014;383(9920):911-22.
7. Siddiqi N, House AO, HolmesJ D. Occurrence and outcome of delirium in medical in-patients: a systematic literature review. Age Ageing. 2006;35: 350-64.
8. Inouye SK, Charpentier PA. Precipitating factors for delirium in hospitalized elderly persons. Predictive model and interrelationship with baseline vulnerability. JAMA. 1996;275:852-7.

9. Inouye SK. Predisposing and precipitating factors for delirium in hospitalized older patients. Dement Geriatr Cogn Disord. 1999;10:393-400.

10. George J, Bleasdale S, Singleton SJ. Causes and prognosis of delirium in elderly patients admitted to a district general hospital. Age Ageing. 1997;26:423-7.

11. Burns A, Gallagley A, Byrne J. Delirium. J Neurol Neurosurg Psychiatry. 2004;75:362-7.

12. Saxena S, Lawley D. Delirium in the elderly: a clinical review. Postgrad Med J. 2009;85:405-13.

13. Flaherty JH. Psychotherapeutic agents in older adults. Commonly prescribed and over-the-counter remedies: causes of confusion. Clin Geriatr Med. 1998;14:101-27.

14. Mintzer J, Burns A. Anticholinesterase side-effects of drugs in elderly people. J R Soc Med. 2000;93:457-62.

15. Blackburn T, Dunn M. Cystocerebral syndrome: acute retention presenting as confusion in elderly patients. Arch Intern Med. 1990;115:2577-8.

16. Inouye SK, van Dyck CH, Alessi CA, et al. Clarifying confusion: the confusion assessment method. A new method for detection of delirium. Ann Intern Med. 1990;113:941-8.

17. Cunningham C. Systemic inflammation and delirium: important co-factors in the progression of dementia. Biochem Soc Trans. 2011;39:945-53.

18. Maldonado JR. Pathoetiological model of delirium: comprehensive understanding of the neurobiology of delirium and an evidence-based approach to prevention and treatment. Crit Care Clin. 2008;24:789-856.

19. Hshieh TT, Fong TG, Marcantonio ER, et al. Cholinergic deficiency hypothesis in delirium: a synthesis of current evidence. J Gerontol A Biol Sci Med Sci. 2008;63:764-72.

20. Lipowski ZJ. Transient cognitive disorders (delirium, acute confusional states) in the elderly. Am J Psychiatry. 1983;140:1426-36.

21. O'Keeffe ST, Lavan JN. Clinical significance of delirium subtypes in older people. Age Ageing. 1999;28:115-19.

22. Stagno D, Gibson C, Breitbart W. The delirium subtypes: a review of prevalence, phenomenology, pathophysiology and treatment response. Palliat Support Care. 2004;2:171-9.

23. Fong TG, Tulebaev SR, Inouye SK. Delirium in elderly adults: diagnosis, prevention and treatment. Nat Rev Neurol. 2009;5:210-20.

24. Wong CL, Holroyd-Leduc J, Simel DL, et al. Does this patients have delirium? Value of bedside instruments. JAMA. 2010;304:779-86.

25. Cole MG. Delirium in elderly patients. Am J Geriatry Psychiatry. 2004;12: 7-21.

26. Meagher DJ, Moran M, Raju B, et al. Phenomenology of delirium: assessment of 100 adult cases using standardized measures. Br J Psychiatry. 2007;190:135-41.

27. Folstein MF, Folstein SE, McHugh PR. "Mini-mental state." A practical method for grading the cognitive state of patients for the clinician. J Psychiatr Res. 1975;12:189-98.

28. Nasreddine ZS, Phillips NA, Bedirian V, et al. The Montreal Cognitive Assessment, MoCA: a brief screening tool for mild cognitive impairment. J Am Geriatr Soc. 2005;53:695-9.

29. Wei LA, Fearing MA, Sternberg EJ, Inouye SK. The confusion assessment method: a systematic review of current usage. J Am Geriatr Soc. 2008;56: 823-30.

30. Trzepacz PT, Mittal D, Torres R, et al. Validation of the delirium rating scale-revised-98: comparison with the delirium rating scale and the cognitive test for delirium. J Neuropsychiatry Clin Neurosci. 2001;13: 229-42.

31. Ely EW, Margolin R, Francis J, et al. Evaluation of delirium in critically ill patients: validation of the confusion assessment method for the intensive care unit (CAM-ICU). Crit Care Med. 2001;29:1370-9.

32. Bergeron N, Dubois MJ, Dumont M, et al. Intensive care delirium screening checklist: evaluation of a new screening tool. Intensive Care Med. 2001;27: 859-64.

33. Jenssen S. Electroencephalogram in the dementia workup. Am J Alzheimers Dis Other Demen. 2005;20:159-66.

34. Inouye SK. Delirium in hospitalized older patients. Clin Geriatr Med. 1998;14:745-64.

35. Hufschmidt A, Shabarin V. Diagnostic yield of cerebral imaging in patients with acute confusion. Acta Neurol Scand. 2008;118:245-50.

36. Elie M, Cole M, Primeau F, et al. Delirium risk factors in elderly hospitalized patients. J Gen Intern Med. 1998;13:204-12.

37. Fick DM, Agostini JV, Inouye SK. Delirium superimposed on dementia: a systematic review. J Am Geriatr Soc. 2002;50:1723-32.

38. Witlox J, Eurelings LS, de Jonghe JF, et al. Delirium in elderly patients and the risk of post discharge mortality, institutionalisation, and dementia: a meta-analysis. JAMA. 2010;304:443-51.

39. Fong TG, Jones RN, Shi P, et al. Delirium accelerates cognitive decline in Alzheimer disease. Neurology. 2009;72:1570-5.

40. Meagher DJ, Leonard M, Donnelly S, et al. A comparison of neuropsychiatric and cognitive profiles in delirium, dementia, comorbid delirium-dementia and cognitively intact controls. Neurol Neurosurg Psychiatry. 2010;8: 876-81.

41. Cole MG, Ciampi A, Belzile E, et al. Persistent delirium in older hospital patients: a systematic review of frequency and prognosis. Age Ageing. 2009;38:19-26.

42. Kiely DK, Marcantonio ER, Inouye SK, et al. Persistent delirium predicts greater mortality. J Am Geriatr Soc. 2009;57:55-61.

43. Ely EW. Confusion assessment method for the ICU (CAM-ICU): the complete training manual. Revised edition: 2010. Vanderbilt University.

44. Sessler CN, Gosnell MS, Grap MJ, et al. The Richmond Agitation-Sedation Scale: validity and reliability in adult intensive care unit patients. Am J Respir Crit Care Med. 2002;166:1338-44.

45. Ely EW, Truman B, Shintani A, et al. Monitoring sedation status over time in ICU patients: reliability and validity of the Richmond Agitation-Sedation Scale (RASS). JAMA. 2003;289:2983-91.

46. Lin SM, Liu CY, Wang CH, et al. The impact of delirium on the survival of mechanically ventilated patients. Crit Care Med. 2004;32:2254-9.

Chapter 9

Approach to a Patient with Intellectual and Memory Impairment

Shyamal K Das, Sandip Pal, Malay K Ghosal

INTRODUCTION

An increasing aging population multiplies the disease burden of geriatric disorders in the society. Cognition-related disorders such as mild cognitive impairment (MCI) and dementia are noteworthy among various geriatric ailments. Memory is an important component of cognition besides attention, language function, executive function, visuospatial, and visuoconstructional ability. Approach to a person with cognitive dysfunction needs clinical evaluation followed by neuropsychological assessment and neuroimaging.

ATTENTION SPAN

For neuropsychological evaluation, initial determination of attention span is important. Attention is a measure of patient's ability to attend to a specific stimulus over an extended period. The basic anatomic structures responsible for maintaining an alert state are the brain-stem reticular activating and the diffuse thalamic projection systems[1] (Fig. 9.1). Selectively focusing attention requires a widespread network of cortical neurons, particularly the prefrontal lobe, posterior cingulate gyrus, inferior parietal cortex, and medial temporal/occipital cortices. Attention is clinically evaluated by digit-repetition test and sustained attention by "A" random-letter test. Normal attention span is a prerequisite for further detailed mental-function testing.

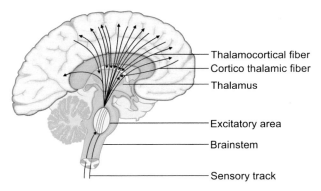

Fig. 9.1: Showing reticular activating system responsible for alerting mechanism.

Labels: Thalamocortical fiber; Cortico thalamic fiber; Thalamus; Excitatory area; Brainstem; Sensory track

MEMORY

Memory is a mental process that allows the individual to store information for later recall. This process consists of three stages. In the first stage, the information is received by a particular sensory modality (say, touch, auditory, or visual). The second stage consists of storing the information. The storage process is enhanced by rehearsal or by association with pre-existing information already in storage through past experience. The final stage is the recall or retrieval. The retrieval is an active process of mobilizing stored information on request or as necessary. This recall is also known as declarative memory. Studies on memory have documented that each aspect of memory involves separate neurobiological substrates or systems. Definitions of different types of memory have been provided in (Table 9.1).

Clinically, memory is subdivided into three types based on the time span between stimulus presentation and memory retrieval. The terms immediate, recent and

TABLE 9.1: **Definitions of different memory types[2-3]**

Term	Definition
Verbal	Memory encoded verbally
Nonverbal memory	Memory not encoded verbally, e.g., visual memory
Immediate recall	It is a process that does not require any long-term storage of information but does require initial registration, short-term holding, and verbal repetition
Short-term memory or working memory	It is characterized by short-term retention of information and important for tasks that require mental manipulation of information such as multistep arithmetic problem or briefly holding information of a telephone number. It does not require medial temporal lobe for recall
Recent memory or new learning	Recent memory is a system for temporarily storing and managing the information over hours and days. This process includes encoding or registration, storing, and retrieving data. One test of recent memory is memory span, the number of items, usually words or numbers that a person can hold onto and recall. Certain limbic structures are required to ensure storage and retrieval. The medial temporal lobe, the mammillary bodies, and the dorsal medial nuclei of the thalami are important subcortical links in the storage and retrieval of both verbal and nonverbal memories
Remote memory	Remote memory typically refers to memory for the distant past, measured on the order of years, or even decades. It includes episodic (autobiographical), personal semantic, and general semantic memory involving historical people and events. Old memories are stored in the appropriate association cortex
Explicit memory	It is the conscious, intentional recollection of previous experiences, and information. People use explicit memory throughout the day, such as remembering the time of an appointment or recollecting an event from years ago
Implicit memory	It is a type of memory in which previous experiences aid in the performance of a task without conscious awareness of these previous experiences. In daily life, people rely on implicit memory every day in the form of procedural memory, the type of memory that allows people to remember how to tie their shoes or ride a bicycle without consciously thinking about these activities[4]
Procedural memory	It is the kind of implicit memory involved in skill learning and other cognitive functions. It is a memory system that is not accessible in terms of specific facts, data, or spatio-temporal events
Semantic	This refers to the knowledge of words and their meanings, of concepts and facts, of symbols and rules to manipulate symbols. It enables the acquisition and retention of factual information about the world in broadest sense. It is equivalent to dictionary memory
Episodic memory	This memory system is involved in remembering specific episodes of one's own past (Tulving 1983). Often it is the earliest symptom of AD dementia. It is equivalent to historical memory
Autobiographic	This memory system consist of episodes recollected from an individual's life, based on a combination of episodic (personal experiences and specific objects, people and events experienced at particular time and place) and semantic (general knowledge and facts about the world) memory[5]
Recognition memory	It is a type of declarative memory. Essentially, recognition memory is the ability to recognize previously encountered events, objects, or people. It can be subdivided into two component: recollection and familiarity. It measure visual and verbal memory allowing clinicians to quickly distinguish between right- and left-hemisphere brain damage and to make judgments about localization[3]
Mild cognitive impairment	MCI is defined as a condition of measurable memory loss, inappropriate for age, and educational background, without core features of dementia.[1] As research on MCI progresses, several clinical subtypes of MCI have been recognized.[6] These include the amnestic or single-domain memory type, multiple domain type, and single nonmemory domain type[7]

AD, Alzheimer's disease; MCI, mild cognitive impairment.

TABLE 9.2: **How to test for various types of memory**[1]

Type of memory	How to test
Immediate	Digit repetition
Working memory	Backward digit repetition or utterance of a telephone number
Recent	In a typical test of memory span, an examiner reads a list of random numbers/words aloud at about the rate of one number per second. At the end of a sequence, the person being tested is asked to recall the items in order. The average memory span for normal adults is seven items.
Remote memory	Evaluate the patient' on place of birth, school information, vocation and marriage date, family information
Visual memory (hidden objects)	Here examiner uses five common small objects (say pen, comb, keys, coin, and spoon) while patient is watching. After engaging the subject with other conversation or cognitive task, the patient was asked to locate and name of the objects after 5 minutes.
Recognition memory	The test consists of two simple subtests: recognition memory for words (verbal) and recognition memory for faces (visual)

remote are commonly used.[1] These terms are nonspecific and the time span in each stimulus is not well-defined. Immediate memory is used to recall a memory trace after an interval of a few seconds. Short-term memory (STM) is part of immediate memory system. Recent memory is the ability to learn new material and retrieve that material after an interval of minutes, hours, or days. Remote memory refers to recall of facts or events that occurred months, years, or decades ago. Memory testing has been provided in Table 9.2. The immediate recall requires initial registration, short-term holding, and verbal repetition. The entire process can be performed by the language cortex surrounding the sylvian fissure. However, the exact mechanism by which these STMs are maintained within the language system is not known. The most common cause of failure on STM tasks is possibly inadequate attention. Immediate memory does not require the limbic system for storage and retrieval. For recent memory, certain limbic structures are required to ensure storage and retrieval. The medial temporal lobe, mamillary bodies and the dorsal medial nuclei of the thalami are subcortical links in the storage and retrieval of both verbal and nonverbal memories (Fig. 9.2). Old or remote memories are stored in the appropriate association cortex, for example, language association cortex for verbal material.

NEUROPSYCHOLOGICAL ASSESSMENT

Neuropsychological assessment is carried out through initial mini-mental status examination (MMSE) testing

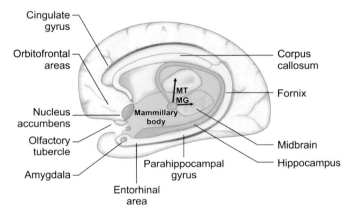

Fig. 9.2: Schematic diagram showing hippocampal formation and Papez circuit for memory.

followed by detailed application of available cognitive test batteries (Table 9.3). The cognitive test batteries should be administered by a trained neuropsychologist. Box 9.3 shows the MMSE validated in these local languages (i.e., Hindi, English, and Bengali) for the urban population. Figures 9.1 and 9.2 show the attentional and memory circuits, and the knowledge of which is essential for conceptual framework. Two case vignettes are presented in Case studies 1 and 2. These vignettes form a template for discussing the approach to an individual with cognitive problems. Since, dementia patient tend to consult of both the neurologists and the psychiatrists, two different cases of different presentations have been described here.

TABLE 9.3: Neuropsychological batteries available in India

Name of batteries	Domain tested/application of test	Comments
NIMHANS neuropsychological batteries[8]	Several Western tests and a few indigenous tests	Based on principles of cerebral localization and lateralization
NIMHANS neuropsychological batteries for adults[9]	Finger tapping, digit substitution, controlled oral word association test, animal naming test, N-back test, Tower of London, Wisconsin card sorting test, Rey auditory verbal learning test, Rey complex figure test, visuospatial functions	Useful for evaluation of head injury, movement disorders, and refractory epilepsy
NIMHANS neuropsychological battery for children[10]	The child version consists of Western tests to evaluate different domains of cognitive functions such as attention, executive functions, memory, comprehension, and visuospatial skills	
Comprehensive neuropsychological battery (AIIMS) battery[11]	This battery was developed in Hindi and includes motor, tactile, visual, receptive speech, expressive speech, reading, writing, arithmetic, memory, and intellectual processes	Based on Luria's functional approach
PGI battery of brain dysfunction[12]	This battery consists of PGI memory scale, Bhatia's short battery of performance—revised, verbal adult intelligence, and Bender-Gestalt test	This battery is compilation of individual tests of memory, intelligence and visual perception in Indian population
Hindi Mental State Examination (HMSE)[13]	HMSE total, calculation, word list learning, recall and recognition, object Naming, verbal fluency (category—animals and fruits), constructional, praxis	Has been used in rural community study in Hindi belt
Kolkata cognitive screening battery[14]	This battery consisted of the object naming test, verbal fluency (category—animals and fruits), mental state examination (similar to MMSE), calculation tests, visuoconstructional ability, and memory (immediate, delayed, and recognition)	This battery is useful for cognitive assessment of persons of aged equal to or above 50 years in urban community setting

MMSE, Mini-Mental Status Examination; NIMHANS, National Institute of Mental Health and Neurosciences, Bangalore; AIIMS, All India Institute of Medical Science; HMSE, Hindi Mental State Examination; PGI, Post Graduate Institute of Medical Science and Research, Chandigarh.

CASE STUDY 1

DKD, a 64-year-old right-handed male, graduate in engineering, retired from personal business presented with forgetfulness in 2012. The symptoms started gradually since 2006. Initially, he used to experience difficulty recalling names of people, following certain banking procedures, conveying messages, forgetting items he just ate, etc. The family members also noticed a change in personality from an active and motivated person to an indifferent and aloof person. Loss of interest in daily activities and an inability to feel pleasure in anything seemed evident with the passage of time. Repetition of the same words was becoming more frequent by the end of 2010. He was experiencing increasing difficulties in judgment and problem solving related to household or business activities. He faced difficulty in financial management of his business and had problems in sequencing and prioritization. By late 2011 and early 2012, the patient was found to have poor attention and concentration, difficulty in initiating and completing tasks, had slowing of psychomotor activities. The family members also noticed disorientation with respect to time and place. At times, he would go to the kitchen instead of the bathroom and frequently could not locate his home on return from his routine walk.

He became gradually withdrawn and stopped meeting his friends and his neighbors. He stopped attending cultural and social functions. Late in the course, he also failed to recognize his friends and close relatives.

He has no prior history of hypertension, hyperlipidemia, or diabetes. The family members did not give any history of epilepsy, thyroid disease, chronic kidney, or hepatic disease. Personal information revealed that the patient had been consuming alcohol (about 1–2 ounce daily) and tobacco over last 35–40 years and also indulged in substance abuse (alprazolam). He had no past history of head trauma. He was a nonvegetarian. Family history of stroke, hypertension, and alcohol and substance abuse was present.

His general physical examination did not reveal any abnormality. His blood pressure was 110/70 mmHg. His neurological examination did not reveal any focal deficit. His eye-movement was normal. His tone, power, deep tendon reflexes and plantar were normal. His frontal lobe release signs were present and exaggerated jaw jerks were also present. The patient had neither any extra pyramidal signs nor any cerebellar features. His gait was normal.

Continued

Continued

During the *clinical interview*, he was observed to be indifferent and aloof. He was disoriented with respect to the city (he said it was his hometown Ranchi and not Kolkata, though knowing fully well that he travelled by train to reach Kolkata), but he was aware that he was in a hospital for clinical assessment. Rapport with the examiner was established after much pursuance but eye contact could be maintained. He had only partial insight into his problems. Speech output was very low, but volume of speech was within normal limits. He seldom spoke spontaneously. Reaction time was delayed. Repetitive speech was present. The patient lacked volition. His target orientation and initiative-taking behavior were poor. He was also observed to have difficulty in following a sequence. He failed to attend a task until completion and required prompts to continue. Perseveration was observed.

On *neuropsychological testing*, his MMSE was 14. He had reduced alertness and difficulty in focusing and sustaining attention. He had slowed mental speed, disorientation with respect to time, place and person (inconsistent). On language assessment, spontaneous speech was reduced (affluency), he had difficulty in understanding complicated or multistep instructions; confrontational naming and writing were compromised. Mild compromise was also observed on reading and repetition tasks.

Gross impairment in the patient's visuoconstructional and visuospatial ability, as well as in the higher cognitive functions (like his capacity to acquire and retain a general fund of information, comprehend and judge social situations, to calculate, and think abstractly) were observed. Marked compromise in executive functioning (inhibition of irrelevant responses, sequencing, executive control of attention, capacity to abstract and judge, sustain attention and generate responses in a regulated manner) was also evident from the neuropsychological findings.

In the memory domain, immediate free recall for digits, words and sentences was compromised. New learning ability in both verbal and visual modalities was impaired; retrieval did not improve through the recognition procedure. Autobiographical memory for remote information was preserved. Recent episodic (personal experiences) memory was also compromised. Both immediate and delayed recall in logical memory was impaired. Confabulation was present. Praxis was preserved, but gnosis was affected. Deterioration in execution of instrumental activities of daily living (IADL) and qualitative deterioration of certain basic ADL were observed. On assessment, symptoms of depression, apathy and indifference were prominent. The Clinical Dementia Rating score (spouse being the rater) was 2. *Neuroimaging* (December 2010) revealed mild diffuse cerebral atrophy and multiple old small infarctions in both centrum semiovale. The patient was suffering from probable dementia either of the *Alzheimer's type* at the *moderate stage of severity* or mixed dementia considering the neuroimaging findings.

CASE STUDY 2

A 78-year-old, retired, right-handed, railway employee, who was previously reserved, well adjusted, responsible, and reasonable by nature developed talkativeness, pressure of speech, elated mood, grandiosity, decreased need for sleep and increased energy with unnecessary excess in activity. Mini-Mental Status Examination was found to be almost normal. The CT scan of the brain showed age-related mild cerebral atrophy. He was diagnosed as a case of bipolar disorder and put on valproate. He was partially controlled but over a period of three months, subsequently developed slow shuffling gait with frequent falls. Over a period of another two months, he developed forgetfulness and started making mistakes in calculation, banking transactions and other day-to-day activities. Ultimately, he was diagnosed as a case of behavioral variant of frontotemporal disorder (FTD).

This case is an example of initial behavioral problems progressively turning into dementia. The behavioral problems were followed by gait disturbances with repeated falls suggestive of extra pyramidal features, and finally dementia.

▌ BASED ON FIRST CASE....

Q.1. What is the problem of the patient?

Ans.1: The patient has significant problem in cognition. *Cognition* refers to a set of mental processes that includes attention, memory, language, learning, reasoning, problem solving, and decision making. Disturbances of cognition might be either physiological (e.g., age related) or pathological including MCI and dementia especially when activities of daily living (ADL) are involved. Our patient had attentional deficit, impaired memory, language dysfunction, impairment of visuospatial and visuoconstructional ability, and executive dysfunction indicating involvement of bilateral attention circuits comprising the dorsolateral prefrontal cortex (DLPFC), posterior parietal cortex and thalamus, memory circuits consisting of hippocampus along with other constituents of Papez circuit (Fig. 9.2). The language dysfunction indicates involvement of language circuit comprising the inferior frontal and temporoparietal areas within the dominant side, and nondominant parietal lobes (visuospatial and visuoconstructional ability), executive dysfunction (prefrontal cortex), and recognition problems (occipitotemporal cortex).[1,6] Thus, he demonstrated diffuse bilateral involvement of the brain. Though, imaging showed small infarcts, the size and location of the infarcts could not explain his disability. So, he might have more involvement that could only be revealed by functional imaging studies, or biopsy, or on autopsy. He had no risk factors for stroke. Overall, there was a gradual and relentless progression of the neurological deficits instead of a stepwise progression, and clinically, the subject had no evidence of focal deficits. Hence, although imaging demonstrated features of vascular disease, it is less likely that he suffered from vascular dementia. Clinically, he might be suffering from either degenerative dementia or mixed dementia. Of course, the final ultimately final diagnosis would depend on autopsy study.

Q.2. How to arrive at the diagnosis?

Ans.2: Diagnosis depends considerably on history, examination, and neuropsychological assessment. According to DSM-IV-TR criteria (Table 9.4), people who have involvement of cognitive functions in two or more domains, associated with impairment in ADL and lack of social interaction, are suffering from dementia. The symptoms should be progressive in nature and there is a significant decline from a previous level of functioning. This patient had involvement of multiple cognitive domains including memory, impairment of ADL, and deterioration of social functioning. Hence, according to the DSM-IV-TR criteria, he might be assigned a diagnosis of dementia.

TABLE 9.4: **Criteria for different subtypes of dementia**

Type	Criteria	

Dementia	DSM-IV TR (Diagnostic and Statistical Manual of Mental Disorders 1994)[8]	• The development of multiple cognitive deficits manifested by both
		  ○ Memory impairment and
		  ○ One (or more) of the following cognitive disturbances: aphasia, apraxia , agnosia, disturbances in executive function
		• Significant impairment in social or occupational functioning and represent a significant decline from a previous level of functioning
		• Gradual onset and continuing cognitive decline
		• The cognitive deficits are not due to any other CNS or systemic causes or substance abuse
		• The deficits do not occur exclusively during the course of a delirium
		• The disturbance is not better accounted for by another axis I disorder, e.g., major depressive disorder, schizophrenia
		• DSM-V now recognizes a less severe level of cognitive impairment, mild NCD (neurocognitive disorder), which is a new disorder that permits the diagnosis of less disabling syndromes that may nonetheless be the focus of concern and treatment

Alzheimer dementia	NINCDS-ADRDA (National Institute of Neurological and Communicative Disorders and Stroke and the Alzheimer's Disease and Related Disorders Association (1984) (recent diagnosis has been supplemented by a biological marker, 2011)[15]	• Definite Alzheimer's disease: The patient meets the criteria for probable Alzheimer's disease and has histopathological evidence of AD via autopsy or biopsy • Probable Alzheimer's disease: Dementia has been established by clinical and neuro-psychological examination. The onset of the deficits is between the ages of 40 and 90 years and finally there must be an absence of other diseases capable of producing a dementia syndrome • Possible Alzheimer's disease: There is a dementia syndrome with an atypical onset, presentation or progression; and without a known etiology; but no comorbid diseases capable of producing dementia • Unlikely Alzheimer's disease: The patient presents with a dementia syndrome with a sudden onset, focal neurologic signs, or seizures or gait disturbance early in the course of the illness[16,17]

Continued

Continued

Type	Criteria	
Vascular dementia	NINDS-AIREN (National Institute of Neurological Disorders and Stroke—Association Internationale pour la Recherché et l'Enseignement en Neurosciences, 1993)[18,19]	The criteria for the clinical diagnosis of probable vascular dementia include all of the following • Dementia established by clinical examination and documented by neuropsychological testing; CVD, defined by the presence of focal signs on neurologic examination, consistent with stroke (with or without history of stroke), and evidence of relevant CVD by brain imaging (CT or MRI) including multiple large vessel infarcts or a single strategically placed infarct (angular gyrus, thalamus, basal forebrain, or posterior or anterior cerebral artery territories), as well as multiple basal ganglia and white matter lacunes, or extensive periventricular white matter lesions, or combinations thereof • A relationship between the above two disorders manifested or inferred by the presence of one or more of the following ○ Onset of dementia within 3 months following a recognized stroke ○ Abrupt deterioration in cognitive functions; or fluctuating, stepwise progression of cognitive deficits • Clinical features consistent with the diagnosis of probable vascular dementia include the following ○ Early presence of gait disturbance ○ History of unsteadiness and frequent, unprovoked falls ○ Early urinary frequency, urgency, and other urinary symptoms not explained by urologic disease ○ Pseudobulbar palsy ○ Personality and mood changes, abulia, depression, emotional incontinence, or other subcortical deficits including psychomotor retardation and abnormal executive function • Features that make the diagnosis of vascular dementia uncertain or unlikely include early onset of memory deficit and absence of corresponding focal lesions on brain imaging • Clinical diagnosis of possible vascular dementia may be made in the presence of dementia with focal neurologic signs in patients in whom imaging evidence of definite CVD are missing; or in the absence of clear temporal relationship between dementia and stroke; or in patients with subtle onset and variable course (plateau or improvement) of cognitive deficits and evidence of relevant CVD • Criteria for diagnosis of definite vascular dementia are ○ Clinical criteria for probable vascular dementia ○ Histopathologic evidence of CVD obtained from biopsy or autopsy ○ Absence of neurofibrillary tangles and neuritic plaques exceeding those expected for age ○ Absence of other clinical or pathological disorder capable of producing dementia
Fronto-temporal dementia (FTD)	Neary consensus criteria (Clinical) (1998)[20]	• Core diagnostic features ○ Insidious onset and gradual progression ○ Early decline in social interpersonal conduct ○ Early impairment in regulation of personal conduct ○ Early emotional blunting ○ Early loss of insight • Supportive diagnostic features ○ Behavior disorder ○ Speech and language disorder ○ Physical signs (primitive reflexes, incontinence, akinesia, rigidity, tremor and low and labile pressure) ○ Investigation (neuropsychology, EEG, brain damage)
Diffuse Lewy body dementia (DLBD)	Clinical and patho-logical diagnosis of dementia with Lewy bodies, 1996[21]	• Central feature: progressive cognitive decline of sufficient magnitude interfering with normal social and occupational function • Two of the following core features are essential for a diagnosis of probable DLB and one is essential for possible DLB: ○ Fluctuation of cognition with pronounced variation in attention and alertness ○ Recurrent visual hallucinations that are typically well formed and detailed ○ Spontaneous features of Parkinsonism • Features supportive of diagnosis: repeated falls, syncope, transient loss of consciousness, neuroleptic sensivity, systematized delusion, hallucinations in other modalities, REM sleep behavior disorders, depression

CNS, central nervous system; AD, Alzheimer disease; EEG, electroencephalography; DLB, dementia with Lewy bodies; REM, rapid eye movement; CT, computed tomography; MRI, magnetic resonance imaging; CVD, cerebrovascular disease.

Q.3. What would be the next steps?

Ans.3: The next step would be the establishment of type of dementia that may be reversible or nonreversible and degenerative (Alzheimer type) or nondegenerative (vascular dementia).The causes of reversible dementia are provided in Box 9.1.[6,22] Exclusion of these causes is essential. The causes of progressive dementias have been elucidated in Box 9.2.

> **Box 9.1: Causes of transient memory loss (potentiality reversible)**
>
> - Iatrogenic: antidepressants, antihistamines, anti-anxiety medications, muscle relaxants, tranquilizers, sleeping pills, and pain medications
> - Nutritional: vitamin B1 and B12 deficiency
> - Toxic: alcohol, tobacco
> - Trauma: head injury leading to concussion
> - Stroke involving strategic sites such as thalamus, hippocampal formation, transient global amnesia
> - Infection: HIV, tuberculosis, meningoencephalitis
> - Psychological-depression, anxiety, and stress
> - Metabolic: hypothyroid, liver failure, kidney failure
> - Sleep deprivation, sleep apnea
> - Postseizure
> - Surgical: subdural hematoma, hydrocephalus, operable extra-axial brain tumor

> **Box 9.2: Causes of progressive memory loss**
>
> - Neurodegenerative: Alzheimer's disease, extrapyramidal (Lewy body disease, Parkinson's disease and Parkinson plus syndrome—progressive supranuclear palsy, Huntington's disease), Frontotemporal dementia
> - Slow virus disease: Creutzfeldt–Jakob disease
> - Nutritional: subacute combined degeneration, alcohol
> - Metabolic-endocrinal-hypothyroidism, hypercalcemia, chronic liver failure, chronic renal failure
> - Neoplastic: brain tumor, paraneoplastic
> - Postradiation
> - Infection: HIV, tuberculosis, neurocysticercosis, neurosyphilis, neurolyme
> - Toxic: alcohol, heavy metal
> - Inflammatory: multiple sclerosis, central nervous system vaculities
> - Iatrogenic: antidepressants, antipsychotic, anticholinergic
> - Surgical, normal pressure hydrocephalus, head trauma, brain tumor

Q.4. What is the rationale for undertaking the investigations?

Ans.4. The first investigation should be a detailed evaluation by a neuropsychologist followed by neuro-imaging.

Neuropsychological evaluation in typical cases shows disproportionate deterioration in memory as compared to age, sex, and education. The initial assessment is done with a brief cognitive battery called the MMSE. Folstein MMSE is used in many countries globally, but needs to be validated in local cultural sensitivity. In India, this has been validated in Hindi by Ganguly and Chandra for Hindi-speaking rural people, and subsequently modified and validated in Bengali and Hindi for the urban nondemented aging population (Box 9.3). Further, there are many neuropsychological batteries available to assess the cognitive functions. Neuropsychological assessment helps to differentiate between a case of true dementia and pseudodementia secondary to anxiety and depression, and also helps in localization of the underlying lesion. Dichotomy between history and neuropsychology, inconsistencies during multiple trials of neuropsychological assessment, improvement with suggestion and motivation may indicate the presence of pseudodementia. In early period of the disease, it also helps to evaluate the different domains involved and determine the subtype of dementia. Memory testing is very important and should be done in all cases as elaborated in Table 9.2. It provides a baseline objective measure in terms of scores by which evaluation of change over time can be recorded. This helps in management and prognostication.

The most important modality of imaging of brain is magnetic resonance imaging (MRI; Figs 9.3 to 9.5), but CT scan of brain may be done where MRI facility is not available. Primarily, the CT scan helps to exclude space-occupying lesions, hydrocephalus, and granulomas. In certain cases of subtyping, the role of nuclear imaging such as single-photon emission computed tomography (SPECT) and positron emission tomography (PET) is helpful.[23] AD may reveal hypometabolism or hypoperfusion in posterior temporoparietal cortex and hippocampal region. The typical radiological features of the different subtypes of dementia have been provided in Table 9.5 and Figs 9.3 to 9.5.

However, the primary role of imaging is to exclude any space-occupying lesions (primary or secondary neoplasm), normal pressure hydrocephalus, diffuse white

Box 9.3: Mini-Mental Status Examination

(Based on Hindi version of Mini-Mental Status Examination by Ganguly and Chandra, the following scale has been validated in Hindi and Bengali version in an urban setting, and normative data has been evaluated based on age, gender, and education.[14]

This test consists of 23 items that test differentiates components of intellectual capability. The items cover several areas of cognitive functioning such as orientation to time, place, memory, attention and concentration, recognition of objects, language function, both comprehension and expressive speech, motor functioning and praxis. It is relatively simple to administer and provides quick brief index of the subjects' current level of functioning.

Name: _____   Age: _____   Sex: _____   Education:_____   Occupation:_____

Score 1= correct response; 0 = incorrect response

1. "Is it morning or afternoon or evening"?
2. "What day of the week is it today?"
3. "What date is it today?"
4. "Which month is this? You can tell me either the Bengali or the English month".
5. "What season of the year is this? "
6. "What is the name of this place/locality?"
7. "In which city does this locality fall under?"
8. "Which state is this?"
9. "What is the name of this country?"
10. "Which place/house is this?"
11. Registration of three objects
   - Mango
   - Chair
   - Coin
   (Tell the subjects: "Remember the names of the three words")

12a. Days of the week forward (from Sunday).
   Say: "Now can you tell me the names of the days of the weeks starting from Sunday?"

   _____   _____   _____   _____   _____

   1= correct sequence (regardless of which attempt or if with self-correction)
   2= incorrect sequence even after 3 attempts (NOT INCLUDED IN TOTAL SCORE)

12b. Days of the week backward
   "Now can you tell me the names of these dates backward?"

   _____   _____   _____   _____   _____

   Give 1 point for each correct response; total = 5.

13–15. Delayed recall of objects
   (Names of previous three things given for registration)

16. Ability to see watch and pen
   Show the subject, the wrist watch and pen and ask: "Can you see these objects?"
   If YES, items 17 and 18 should be completed, if the subject is unable to see the objects, allow the subject to hold them.
   If NO, items 17a and 18a apply.

17. Identification of watch (visual recognition)
   If the subject is ABLE to see the objects—show him the wrist watch and say: "What is this?"

17a. (If necessary) *Identification of watch by touching*
   If the subject is UNABLE to see the objects—give the wrist watch to the subject and ask him how to feel it and ask: "What is this?"

18. Identification of pen (visual recognition): If the subject is *able* to see the objects then show him the pen and say: "What is this?"

18a. (If necessary) Identification of pen by touching.
   If the subject is unable to see the objects-Give the pen to the subject and ask him how to feel it and ask: "What is this?"

Continued

Continued

19. Sentence repetition
    Instruction: "Now I am going to say something, listen carefully and repeat it exactly as I say it after I finish".
    Phrase: "Neither this, nor that".
20. Follow command
    Say: "Now look at my face and do exactly what I do". Then close your eyes for 2 seconds and then open your eyes. Watch the subject to see if he follows the action. If he does it correctly then score as Correct.

    "CLOSE YOUR EYES".
21. Three—step command (oral)
    "First, take the paper in your right hand, then with both your hands fold it into half once and then give the paper back to me."
    If the subject's right hand is disabled; ask him to take the paper in his left hand.
22. Sentence construction
    Tell the subject: "Now say a line about your house".
23. Copy figure
    The figure is a simple one, a diamond within a square.

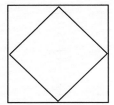

BMSE Score Distribution

Subtest	Task	Score	Total score
Orientation	• Time orientation—time of the day, day, date, month, and season • Place orientation—locality, city, state, country, place/house	5 5	10
Registration	Mango, chair, coin	3	3
Attention and concentration	• Days forward • Days backward OR • Bus fare (best of two scores)	5 5	Not included in total score 5
Recall	Mango, chair, coin	3	3
Naming	Watch, pen	2	2
Repetition	Sentence	1	1
Follow command	Close your eyes	1	1
Three step command		3	3
Sentence construction	Generate a sentence	1	1
Copying figure		1	1
		Total BMSE score	**30**

In validation study among 745 subjects, mean score was 28.7(± 2.1); 10 percentile score—26 and 90 percentile score is 30. When the score is below 10 percentile it is abnormal.

matter disease, granuloma, infection, and stroke that can present with dementia.[24] Presence of generalized cortical atrophy, and selective or regional atrophy may be helpful in subtyping of dementia (Table 9.5 and Figs 9.3 to 9.5). Early hippocampal atrophy may suggest Alzheimer type of dementia. Frontotemporal, frontal, and neocortical temporal (anterior, lateral, and inferior) atrophy may

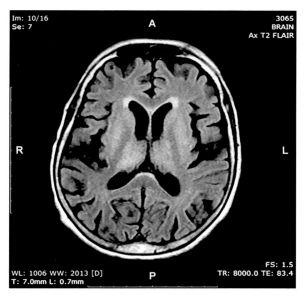

Fig. 9.3: Showing axial image in T2 flair in a case of probable Alzheimer's disease.
Courtesy: Dr MK Ghosh, Associate Professor, Department of Radiology, Burdwan Medical College, Bardhaman, West Bengal, India.

suggest frontotemporal type of dementia. In contrast, more white matter changes and less temporal lobe atrophy are seen in vascular dementia (Figs. 9.5A and B).

In some, signal abnormalities in the basal ganglia may suggest Creutzfeldt–Jakob disease (CJD). Electro-encephalogram (EEG) is useful for detecting CJD, subacute sclerosing pan encephalitis (SSPE), and also in metabolic encephalopathy mimicking dementia. Electro-encephalogram in CJD shows periodic short-duration bursts, and in SSPE the bursts are of long duration with postburst suppression.

Biochemical investigations should be done to establish, and also to exclude the reversible causes of dementia. Recently, diagnosis has been made possible by estimation of fractions of amyloid protein in cerebrosipinal fluid (CSF). The CSF-Aβ_{42} is low in subjects with AD, because it is increasingly consumed to form the amyloid plaque, but tubular associated protein (TAU) may be increased.[6,22] Low CSF-Aβ_{42} or low ratio of Aβ to TAU may help in diagnosis of Alzheimer's disease. These protein fragments may act as biomarkers of Alzheimer's disease. Sensitivity of the test is about 60%. To exclude the reversible causes of dementia, one should measure the metabolic parameters, particularly serum folate and vitamin B12 levels. The CSF estimation of a particular peptide fragment of normal brain protein (14-3-3) by immunoassay is important for diagnosis in CJD disease.[22]

Genetic study is important for those who have positive family history, Down syndrome, and young onset dementia. Presence of mutation of presenilin gene-1 and

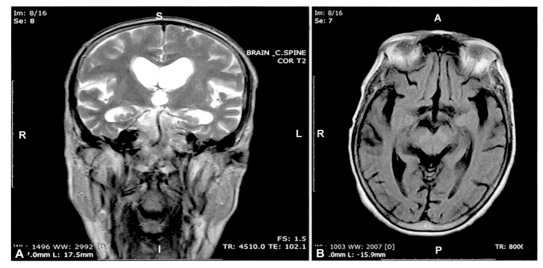

Figs 9.4A and B: Dilatation of temporal horn due to hippocampal atrophy. **(A)** Coronal view (T2 image); **(B)** Axial view (T1 image).
Courtesy: Dr MK Ghosh, Associate Professor, Department of Radiology, Burdwan Medical College, Bardhaman, West Bengal, India.

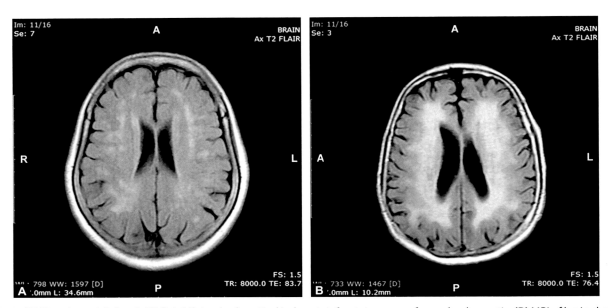

Fig. 9.5: **(A)** Showing axial view in T2 flair-bilateral subcortical ischemic infarcts in a case of vascular dementia; **(B)** MRI of brain showing axial T2 flair. Image showing multiple subcortical infarctions and periventricular ischemic demyelination in vascular dementia.
Courtesy: Dr MK Ghosh, Associate Professor, Department of Radiology, Burdwan Medical College, Bardhaman, West Bengal, India.

TABLE 9.5: Radiological features in different types of dementia

Alzheimer type disease	Global atrophy, hippocampal atrophy, and temporal lobe predominance
Frontotemporal dementia	Frontal and temporal atrophy (anterior)
Creutzfeldt–Jakob disease	Frontal dominance, abnormal intensity of basal ganglia, and thalami
Vascular or multi-infarct dementia	White and deep gray lacunae, stroke of different ages
Lewy body dementia	Brainstem, substantia nigra, cortical atrophy

presenilin-2 gene has been noticed with history of familial dementia cases that generally have early onset (below 60 years). In adult-onset sporadic dementia, Apo-E4 in homozygous state indicates high chance of developing Alzheimer dementia.

Q.5. What do you mean by clinical dementia rating (CDR) scale and how does it help?

Ans.5: The CDR scale covers six domains: memory, orientation, judgment, and problem solving, community affairs, home and hobbies, and personal care. It is a 5-point scale where CDR score of zero indicates no dementia, 0.5 indicates questionable dementia, and scored 1, 2, and 3 indicate mild, moderate, and severe dementia, respectively.[23] This scale helps to estimate the severity of cognitive dysfunction.

The Case study 2 explains that sometimes a case of dementia may present with psychiatric problems that is particularly true of behavioral variant frontotemporal dementia (FTD).

Whenever any person with intellectual or memory impairment comes to a clinician, the clinician needs to answer certain preliminary questions before further enquiry. Has the person come by himself or is being brought by someone else? In the first case, the chance of dementia is less than the second one. Next is to enquire about whether the person is suffering from some organic problem or some functional psychiatric problem? If the problem is organic, is it acute or chronic? In each case, one has to ascertain whether this is due to some diffuse lesion or some focal lesion.

Q.6. How will you approach a case of transient versus progressive memory loss?

Ans.6: This is based on history, examination, neuro-psychological assessment, biochemical investigations, and imaging findings (Boxes 9.1 and 9.2).

Q.7. What are the causes of reversible dementia?

Ans.7: Since, reversible causes are treatable, these need to be differentiated urgently. A detailed clinical history, associated neurological examination, imaging and biochemical findings help to differentiate the reversible versus irreversible dementia.

Q.8. How will you approach a case of intellectual impairment or cognitive dysfunction?

Ans.8: In a patient with cognitive impairment, a detailed history about the onset, duration, and tempo of the progression of the disease is very important. If a person has acute onset or he/she can tell the onset with certainty, then in all probability we are not dealing with a case of Alzheimer's disease. If all the manifestations are consistent with AD, but history is too short or relatively acute in onset, the trick is as follows: ask the family members about the usual work that he/she could do in the past and since when he stopped doing it (e.g., cooking, marketing, financial transactions, and rituals). Many a times, this is ignored by the family members as they take it normal at this age and complain only when things have aggravated, for instance, in the presence of fever or cataract surgery simulating an acute onset-disease. An acute-onset (minutes to hours) suggests delirium and differential diagnosis of delirium should be considered.[6,22,23] If the symptoms are progressive one should consider degenerative or progressively expanding space-occupying lesion; if they are stepwise, repeated vascular events should be considered; if they are relapsing and remitting a demyelinating or inflammatory cause should be searched for and if they are remitting, then transient vascular events or metabolic causes could be the underlying reason.[26] A different approach is required for rapidly progressive dementia which will be dealt in detail later.

The next important question faced by the clinician is whether the condition is at least partially treatable or reversible (Boxes 9.1 and 9.2).

EARLY DIAGNOSIS IN DEMENTIA

The importance of early diagnosis in dementia cannot be overemphasized (Box 9.4).

Barriers to early diagnosis of dementia are many.[27] Most of the patients with MCI and dementia have poor insight, and they present to the doctor at an average of 3.5 years after the actual initiation of cognitive impairment. Moreover, subtle cognitive changes are often missed by the physicians in their routine examination in the absence of proper infrastructural facilities such as neuropsychological assessment. Other reasons for in-adequate dementia care in India are stigma, lack of awareness, lack of funding, lack of policy initiatives, and inadequate training.[28]

Risk Factors and Medical History[29]

The medical history-taking of the patient should carefully look into the risk factors that may predispose a person to cognitive impairment (Box 9.5).

Is Memory Always Affected in Dementia or Other Cognitive Dysfunction?

Though, memory is the predominant complaint in a significant number of the cases, it may remain unaffected or subtly affected in some types of dementias, e.g., FTD. Mini-Mental Status Examination (MMSE) may not be appropriate to pick up early cases FTD where patients

> **Box 9.4: Benefits of early diagnosis of dementia**
> - It decreases hospital admissions or emergency room visits
> - Improves the quality of life of the patients as well as the caregivers
> - Disease modifying agents will be expected to be available shortly
> - Reduces the consequences due to a patient's poor judgment with finances, insurances, driving, medication-use, etc.
> - Legal and ethical issues related to property transfer can be timely and judiciously settled
> - Unnecessary consultation (e.g., the ophthalmologists in case of consulted several times for posterior cortical atrophy)

> **Box 9.5: Risk factors for dementia**
> - Diabetes, hypertension, dyslipidemia or other vascular risk factors
> - Any family history of dementia
> - Any history of head injury, epilepsy, stroke
> - Use of drugs that may affect memory functions, e.g., benzodiazepines and anticholinergic drugs
> - Use of illicit drugs and alcohol
> - Exposure to environmental toxins, e.g., fuels or solvents
> - Any associated comorbidity like cardiovascular disease, infection, pulmonary, hepatic, or renal insufficiency
> - Any accelerated weight loss, late life depression, gait disturbance, or physical frailty

usually present with personality and behavior changes. Similarly in cases with mild cognitive impairment, there is a nonamnestic type where memory is not affected.

There are some types of dementia where the initial brain damage in more focal, later progressing to being more and more diffused, as in the case of semantic dementia.

Besides memory, other cognitive functions (language, apraxia, agnosia, and executive functions) are also important components of a comprehensive dementia assessment.[30]

Language abnormality is manifested by word finding problem, naming problem, incoherence (jargon aphasia), paraphasic errors, or reading problems, when the patient takes more time to read, cannot read fluently, and may have to read letter by letter. In writing, one shows spelling mistakes and paragraphic errors. Loss of prosody is a common feature of right hemisphere dysfunction.

Apraxia is manifested by problems in using day-to-day objects, e.g., tooth brush, comb, spoon, etc., in the absence of any motor, sensory, or coordination difficulties. There may also be difficulties in dressing, buttoning, opening locks with keys, etc.

Agnosia is sometimes confused with naming problem or semantic loss. In visual agnosia, one cannot name an object presented visually but if placed in a different modality (e.g., on the hand), the patient can recognize the object through touch and pressure sensation.

Executive dysfunction is presented through myriad of ways. Executive functions are defined as "the higher level cognitive functions, believed to be mediated through the left prefrontal cortex (LPFC), that are involved in the control and direction (planning, organizing, monitoring, sequencing, switching, inhibition) of lower automatic functions".[31] The patients cannot manage their day-to-day activities, keeping things haphazardly, taking extra time to do some work (e.g., cooking), unable to continue conversations efficiently, unable to give their opinion in family matters, unable to manage the household efficiently, eating without maintaining the normal sequence (e.g., mixing everything), etc.

Ultimately, all of the above will lead to impairments of ADL which may be basic or instrumental, as well as social interaction. However, MCI, there is generally no impairment in ADLs and social interaction, an important difference between dementia and MCI.[7]

Neurological examination is imperative in every patient and some important clinical pointers to diagnosis are presented in Box 9.6.

> **Box 9.6: Clinical pointers to dementia**
>
> - Alzeimer's disease does not have motor abnormality until late
> - Hemiparesis or focal neurological deficit indicates vascular dementia, or space-occupying lesion, or subdural hematoma
> - Frontotemporal dementia, supranuclear gaze palsy, Parkinsonian features, or features of amyotrophic lateral sclerosis
> - Diffuse Lewy body disease—initial parkinsonism features
> - CBGD (cortico basal ganglia degeneration)—asymmetric Parkinsonian features, dystonia, myoclonus, apraxia, alien hand syndrome
> - Normal pressure hydrocephalus—gait problem, urinary incontinence
> - Progressive supranuclear palsy—unexpected falls, axial rigidity, vertical gaze palsy, and dysphagia
> - Creutzfeldt–Jakob disease—diffused rigidity, akinetic state and myoclonus
> - Dementia with myelopathy or neuropathy—alcohol or other vitamin deficiency or heavy metal intoxication

Cortical versus Subcortical Dementia

A traditional way of differentiating dementia is cortical from subcortical dementia, though there may be an admixture of symptoms. In cortical dementia, cortical symptoms like amnesia, aphasia, agnosia, and apraxia predominate, whereas in subcortical dementia, cognitive slowness, retrieval deficits, mood symptoms and movement disorders take the precedence. In subcortical dementia, the frontal subcortical circuit is implicated. All of them start from the prefrontal cortex and then goes to different parts of striatum, then to thalamus and coming back to the prefrontal cortex in a closed loop [the cortico-striato-thalamo circuit (CSTC)]. There are three important CSTCs, the DLPFC, the orbitofrontal cortex (OFC), and the anterior cingulate cortex (ACC). Dorsolateral prefrontal cortex damage with executive dysfunction, OFC damage is associated with disinhibitory behavior and emotional disturbance, and ACC damage is associated with apathy.[32] The prototype of cortical dementia is AD, and the prototypes of subcortical dementia are Huntington's disease, Parkinsonism plus syndrome, CJD, and AIDS dementia complex. Subcortical dementia is characterized by the presence of slowness along with frontal executive dysfunction and depression; however, pure cortical symptoms like memory may also be present and which is explained by the circuit theory rather than isolated module involvement.

Differences between Dementia and MCI

Mild cognitive impairment is differentiated from dementia by preserved ADL and intact social interaction. Cognitive dysfunction in MCI is disproportionate to the patient's age and education. Each year about 10–20% of patients with MCI progresses to dementia. However, it is also possible that many cases with MCI may revert to normal.

Approach to Early Onset Dementia

It is very difficult to differentiate between MCI and early-onset dementia. If the symptoms are progressive and associated with impairment of performance of daily activities and social functioning, dementia is considered. The CDR score, sometimes, might be helpful. This stage of dementia is very important as intervention is often considered to prevent progression of dementia.

Approach to Rapidly Progressive Dementia

One should consider rapidly progressive dementia (RPD) if any one of the following is there: rapid onset, presence of myoclonus, and associated systemic symptoms. Under this category, Creutzfeldt–Jakob disease should primarily be considered. This condition is characterized by rapid onset dementia and myoclonus. The survival after diagnosis is <1 year. Other conditions associated with similar rapid-onset dementia and myoclonus are Hashimoto encephalopathy, lithium intoxication, Whipple's disease, intravascular lymphoma, and carcinomatous meningitis.[6,22] In young age, sometimes SSPE and lipidosis can also present with a similar picture.

Differentiation between Different Degenerative Dementias

It is sometimes difficult to differentiate AD from FTD. In FTD, there is an early loss of social and interpersonal behavior and loss of insight.[20] Another way to differentiate is to find out the ratio of the score of verbal fluency plus language to orientation plus memory (VL/OM). VL/OM ratios of <2.2 differentiate FTD from non-FTD and VL/OM ratios >3.2 differentiate AD from non-AD.[33]

Environmental dependency behavior which includes imitation behavior and utilization behavior if present also helps to distinguish FTD from AD.[34] In Diffuse Lewy body disease, apart from an early appearance of Parkinsonian features, fluctuating cognition, formed visual hallucinations, and visuospatial impairment also predominate.[21] The presentation of vascular dementia depends on the area of vascular involvement and may be primarily cortical, primarily subcortical, or a combination of the two.[35] There are consensus guidelines for diagnosis of different types of dementias, e.g., NINCDS-ADRDA,[16] NINDS-AIREN,[18,19] DSM-IV-TR,[36] and Neary consensus criteria[13] (Table 9.4). Recently, there have been efforts to incorporate biomarkers in the diagnosis of AD and MCI but at the research level criteria.[14,17]

Aphasia and Dementia

It is difficult to assess a patient with aphasia presenting with dementia features. This is particularly important in poststroke patients. Most of the studies exclude aphasia patients when studying cognitive dysfunction for difficulties in assessment of mental status with language dysfunction. If possible, nonverbal memory may be tested, further one has to use clinical judgment, e.g., whether the ADLs are proportionately impaired or not. If the impairment of ADLs cannot be explained by the language dysfunction, one can have a strong intuition that the person may be suffering from some underlying dementia.

Thus, the discussion on these two patients will give a glimpse of the approach to a patient who presents with intellectual deterioration to a neurologist or a psychiatrist.

REFERENCES

1. Strub RL, Black FW. The mental status examination in neurology, 4th edition. New Delhi: Jaypee Brothers Medical publishers (P) Ltd; 2003.
2. Schacter DL. Implicit memory: history and current status. J Exp Psychol Learn Mem Cogn. 1987;13:501-18.
3. Medina JJ. The biology of recognition memory. Psychiat Times. 2008.
4. Tulving E, Schater D. Priming and human memory systems. Science. 1990;247:301-6.
5. Williams HL, Conway MA, Cohen G. Autobiographical memory. In: Cohen G, Conway MA (Eds). Memory in the Real World, 3rd edition. Hove: Psychology Press; 2008. pp. 21-90.
6. Longo DI, Fauci AS, Kasper DL, et al. New York: Harrison's Principles of medicine (Vol. 2); 18th edition. McGraw Medical; 2012.
7. Petersen RC, Doody R, Kurz A, et al. Current concepts in mild cognitive impairment. Arch Neurol. 2001;58:1985-92.
8. Mukundan CR, Murthy MN. lateraling and localizing cerebral lesions by a battery of neuropsychological tests. Paper presented at the joint conference of Neurology, Psychiatry. Clinical psychology and psychiatric social work societies of India, NIMHANS, Bangalore, India, 1979.
9. Rao SL, Subbakrishna DK, Gopukumar K. NIMHANS Neuropsychological Battery Manual. Bangalore, India, 2004.
10. Kar BR, Rao SL, Chndramouli BA, et al. NIMHANS Neuropsychological Battery from Children Manual. Bangalore, India: NIMHANS Publication; 2004.
11. Gupta S, Khadelwal S, Tandon P. AIIMS Comprehensive Neuropsychological Battery in Hindi (adult form). J Pers Clin Stud. 2000;16:75-102.

12. Pershad D, Verma SK. Handbook of PGI Battery of Brains Dysfunction (PGI-BDD). Agra, India: National Neuropsychological Corporation; 1990.

13. Ganguli M, Ratcliff G, Chandra V, et al. A Hindi Version of MMSE: the development of a cognitive screening instrument for a largely illiterate rural elderly population in India. Int J Geriatr Psychiatry. 1995;10:367-77.

14. Das SK, Banerjee TK, Bose P, et al. An urban community based study study of cognitive function among non-demented population in India. Neurology Asia. 2006;11:37-48.

15. Jack CR (Jr), Albert MS, Knopman DS, et al. Introduction to the recommendations from the National Institute on Aging and the Alzheimer's Association Workgroup on Diagnostic Guidelines for Alzheimer's Disease. Alzheimers Dement. 2011;7(3):257-62.doi:10.1016/j.jalz.2011.03.004.

16. McKhann G, Drachman D, Folstein M, et al. Clinical diagnosis of Alzheimer's disease: report of the NINCDS-ADRDA Work Group under the auspices of Department of Health and Human Services Task Force on Alzheimer's disease. Neurology. 1984;34:939-44.

17. Albert MS, DeKosky ST, Dickson D, et al. The diagnosis of mild cognitive impairment due to Alzheimer's disease: recommendations from the National Institute on Aging and Alzheimer's Association workgroup. Alzheimers Dement. 2011;7(3):270-79. doi:10.1016/j.jalz.2011.03.008.

18. Roman GC, Tatemichi TK, Erkinjuntti T, et al. Vascular dementia: diagnostic criteria for research studies: report of the NINDS-AIREN international workshop. Neurology. 1993;43:250-60.

19. Drachman D, Folstein M, Katzman R, et al. Clinical diagnosis of Alzheimer's disease: report of the NINCDS-ADRDA Work Group under the Auspices of Department of Health and Human Services Task Force on Alzheimer's Disease. Neurology. 1984;34:939-44.

20. Neary D, Snowden JS, Gustafon L, et al. Frontotemporal lobar degeneration: a consensus on clinical diagnostic criteria. Neurology. 1998;51;1546-54.

21. McKeith IG, Dickson DW, Lowe J, et al. Diagnosis and management of dementia with Lewy bodies. Neurology. 2005;65:1863-72.

22. Ropper AH, Samuels MA, Adams V. Principles of Neurology, 9th edition. New York: McGraw-Hill Medical; 2009.

23. Das SK (Ed.). Understanding Dementia: Disease, Treatment and Care. Connectiva, Kolkata, ARDSI, 2009.

24. Yousem DM, Grossman RI. Neurodegenerative Disorders and Hydrocephalus from Neuroradiology—the Requisites, 3rd edition. Philadelphia: Mosby Elsevier; 2010. pp. 249-78.

25. Morris JC. The clinical dementia rating (CDR): current version and scoring rules. Neurology. 1993;43:2412-14.

26. David A. Basic concepts in neuropsychiatry in Lishman's organic psychiatry A textbook of neuropsychiatry. In: David A, Fleminger S, Kopelman MD, Lovestone S, Mellers JDC (Eds), 4th edition. Wiley-Blackwell; 2009.

27. Barker WW, Luis C, Harwood D, et al. The effect of a memory screening program on the early diagnosis of Alzheimer disease. Alzheimer Dis Assoc Disord. 2005;19:1-7.

28. Dementia India Report 2010 prevalence, impact, cost and service for dementia. Alzheimer's and related disorder society of India; 2010.

29. Lipton AM, Rubin CD. Medical evaluation and diagnosis in Alzheimer disease and other dementia. In: Weiner MF, Lipton AM (Eds). American Psychiatric Press; 2009.

30. Galvin JE, Sadowsky CH. Practical guidelines for the recognition and diagnosis of dementia. J Am Board Fam Med. 2012;25:367-82.

31. Stuss DT. New approaches to prefrontal lobe testing. In: Miller BL, Cummings JL (Eds). The Human Frontal Lobes Functions and Disorders, 2nd edition. New York: The Guilford Press; 2007.

32. Cummings JL. Frontal subcortical circuit and human behaviour. Arch Neurol. 1993;50:873-80.

33. Mioshi E, Dawson K, Mitchell J, et al. The Addenbrooke's Cognitive Examination Revised (ACE-R): a brief cognitive test battery for dementia screening. Int J Geriatr Psychiatry. 2006;21:1078-85.

34. Ghosh A, Dutt A, Bhargava P, et al. Environmental dependency behaviour in frontotemporal dementia: have we been underrating them. J Neurol. 2013;260:861-8.

35. Braaten AJ, Parsons TD, McCue R, et al. Neurocognitive differential diagnosis of dementing diseases: Alzheimer's dementia, vascular dementia, frontotemporal dementia and major depressive disorder. Int J Neurosci. 2006;116:1271-93.

36. Diagnostic and Statistical Manual of Mental Disorders, 4th Edition. Text Revision; American Psychiatric Association, 2000.

Chapter 10

Approach to Global Development Delay and Developmental Regression

Pratibha Singhi, Naveen Sankhyan

INTRODUCTION

Global developmental delay (GDD) is an umbrella term widely used by clinicians while imparting clinical care to a young child with developmental delay. GDD is not a diagnosis by itself and so it should be used only as a basis for reaching a diagnosis. It is widely accepted that this term implies significant delay in two or more areas of developmental performance: defined as gross/fine motor, speech/language, cognition, social/personal, and activities of daily living. Significant delay is defined as developmental level two standard deviations or more below the mean on age-appropriate, standardized norm-referenced tests.[1] Conventionally, the term developmental delay is reserved for children below 5 years of age. The term mental retardation (MR) or more appropriately "intellectual disability" is usually applied to older children (>5 years) when IQ testing is valid and reliable.[2] The prevalence of intellectual disability is estimated to be around 1–3% of the population.[3]

DIAGNOSTIC APPROACH

The essential components of the diagnostic evaluation of a child with GDD or intellectual disability include the following:

- Clinical history (including prenatal and birth history), family history and construction of a pedigree of three generations
- Physical and neurologic examination
- Psychological evaluation
- Laboratory tests, including metabolic, genetic testing, and imaging.

CLINICAL ASSESSMENT

A thorough history is essential to elicit antenatal and perinatal risk factors for GDD/ID. Particular emphasis on maternal health during the first trimester of pregnancy including fever, drug intake, etc., is important. Evidence for adverse events or toxin exposures and clues to intrauterine difficulties (oligohydramnios, preeclamptic toxemia, poor growth, antenatal bleeding, reduced fetal movements, etc.) should be enquired for. Timing and mode of delivery, birth weight, Apgar scores, head circumference at birth, time to independent feeding, and duration of postnatal hospital stay are important objective markers of newborn health status. One needs to remember that a mere history of delayed cry, although an important clue, is insufficient to conclude perinatal insult, unless there is definite suggestion of neonatal encephalopathy (e.g., excessive lethargy, seizures, feeding difficulties requiring oro/nasogastric feeding). Postnatal insults such as neuro-infections are common in resource-poor countries and account for a large number of children with GDD/ID. A detailed developmental history and past history should be elicited for presence of seizures, hospitalizations, and other acute or chronic conditions. A family history of ID can point toward a genetic cause of GDD/ID, e.g., fragile-X syndrome or other X-linked mental retardation syndromes. Family history may also point toward an unrecognized metabolic

After the history, the clinician should have clear idea of the following:[4]

- Whether it is a static or progressive disorder
- The developmental and functional level of the child
- Timing of the possible underlying cause
- An obvious etiologic cause
- The associated comorbid medical or behavioral conditions (e.g., epilepsy and attention-deficit hyperactivity disorder)
- The socioeconomic and sociocultural milieu of the child

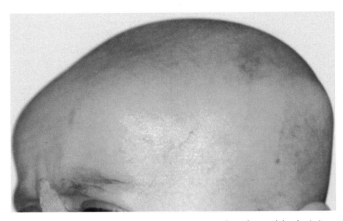

Fig. 10.1: Note the sparse, hypopigmented curly, stubby hair in a child with *Menkes' disease.*

disorder such as phenylketonuria. To recognize patterns of inheritance, it is essential that a carefully elicited history is used to construct a three-generation pedigree and identify consanguinity. In relevant cases, a history of toxin exposure should also be elicited, e.g., lead intoxication (Box 10.1).

The examination of child with GDD/ID is primarily aimed at the evaluation for dysmorphic features. Special attention is to be paid to the size and shape of head, faces, eyes, hearing, hair (Fig. 10.1), stature, skin (Figs 10.2 and 10.3), and presence of organomegaly. The head circumference growth should be assessed over time to understand the trajectory of head growth. In cases of abnormal head size, parental head circumferences should be obtained and plotted. The head shape, sutures, and fontanelles should be noted in an infant.

In cases where an obvious cause is eluding, a dysmorphologic examination and syndrome recognition by an experienced clinical geneticist is helpful. A diagnosis is significantly more likely when a child is noted to have an unusual appearance with the presence of specific features suggestive of a diagnosis (Fig. 10.4).

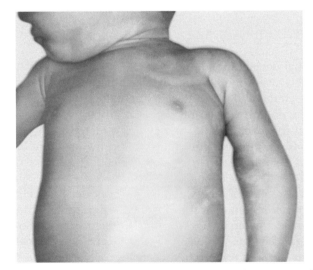

Fig. 10.2: Multiple streaky hypopigmented skin lesions over the back of the child with hypomelanosis of Ito.

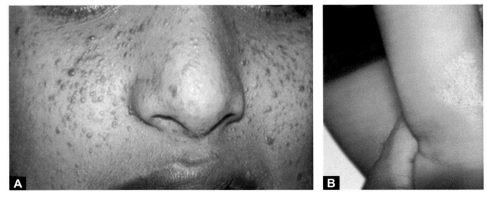

Figs 10.3A and B: Skin findings in tuberous sclerosis. **(A)** Adenoma sebaceum; **(B)** Ash leaf spots.

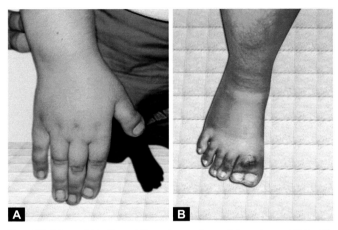

Figs 10.4A and B: Broad thumbs and great toes in a child with Rubinstein–Taybi syndrome.

TABLE 10.1: Selected red flags for development in childhood

Age at which assessed	Observation
Any age	• Failure to gain/loss of previously acquired milestones • Persistent squint • Lack or loss of response to noises • Strong parental concerns • Poor interaction with adults or children • Markedly stiff or loose limbs
0–3 months	• Persistent fisting • No visual fixation • Fails to alert to stimuli
4–6 months	• Floppy head or lack of head control • Absence of social smile
6–12 months	• Unable to reach for toys • Unable to localize sounds • No babbling • No mouthing of objects
12–24 months	• Hand dominance • Lack of interest or interaction with others • Lack of imitation (after 18 months) • Does not respond to name • Does not walk alone (after 18 months)

The history and examination provide essential clues to the diagnosis, which can be later confirmed by additional studies, e.g., in patients with fragile-X syndrome, the history and examination may be contributory to the diagnosis and the molecular genetic analysis confirms it. A detailed neurological evaluation is of importance to identify children with cerebral palsy, muscle weakness, spasticity, paresis, epilepsy, and microcephaly. Such abnormalities on neurologic examination assist in determining the need for additional investigations such as electroencephalography, neuroimaging or molecular genetic testing, or referral to other specialists, such as psychologists and geneticists for further assessment.

DEVELOPMENTAL ASSESSMENT

The clinical history can be supplemented with standardized testing by a developmental or a clinical psychologist; this psychological evaluation will provide a much better assessment of the child's developmental abilities. Standardized tools would include screening tests such as the Denver's Developmental Screening Test, the Ages and Stages Questionnaire, and the more detailed tests such as the Developmental Assessment Scale for Indian Infants, Developmental profile-3, and the Bailey's Developmental Scales.

When there is concern about developmental delay in a child, a developmental quotient should be calculated for each developmental stream. It is a means to simply express a developmental delay in quantifiable terms. The developmental quotient is the ratio of the child's developmental age over the chronological age

(Table 10.1). Typical development is a developmental quotient >70%, and atypical development is a developmental quotient <70%.

INVESTIGATIONS

The choice and the sequence of investigations should be guided by the clinical evaluation (Fig. 10.5).[3] Some investigations form a part of holistic evaluation (vision, hearing testing, ultrasound, skeletal X-rays), while others offer means to establish a diagnosis (genetic, metabolic testing). In the absence of a universal thyroid screening, thyroid function tests must be done in all children with GDD/ID. Keeping in mind that large numbers of children in resource-poor countries have acquired causes for GDD/ID, it is prudent to opt for imaging studies as the initial diagnostic testing. Magnetic resonance imaging (MRI) is clearly the imaging modality of choice, given the higher resolution and better pickup of dysgenesis and white matter abnormalities.

Genetic Testing

It is preferable to involve experts in clinical genetics whenever possible for the genetic evaluation of GDD/ID.

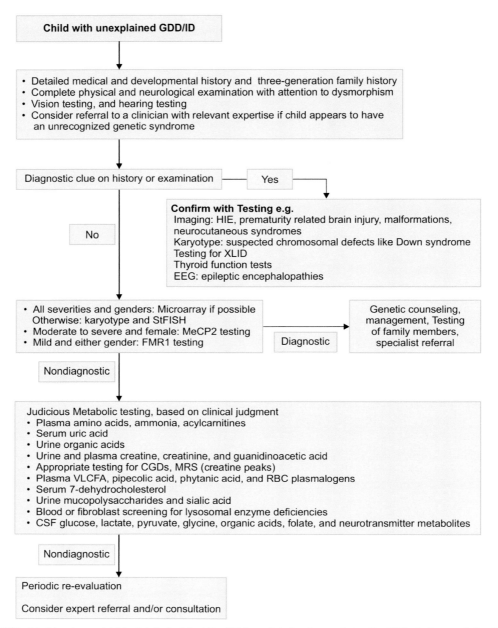

Fig. 10.5: Diagnostic approach to a child with global developmental delay/intellectual disability.[4]

Cytogenetic Studies

The reported frequency of chromosomal anomalies detected by high-resolution karyotyping (i.e., 550 bands) in patients evaluated for intellectual disability or developmental delays is around 10%.[5] This test is reported to be a valuable initial test for evaluation of GDD. Chromosome abnormalities are found in all categories of intellectual disability, mild to profound, and in both sexes.[5]

Fluorescent in situ Hybridization (FISH) Testing

About half of all structural chromosome abnormalities include the telomere of the chromosome. Many of these abnormalities may be missed by the standard karyotype. Fluorescent in situ hybridization techniques have been applied to examine the subtelomeric regions of each chromosome for abnormalities that are known to cause intellectual disability.[6] The yield for subtelomeric abnormalities in GDD/ID detected by FISH is about 6%.[6] The presence of major and minor physical anomalies does not affect the yield; however, the yield is higher among familial cases as compared with sporadic cases.

Comparative Genomic Hybridization Techniques (aCGH)

It is a better technique to evaluate chromosomal abnormalities. It identifies deletions and/or duplications of chromosome material with a high degree of sensitivity in a more efficient manner than FISH techniques.[6] Furthermore, the FISH test is predominantly used to confirm a clinical diagnosis, whereas the aCGH does not require an expert clinician to suspect a specific diagnosis. However, it is expensive and currently not available at most centers.

Metabolic Testing (Box 10.2)

Metabolic testing is expensive and exhaustive; hence, its judicious use is warranted. In such situations, it would be wise to obtain an expert consultation before proceeding with these tests.

> **Box 10.2: Indications for screening for inborn errors of metabolism in children with GDD/ID**
>
> Clinical situations that suggest a possible inborn error of metabolism and should prompt careful and detailed metabolic testing include the following:[7]
> - *Pregnancy*: A history of maternal acute fatty liver of pregnancy or hemolysis, elevated liver enzymes, and low platelets are associated with several fatty acid oxidation disorders
> - *Family history*: Parental consanguinity, unexplained neonatal, or infant deaths
> - *Others*: Unexplained hypoglycemia, recurrent encephalopathy, protein aversion, multisystem involvement, possible white matter involvement[4]

DEVELOPMENTAL REGRESSION

Developmental regression in children usually implies loss of previously acquired developmental milestones. It may be associated with loss of memory, ability to think, understand and recognize along with personality changes or distressing behavior. Loss of vision, deafness, abnormalities in tone, loss of motor abilities, and seizures are commonly associated. This neurological deterioration should not be secondary to any other concurrent systemic illness (Box 10.3).

An accurate diagnosis is crucial for genetic counseling, prognostication, initiating prevention strategies, prenatal diagnosis and may rarely lead to specific therapeutic interventions. A structured and systematic clinical approach to a child with neuroregression allows more selective diagnostic testing.

EPIDEMIOLOGY

The true incidence of childhood regression in India remains unknown. Most of the common neurodegenerative diseases have been reported from India in various published case reports or series.[8-12] Certain types of white matter degenerations like, "megalencephalic leukodystrophy with subcortical cysts," are common in India.[13]

APPROACH TO DIAGNOSIS

The first step in the evaluation of a child with neuroregression is to be sure that there is true developmental regression. For this, causes of pseudoregression should be excluded in all children with regression of milestones (Box 10.4).

Apart from the above causes of pseudoregression, a few other causes need to be kept in mind. These include hypothyroidism, chronic infections (HIV, SSPE), toxin exposure (lead), nutritional deficiency states (infantile tremor syndrome), and structural causes (progressive hydrocephalus, or vertebral anomalies and spinal compression).

> **Box 10.3: Key point**
>
> Occasionally, the degenerative process may be slower than the developmental progression of the child. In such cases, there may not be any apparent loss of developmental milestones and the child may present with slow acquisition of milestones or with no gain in development over a period of time

TABLE 10.2: **Clinical features of gray and white matter diseases[19]**

Feature	Gray matter	White matter
Dementia	Early	Late
Seizures	Early and prominent	Late
Psychological symptoms	May be present	Uncommon
Basal ganglia signs and symptoms	Often present	Absent
Retinitis pigmentosa	May be present	Absent
Primary optic atrophy	Rare	May be seen
Primary neuropathy	Rare	May be seen
Imaging (MRI)	Cortical atrophy, abnormalities in basal ganglia, cerebellum	Clearly identifies abnormalities in white matter
Electroretinogram (ERG)	May be abnormal	Normal
Visual-evoked response (VER)	May be abnormal	Normal
Brainstem auditory-evoked responses (BAER)	Usually normal	Abnormal

Box 10.4: Conditions associated with pseudoregression

The common causes of pseudoregression in children include the following:[14]
- Uncontrolled seizures
- Overmedication with anticonvulsants
- Intercurrent systemic illness
- Secondary complications like joint contractures, movement disorders, etc.
- Depression or other emotional problems especially in older children
- Secondary complications of comorbidities like nutritional deficiencies

The second step in the evaluation is to complete a thorough history and examination to ascertain the age of onset, extent, and evolution of the disease (white matter, gray matter, cerebellum, etc.) (Table 10.2).

HISTORY AND EXAMINATION

A detailed history is crucial to ascertain the age of onset, and the spheres of development affected—motor, cognitive, language, vision, and hearing. A family history of three generations is important to identify the possible modes of transmission and also helps to identify individuals at risk of disease. Sometimes specific clues during the general physical and systemic examination can be obtained that can help to identify the nature of the disorder (Table 10.3). After a careful history and examination if one is able to assign the patient into one of the following groups, then further evaluation becomes easier:
1. Gray matter degenerations—Poliodystrophies
2. White matter degenerations—Leukodystrophies
3. System disorders:
   a. Progressive ataxias
   b. Basal ganglia disorders
4. Multisystem disorders with neuroregression.

REGRESSION IN A CHILD BELOW 2 YEARS[15] (FIGS 10.6 AND 10.7)

A neuroregressive disorder in infancy might manifest as delayed milestones or as nonattainment of milestones. Because the baby has just begun to attain milestones, it is often difficult to ascertain true regression. Infants affected by regression generally lack early developmental milestones such as, poor head control, lack of socialization, lack visual or auditory attention, inability to use hands, etc. Other common features include hypotonia, feeding problems, recurrent vomiting, and/or failure to thrive. "Rett's syndrome" is a distinct neurodegenerative disorder in girls that presents with microcephaly, progressive decline in cognitive abilities starting in infancy, and is associated with loss of purposeful hand movements.[16]

Once a child has attained some recognizable milestones of development, it is easier to ascertain the loss of motor milestones that have been attained. The loss of motor abilities may result either from central causes

TABLE 10.3: Some clinical pointers in hereditary neurodegenerative disorders[19]

Organ/feature	Abnormality	Disorders
Head	Microcephaly	NCL, Krabbe's disease, Rett's syndrome
	Macrocephaly	MPS, Alexander's disease, Canavan's disease, GM1 gangliosidosis, Tay–Sachs disease, MLSC
Hair	Alopecia	Biotinidase deficiency
	Pigmentary changes	PKU, Menkes' syndrome
	Wooly, kinky hair	Menkes' syndrome
Skin	Rash	Biotinidase, holocarboxylase deficiency
	Subcutaneous nodules	Farber's disease
	Angiokeratomas	Fabry's disease
	Fat pads, focal atrophy	Congenital disorders of glycosylation
	Hyperpigmentation	Adrenoleukodystrophy
Eyes	Cataract	Galactosemia, Zellweger's syndrome, Wilson's disease
	Retinitis pigmentosa	Peroxisomal disorders, NCL, mitochondrial encephalomyopathies, MPS, PKAN, ABLP
	Cherry red spot	Tay–Sachs disease, Niemann–Pick disease, GM1 gangliosidosis
	Optic atrophy	NCL, MLD, Krabbe's disease, Canavan's disease, GM2 gangliosidosis
Ears	Deafness	MPS, ALD, mitochondrial disorders
	Hyperacusis	Krabbe's disease, Tay–Sachs disease
Abdomen	Hepatosplenomegaly	MPS, GM1 gangliosidosis, Gaucher's disease, Niemann–Pick disease
	Hernia	GM1 gangliosidosis, MPS
Nervous system	Peripheral neuropathy	MLD, Krabbe's disease, mitochondrial disorders
	Hydrocephalous/raised Intra-cranial pressure	MPS, infantile Alexander's disease
Cardiac	Cardiomyopathy	FAOD, mitochondrial disorders, Friedreich ataxia, AVED, Pompe's disease
	Valvular defects	MPS, Zellweger's syndrome, Fabry's disease

NCL, neuronal ceroid lipofuscinosis; MPS, mucopolysaccharidosis; PKU, phenylketonuria; PKAN, pantothinate kinase associated neurodegeneration; ABLP, abetalipoproteinemia; MLD, metachromatic leukodystrophy; ALD, adrenoleukodystrophy; FAOD, fatty acid oxidation disorder; AVED, ataxia with vitamin E deficiency; MLSC, megalencephalic leukoencephalopathy with subcortical cysts.

like pyramidal, cerebellar, extrapyramidal involvement, or from peripheral nerve involvement. During the second year of life, disorders with gradually increasing dysmorphism, skeletal abnormalities and cognitive decline (mucopolysaccharidosis and mucolipidosis) also become manifest. Apart from this, there is a distinct group of disorders [neuronal ceroid lipofuscinosis (NCL)] that presents with frequent seizures, associated cognitive impairment, and visual loss. Certain neurometabolic disorders present in children with recurrent neurological deterioration interspersed with apparent recovery (organic aciduria, mitochondrial disorders, urea cycle disorders, etc.).

NEUROREGRESSION IN LATER CHILDHOOD AND ADOLESCENCE[15] (FIGS 10.8 AND 10.9)

As the child grows older, it becomes easier to recognize loss of abilities which had already been attained. However in children with slow insidious onset of problems, the recognition of an underlying neurodegenerative process may be delayed. The initial presentation may include only behavioral changes, that may not be recognized as reflective of a degenerative process. Because of the relatively mature nervous system in the older child it is possible to group many of the neuroregressions into categories such as

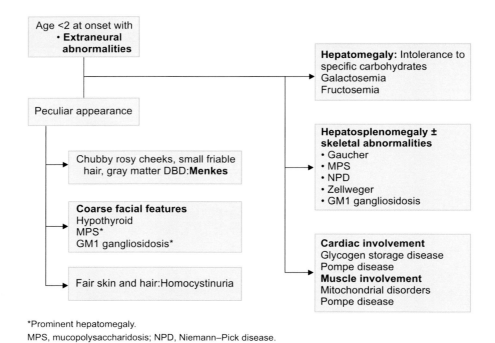

*Prominent hepatomegaly.
MPS, mucopolysaccharidosis; NPD, Niemann–Pick disease.

Fig. 10.6: A simplified approach to a child <2 years with suspected degenerative brain disorder with extraneural abnormalities.[19]

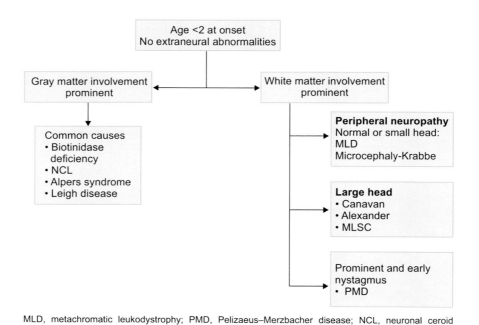

MLD, metachromatic leukodystrophy; PMD, Pelizaeus–Merzbacher disease; NCL, neuronal ceroid lipofuscinosis; MLSC, megalencephalic leukoencephalopathy with subcortical cysts.

Fig. 10.7: A simplified approach to a child <2 years with suspected degenerative brain disorder with no extraneural abnormalities.[19]

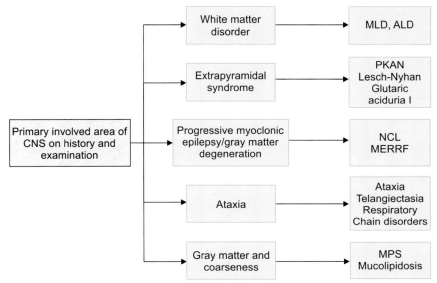

MLD, metachromatic leukodystrophy; ALD, adrenoleukodystrophy; MERRF, myoclonic epilepsy with ragged red-fibers; PKAN, pantothenate kinase-associated neurodegeneration; NCL, neuronal ceroid lipofuscinosis.

Fig. 10.8: Approach to progressive neurological deterioration in 2–5 years of age group.[19]

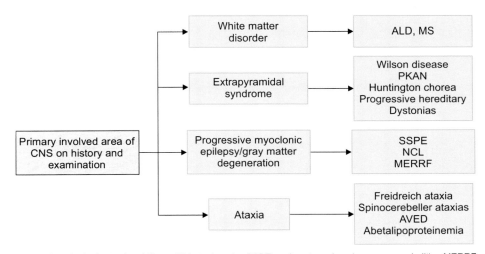

ALD, adrenoleukodystrophy; MS, multiple sclerosis; SSPE, subacute sclerosing panencephalitis; MERRF, myoclonic epilepsy with ragged-red fibers; PKAN, pantothenate kinase-associated neurodegeneration; NCL, neuronal ceroid lipofuscinosis; AVED, ataxia with vitamin E deficiency.

Fig. 10.9: Approach to progressive neurological deterioration in 5–15 year age group.[19]

cerebellar and extrapyramidal syndromes, etc. This allows for easier recognition of the underlying disorder. However, the disorders presenting later in childhood are also characterized by variability in presentation. Apart from hereditary disorders, subacute sclerosing pan-encephalitis (SSPE) is a common cause of neuroregression in resource-poor countries.[17] The diagnosis should be considered in all children with behavioral changes and cognitive deterioration with or without myoclonic jerks.

INVESTIGATIONS[14,15]

A thorough history and examination helps to formulate differential diagnosis and guides the choice of investigations. In resource limited settings, it is prudent to use the investigations judiciously and plan investigations based on results of prior investigations. The initial investigations should be aimed at ruling out any treatable disorders, however, unlikely that may seem. These may include hypothyroidism, tumors or other surgically amenable conditions, infections such as HIV infection or vitamin responsive states such as E, B-12 deficiency.

Imaging

A high-resolution magnetic resonance imaging (MRI) with spectroscopy (MRS) would be the initial investigation in most children. MRI might provide a diagnostic clue, e.g., pantothenate kinase-associated neuro-degeneration with "eye of tiger" sign in globus pallidi (Fig. 10.10), or the typical posterior dominant changes in adrenoleukodystrophy with peripheral contrast enhancement (Fig. 10.11). Spectroscopy helps in the diagnosis of certain disorders such as Canavan's disease, mitochondrial encephalopathies, and creatine-deficiency disorders. If not providing a specific diagnosis, imaging helps to determine the primary area of involvement (e.g., leukoencephalopathy, basal ganglia disease, cerebellar degeneration, gray matter disease,

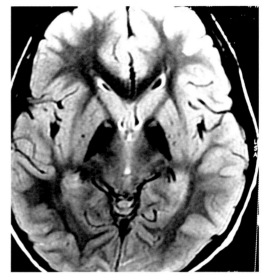

Fig. 10.10: Axial T2W MRI in a child with "pantothenate kinase associated neurodegeneration" showing the bilaterally hypo-intense globus pallidi with an area of central hyperintensity.

etc.). This initial narrowing of possibilities helps to decide the further investigative approach.

Radiographs

Multisystem disorders with neurovisceral storage may be suspected and skeletal survey is important to look for abnormalities thereof. The disorders in which radiographic

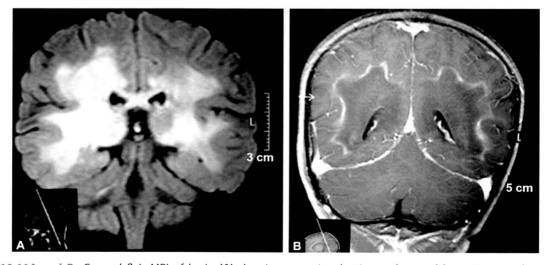

FigS 10.11A and B: Coronal flair MRI of brain **(A)** showing posterior dominant abnormal hyperintense white matter in a child with *adrenoleukodystrophy*. The corpus callosum is also prominently involved. Note the classical peripheral postcontrast enhancement in the areas of active demyelination in the Post-Gad coronal MRI brain **(B)**.

abnormalities may be seen in mucopolysaccharidosis, gangliosidosis, or peroxisomal disorders.

Electrophysiological Tests

These include visual-evoked potentials, auditory-evoked potentials, nerve conduction studies, electromyography, electroencephalography, and somatosensory-evoked potentials. These tests help delineate the extent of central and peripheral nervous system involvement in the patient. This information further helps in narrowing the differential diagnosis. For example, the presence of neuropathy in the setting of white matter neurodegeneration in a 2-year-old would suggest a diagnosis of metachromatic leukodystrophy (Fig. 10.8).

Metabolic Tests

Investigation of a suspected neurometabolic disorder would include an initial assessment of arterial blood gases and acid base status, lactate, pyruvate, ammonia, and urine ketones. This is followed by a urine and blood assay for plasma amino acids, urine organic acids, and blood acylcarnitine levels. The further choice of investigations is guided by the results of these tests.

Histopathological and Ultrastructural Information from Tissue Biopsies

- Bone marrow: This can be useful in demonstrating storage cells that can be seen in Niemann–Pick disease, or Gaucher's disease.
- Conjunctival, skin, or rectal biopsy can help in demonstrating abnormal depositions in NCL
- Hair microscopy: This simple investigation can help in the diagnosis of Menkes' disease (Fig. 10.12)

Other specific investigations may be done based on clues from preceding investigations (Box 10.5).

Box 10.5: Miscellaneous specific investigations in a disorder with neurological regression

- Serology: HIV, SSPE
- Enzyme analysis: Lysosomal storage disorders, biotinidase deficiency
- Plasma very long chain fatty acids, and plasmalogen levels: Peroxisomal disorders
- Urine copper, serum ceruloplasmin: Wilson's disease (Fig. 10.12)
- Urine mucopolysaccharide quantification: Mucopolysaccharidosis
- Urine organic acids: Organic acidemias

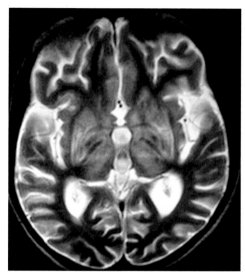

Fig. 10.12: T2W axial MRI in a child with *Wilson's disease* showing the involvement of bilateral basal ganglia.

Mutation Testing

This is generally undertaken when the diagnosis is quite clear. In certain situations it may be an affordable option (e.g., Duchenne muscular dystrophy (DMD) and spinal muscular atrophy). Knowledge about the disease-causing mutations helps in genetic confirmation of the disease. This helps in genetic counseling and prenatal diagnosis. This also helps parents and caregivers to keep track of newer emerging therapies (e.g., exon skipping for DMD).[18]

REFERENCES

1. Williams J. Global developmental delay—globally helpful? Dev Med Child Neurol. 2010;52:227.
2. Schroeder S, Gerry M, Gert G, et al. Final Project Report: usage of the term "Intellectual disability:" Language, Image and Public Education, in American Association of Intellectual disability Resource Network International. Center on Developmental Disabilities; Center for the Study of Family, Neighborhood and Community Policy, University of Kansas, 2001. pp. 1-216.
3. Shevell M, Ashwal S, Donley D, Flint J, et al. Practice parameter: evaluation of the child with global developmental delay—Report of the Quality Standards Subcommittee of the American Academy of Neurology and the Practice Committee of the Child Neurology Society. Neurology. 2003;60:367-80.
4. Sherr EI, Shevell MI. Global developmental delay and mental retardation/intellectual disability. In: Swaiman KF, Ashwal S, Ferriero DM, Schor NF (Eds). Pediatric Neurology: Principles and Practice, 5th edition. Saunders Elsevier; 2012. pp. 554-74.
5. Van Karnebeek CDH, Jansweijer MCE, Leenders AGE, et al. Diagnostic investigations in individuals with mental retardation: a systematic literature review of their usefulness. Eur J Hum Genet. 2005;13:2-65.

6. Battaglia A, Carey JC. Diagnostic evaluation of developmental delay/mental retardation: an overview. Am J Med Genet C Semin Med Genet. 2003;117C(1);3-14.

7. Cleary MA, Green A. Developmental delay: when to suspect and how to investigate for an inborn error of metabolism. Arch Dis Child. 2005;90: 1128-32.

8. Sinha S, Satishchandra P, Gayathri N, et al. Progressive myoclonic epilepsy: a clinical, electrophysiological and pathological study from South India. J Neurol Sci. 2007;252:16-23.

9. Sachin S, Goyal V, Singh S, et al. Clinical spectrum of Hallervorden-Spatz syndrome in India. J Clin Neurosci. 2009;16:253-8.

10. Sharma S, Singh TD, Poojary SS, et al. Analysis of autosomal dominant spinocerebellar ataxia type 1 in an extended family of central India. Indian J Hum Genet. 2012;18:299-304.

11. Bahl S, Virdi K, Mittal U, et al. Evidence of a common founder for SCA12 in the Indian population. Ann Hum Genet. 2005;69:528-34.

12. Shukla P, Vasisht S, Srivastava R, et al. Molecular and structural analysis of metachromatic leukodystrophy patients in Indian population. J Neurol Sci. 2011;301:38-45.

13. Gorospe JR, Singhal BS, Kainu T, et al. Indian Agarwal megalencephalic leukodystrophy with cysts is caused by a common MLC1 mutation. Neurology. 2004;62:878-82.

14. Neurologic syndrome. In: Clarke JTR (Ed). A Clinical Guide to Inherited Metabolic Diseases, 3rd edition. Cambridge: Cambridge University Press; 2006. pp. 28-89.

15. Lyon G, Kolodny EH, Pastores GM. Neurology of Hereditary Metabolic Diseases in Children, 3rd edition. New York: McGraw-Hill Companies; 2006. pp. 65-392.

16. Opitz JM, Lewin SO. Rett syndrome—a review and discussion of syndrome delineation and syndrome definition. Brain Dev. 1987;9:445-50.

17. Prashanth LK, Taly AB, Ravi V, et al. Adult onset subacute sclerosing panencephalitis: clinical profile of 39 patients from a tertiary care centre. J Neurol Neurosurg Psychiatry. 2006;77:630-33.

18. Cirak S, Arechavala-Gomeza V, Guglieri M, et al. Exon skipping and dystrophin restoration in patients with Duchenne muscular dystrophy after systemic phosphorodiamidate morpholino oligomer treatment: an open-label, phase 2, dose-escalation study. Lancet. 2011;378:595-605.

19. Sankhyan N. Neurodegenerative disorders. In: Parthasarathy A (Ed). IAP Textbook of Pediatrics. New Delhi: Jaypee Publishers; 2013. pp. 319-22.

Chapter 11

Approach to a Patient with Speech and Language Disorders

Apoorva Pauranik

INTRODUCTION

Aphasia and related disorders of speech, communication, reading and writing are a significant workload for neurologists (Table 11.1). Aphasia persists as disability in 21–38% of stroke survivors. Community incidence is 43/100,000 per year, and prevalence is 3000 per million.[1] It is more common than many neurological diseases like Parkinsonism, multiple sclerosis, motor neuron disease, and muscular dystrophy combined together. Dementia, head injury, brain tumors, and encephalitis are additional causes of aphasia. Language learning disabilities including dyslexia (prevalence 5%) are a major community problem whose assessment and therapeutic rehabilitation is guided by cognitive neuropsychological principles, similar to those applicable to acquired aphasia and alexia (Table 11.2).

Unfortunately, there is a huge treatment gap for patients suffering from aphasia despite the advent of newer methods of therapy, further amplified by new tools and technologies from computers and communication.

ANATOMICAL AND PATHOLOGICAL SUBSTRATE

Approximately, 90% of people are right handed and 10% are nonright-handed (left-handed and ambidextrous). The planum temporale on the posterosuperior surface of the temporal lobe is larger on the left side in about two-thirds of the population. The left hemisphere controls speech in 98% of the dextral and also in about 50% of the nonright-handed persons, explaining low incidence (2–3%) of crossed aphasia.[2]

TABLE 11.1: The wide range of disorders of speech, language, and communication

Type of disorder	Comment
Disorders of phonation	
Aphonia Dysphonia	• Almost always due to laryngeal dysfunction • Local, nonneurogenic causes • Neurogenic paralysis of vocal cord muscles
Disorders of articulation	

Anarthria Dysarthria	• Non-neurological local causes
	• Neurological causes
	  ○ Muscles: polymyositis
	  ○ Neuromuscular: myasthenia gravis
	  ○ Neuropathic: Guillain-Barre syndrome
	  ○ Brain stem, cerebellum, basal ganglia: cerebrovascular accident, neoplasia, infection, degeneration (Parkinsonism), trauma, developmental

Disorders of fluency	
Stammering (Stuttering) Cluttering	• Usually developmental • No visible underlying pathology in most
Disorder of language	

Aphasia Alexia/ dyslexia Agraphia	• Cortical speech areas, subcortical grey, and white matter
	  ○ Stroke, trauma, central nervous system infections, neoplastic
	• Developmental: mental retardation, cerebral palsy
	• Degenerative
	  ○ Young age: autism, Rett's syndrome, leuko- and polio-dystrophies
	  ○ Old age: Alzheimer's and other dementias

TABLE 11.2: **Community burden of aphasia and other disorders of speech and communication**

Disease Condition	Over all burden	Percentage with aphasia
Stroke	Prevalence 0.5%	25%
Head injury	Prevalence 1.2%	5–10%
Dementia	10% above the age of 60 years	Almost all have variable impairment of language functions depending on severity
Mental retardation	5% (all)1% (severe)	Almost all have variable impairment of language function depending on severity
Learning disabilities (e.g., dyslexia)	5%	All have variable handicap in reading and writing skills
Fluency and articulation disorders: stuttering, stammering, lisping, cluttering, lalling	1%	Variable handicap in all

Clinicopathological correlation, with the help of neuroimaging, is an important step in working up a patient with aphasia. The anatomical substrate of aphasia may be conceptualized along three axes of dichotomy in relation to the clinical picture (Fig. 11.1).

Cardiac embolism, atrial fibrillation and a larger volume of the cerebral lesion are associated with a higher probability of aphasia as well as mortality.

Global aphasia would suggest occlusion of internal carotid artery or stem of middle cerebral artery (MCA) or large deep basal ganglionic plus thalamic hemorrhage. Most aphasia syndromes occur due to infarction in left MCA territory with the exception of transcortical motor aphasia which is due to a lesion affecting anterior cerebral artery (ACA) and pure alexia without agraphia occurs because of a lesion affecting blood supply from the posterior cerebral artery (PCA) (refer to Appendix 1 for glossary of related terms).

Nonfluent aphasia predominates in young patients suggesting an anterior lesion, while in elderly patients, fluent aphasia is often attributed to cardioembolism (up to 40%) in the posterior division of the MCA.[3]

Transcortical aphasia syndromes suggest infarction in watershed territories between ACA-MCA-PCA, thereby disconnecting the core speech centers in the Sylvian region from the more peripheral association cortices in the frontoparietal-occipital regions. Hemodynamic compromises, like those in severe sustained hypotension, reduced cardiac output, and proximal vascular occlusion in aorta and carotid arteries would typically predispose to lesions in watershed areas.

Aphasia after head injury is most commonly associated with right-sided blunt orbitofrontal trauma with a contrecoup left temporoparietal injury. Trauma pathology tends to be less localized than ischemic stroke (except gun-shot wounds); hence, aphasic syndromes are often not pure or classical, but rather mixed with signs of more diffuse pathologies like altered sensorium, delirium, and amnesia. Recovery may be better.

Aphasia due to tumors of left cerebral hemisphere will usually have gradual onset, poor syndromic phenotype, and additional clinical deficits due to cerebral edema and increased intracranial pressure.

In Alzheimer's disease, memory loss and general cognitive deterioration precedes the language dysfunction. Naming and discourse tend to get affected later. Language becomes impoverished in content with loss of abstraction and metaphor. Repetition, oral reading, auditory comprehension, and grammar are preserved till late. From an evolutionary or ontogeny point of view, skills acquired later in life are the first to go, like written expression, reading comprehension and semantics rather than syntax and phonology (articulation). The aphasia profile initially looks like anomic, later transcortical sensory and Wernicke, finally degrading into severely nonfluent output or muteness.

Frontotemporal degeneration is the second most common form of early onset dementia. Behavioral variant accounts for more than half of the cases. The three subtypes of primary progressive aphasias affect language and communication for the initial 2 years or more, without other cognitive derangements. They can be differentiated on the basis of fluency, comprehension, and repetition[4] (Table 11.3).

Aphasias with subcortical lesions have also been identified, particularly left striatocapsular and thalamic pathology. The clinical deficit is more often due to associated reversible cortical hypoperfusion or deactivation. Subcortical aphasias suggest the existence of cortical–subcortical circuits in language, as observed in other forms of cognition.

Dichotomy A: Central sulcus/Rolandic sulcus		Dichotomy B: Lateral sulcus/Sylvian fissure	
Anterior lesions Prerolandic	Posterior lesions Retrorolandic	Perisylvian	Extrasylvian
Non-fluent; dysarthric; Comprehension Normal e.g., Broca, transcortical motor	Fluent: Nondysarthric Comprehension abnormal e.g., Wernicke, transcortical sensory	Repetition is poor e.g., Broca, Wernicke, Conduction	Repetition is preserved e.g., Transcortical aphasias, anomic aphasia. Alexia without agraphia

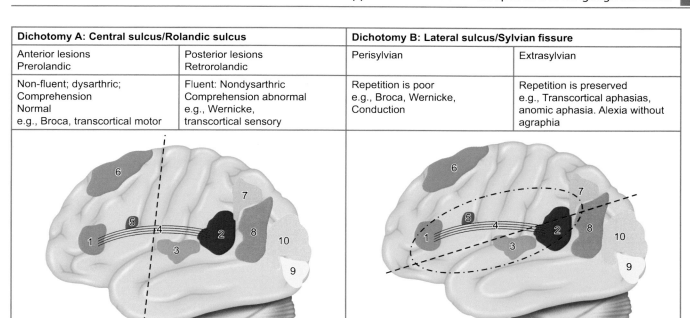

1. Broca's area; 2. Wernicke area; 3. Primary auditory cortex; 4. Arcuate fasiculus; 5. Primary motor area: mouth and tongue; 6. Motor association cortex and supplementary motor area; 7. Supramarginal gyrus; 8. Angular gyrus; 9. Primary visual cortex; 10. Visual association cortex.

1. Broca's area; 2. Wernicke area; 3. Primary auditory cortex; 4. Arcuate fasiculus; 5. Primary motor area: mouth and tongue; 6. Motor association cortex and supplementary motor area; 7. Supramarginal gyrus; 8. Angular gyrus; 9. Primary visual cortex; 10. Visual association cortex.

Dichotomy C: Cortical gray matter and subcortical gray and white matter

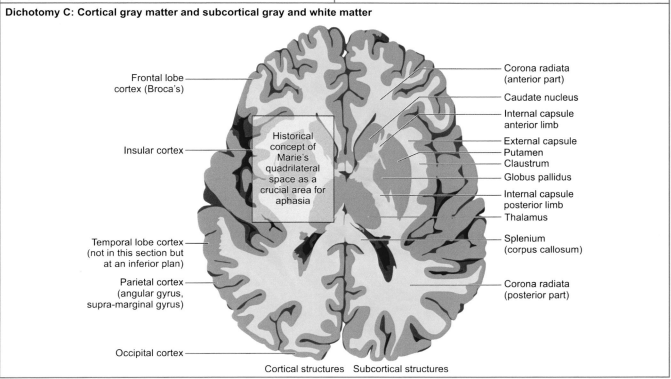

Fig. 11.1: The anatomical substrate of aphasia.

TABLE 11.3: The three types of Primary Progressive Aphasias as variants of Frontotemporal Degeneration

Clinical features	Nonfluent/agrammatic variant	Semantic variant	Logopenic variant
Comprehension (Simple)	Fair	Poor	Fair
Comprehension of complex sentences	Poor	Poor	±
Repetition	Poor	Fair	±
Naming	Fair ±	Poor	±
Object knowledge	Fair	Poor	Fair
Paraphasia	Many	Uncommon	Fairly common
Agrammatism	Severe	Nil	Mild or minimal
Dysprody	Severe	Nil	Nil
Apraxia of speech	Nil	Nil	Mild moderate
Alexia, agraphia	Nil	Severe	Nil
Imaging	Left posterior frontoinsular	Anterior temporal left > right	Posterior perisylvian
Pathology	Tau > TDP43	TDP43	Amyloid plaques, neurofibrillary tangles

TABLE 11.4: Language, experience, and proficiency: a simplified questionnaire

	Mark as	Language A	Language B	Language C
Proficiency in	-/+ / ++/+++/++++			
Speaking				
Understanding				
Reading				
Writing				
Place of use	-/+ / ++/+++/++++			
At home				
At work				
At school				
With friends				
Sequence of acquisition	Serial order of acquisition of that language at different ages			
Over all order of dominant usage	-/+ / ++/+++/++++			

CLINICAL APPROACH

One must begin with patient's educational and working status, language proficiencies (Table 11.4),[5] and handedness (Table 11.5).[6] Multilingualism is common in India, except for illiterate or less-educated monolinguals from rural areas. Aphasia assessment may be required to be done in more than one language for some patients. The clinical profiles may differ across the languages. Illiteracy restricts the range of stimuli and the tasks to be tested, and may have some bearing upon clinic-anatomical correlations. These are challenges as well as opportunities for aphasiologists in India.[7] Associated neurological deficits should be documented.

A brief examination can be completed in 5–10 minutes and will provide basic data about the presence of aphasia, its severity and a tentative diagnosis of the aphasia syndrome. More detailed assessment spanning over one to two hours in one or more sessions will be required in most subjects for comprehensive profiling and planning the rehabilitative speech therapy (Box 11.1).

A large number of testing protocols have been developed for speech and language communication[8] (Table 11.6). Many Indian adaptations are in use but

TABLE 11.5: Handedness questionnaire. Enquire from the patient or caregiver about the preferred use of right or left hand in the following tasks

	Task /object	Left hand	Right hand
1.	Eating		
2.	Writing		
3.	Mopping		
4.	Cutting with a knife		
5.	Brooming		
6.	Lighting a match stick		
7.	Using a spoon		
8.	Using a scissors		
9.	Throwing		
10.	Opening a box (lid)		

Total checks: LH = RH = Cumulative Total CT = LH + RH = Difference D = RH – LH = Result R = (D/CT) 100 = Interpretation (Left handed: R <40) (Ambidextrous: -40 R + 40) (Right handed: R > +40).

their standardization and validation has not been well documented.

ORAL EXPRESSION, ARTICULATION, AND FLUENCY

Listen carefully to the patient and ask questions like, *"Tell me about your illness," "your family," "the work done by you at your job,"* etc. An adequate sample of narrative speech is needed to detect the types of deficits. Efforts are needed to make patients speak, not merely isolated words or gestures but longer phrases and sentences. Patient should be asked to describe the things and actions going on in a picture. The response may be incomplete, halting, sparse, and failing to grasp the totality of the scene despite repeated hints.

Defective articulation and phonation are recognized during conversation or reading or repetition. Keep handy a list of target syllables, words or short phrases for testing articulation. They can be chosen on the basis of Hindi (and other Indian language) (Appendix 2) alphabet which have a fairly scientific arrangement of vowels and consonants into different groups according to the place of production.

Dysarthria is common in nonfluent aphasias. Pure dysarthria can occur in many disorders other than aphasia (Table 11.7). Isolated dysarthria due to cortical lesion in the language zone is rare and has been described as "apraxia of speech" in which consonants are frequently substituted rather than distorted as in dysarthria, more

Box 11.1: The clinical examination of aphasia

Auditory comprehension
- Single words
- Commands, sentences
- Discourse, paragraphs

Articulation
- Recitation, singing
- Simple words
- Complex words
- Sentences

Fluency
- Phrase length
- Agrammatism
- Stereotyped utterance
- Word finding difficulty
- Phonological paraphasias
- Semantic paraphasias
- Neologisms
- Circumlocution

Repetition
- Syllable
- Words—high frequency and high imageability
- Words—low frequency, low imageability
- Phrases

Naming
- Body parts
- Real objects
- Pictures
- Question-based
- Effect of cueing (phonemic and semantic)
- Rejection of wrong answers
- Acceptance of correct answers

Reading
- Matching letters, syllables, words, numerals
- Pointing to letters, syllables, words, numerals
- Reading-aloud letters, syllables, words, numerals
- Sorting words and nonwords
- Word—Picture matching
- Sentence—Picture matching
- Filling in the blanks in sentences
- Reading a paragraph and answering questions

Writing
- Copying letters, syllables, numerals, words, sentences
- Writing to dictation—letters, syllables, numerals, words, sentences
- Signature, name, address, automatic sequences
- Written naming of objects, pictures
- Written description of a picture scene

so with polysyllabic words at initiation. The errors keep changing from one attempt to the next, while the distortion of phonemes is consistent in dysarthria. The output in apraxia of speech is effortful, groping for self-correction and dysprosodic. It is common with Broca's

TABLE 11.6: **Current tests and methods of aphasia assessment**

Clinical bedside examination	Unstructured and variable, as described in various texts
Screening test	Frenchy Aphasia Screening Test (5–10 minutes)
Comprehensive examination	• The Boston Diagnostic Aphasia Examination • The Western Aphasia Battery
Tests of specific aspects of language behavior	• The Boston Naming Test • The Token Test (syntactic comprehension) • Tests for reading and writing
Tests based on cognitive neuropsychological approach	• PALPA (Psycholinguistic Assessment of Language Processing in Aphasia) • PAL (Psycholinguistic Abilities in Language) • CAT (Comprehensive Aphasia Test)
Assessment for functional communication and quality of life	• ASHA functional assessment • Communication activities of daily living • Quality of life scale in stroke—aphasia
Tests for special populations	Infants and children, traumatic brain injury, right hemisphere lesions, the elderly and dementia subjects, multilingual subjects

TABLE 11.7: **Types of dysarthria**

Site of the lesion	Disease example	The type of speech	Label
Bilateral upper motor neuron	Bilateral strokes; tumors, primary lateral sclerosis	Harsh voice; slow rate; strain-strangle, imprecise consonants	Spastic ++
Unilateral upper motor neuron	Stroke, tumor	Consonant imprecision, harsh voice quality, slow rate	Spastic ++
Lower motor neuron	Bulbar palsy, myasthenia gravis	Breathy, nasal voice, imprecise consonants	Flaccid
Upper and lower motor neuron	Amyotrophic lateral sclerosis, multiple strokes	Strain-strangle, hyper nasality, harsh voice, slow rate, imprecise consonants	Spastic and flaccid
Basal ganglia: a	Parkinson's disease	Rapid rate, reduced loudness, monotonous and nonvariable amplitude	Hypokinetic
Basal ganglia: b	Dystonia, Huntington disease	Prolonged phonemes, inappropriate silences, variable rate, voice stoppages	Hyperkinetic
Cerebellum	Stroke, degenerative diseases, multiple sclerosis	Irregular articulatory breakdowns, made apparent on rapid repetition of complex polysyllable, excessive and equal stress	Ataxic

aphasia. Written performance is better than verbal. Dysarthria is not significantly influenced by the type of linguistic material or by the task.

Nonfluent speech is one of the commonest clinical observations in aphasia, more so with anterior or prerolandic lesions. Patients speak in monosyllables or in short sentences. Sometimes only a single utterance is repetitively used in every conversation. These verbal stereotypes are sometimes intoned differently to convey some meaning as in *yes!, yes?, y..y..es?* There may be delay in initiation of a response, increased effort, apparent strain, pauses in between words and sentences and interruptions. Nonfluent speech, as in Broca's aphasia, also exhibits agrammatism in which there is an absence or a paucity of function words. The short phrases are composed of content words only; however, meaning is conveyed somehow in a manner resembling "telegraphic language" as if to economize on words.

Word-finding difficulty, a feature of all types of aphasia, is manifest by repetition of determiners (a, an, the), prepositions (this, that, which, so), other functional or grammatical units (and, yes) and vocal and gestural mannerisms (*"uh,"* pointing towards something), circumlocution, paraphasias, neologisms and jargon.

If one listens to a fluent aphasia from a distance, ignoring the actual content of the speech, it appears effortless, with normal melody, accent, prosody and mannerisms. However, on close observation, the content is empty and abnormal. Phrases and sentences are of normal length, or sometimes, overly lengthy. The patient fails to know when to stop. They may speak excessively (logorrhea), being unaware of the abnormality. There are many paraphasias, circumlocutions and abundance of function words or grammar words whose information load is low. The content words, which carry information, are scarce and are used by flouting the rules of grammar. Jargon is common. Such patients have profound defects in auditory and reading comprehension. A classical example is the Wernicke's aphasia.

AUDITORY COMPREHENSION

If a patient merely shows the tongue on command or nods the head this way or that in response to a question, it does not imply normal comprehension. Further testing is needed through more difficult tasks. Each command must be stated only once, at a fairly slow and regular rate and not repeated piecemeal.

While giving a command, the examiner and by-standers, must not make any gestures. For auditory comprehension at the one-word level, the examiner speaks out the word and asks the patient to point to the corresponding picture or object or body part. The patient's performance is scored in terms of correct answers with respect to help or cues and time latency. Some patients may perform poorly at the single-word level (identification by pointing) but better in sentence comprehension as meanings may be discernible through redundancy of words.

At the sentence level, command comprehension can be made difficult by involving more than one step. Example: "Fold this piece of paper and put it into your pocket," "Pick up the piece of cloth, put it into the glass and then invert the glass on the table." Then simple yes--no questions are asked "Does the stone sink in water?" "Is an elephant larger than an ant?" Not uncommonly, many patients who appeared to perform fairly well in daily household communication through gestures, fail miserably in these formal modes of testing. At the discourse level, a short story is narrated and questions are asked based on it. Picture-sentence matching tasks use one sentence and many picture choices and vice versa (Appendix 3).

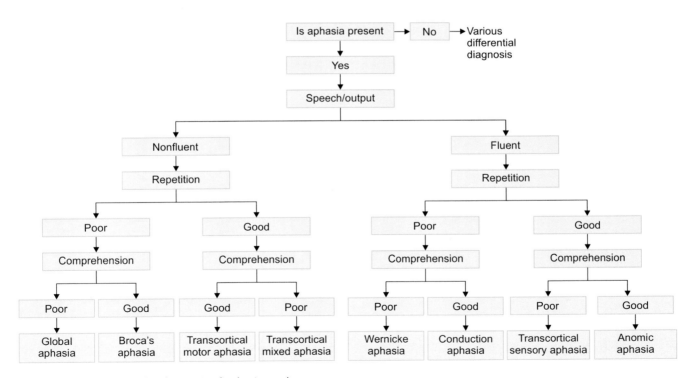

Fig. 11.2: Algorithm for the diagnosis of aphasia syndrome.

REPETITION

The patient is expected to repeat verbatim whatever is uttered by the examiner. Initial stimuli are simple, short and common; later, they are made longer, hard to pronounce and uncommon. The examiner speaks the word or phrase in a clear voice, one at a time at a constant slow speed. The patient may totally fail, remain mute, or come up with the wrong responses. The errors may be sound disorders, incomplete responses, deletions, or paraphasias. Repetition is a relatively simple but important test. As depicted in algorithm (Fig. 11.2), it is a crucial node for syndromic diagnoses.

NAMING

The targets can be chosen from among body parts, persons, real-life articles in the room or objects assembled on the table for the purpose. Drawings or photographs of the objects can be used. The examiner puts her finger on the object or photo and asks the patient to name it. The target should be clear, concise, and nonambiguous. The response may be absent, delayed, or altered. It may be related to the target word either by sound (phonemic paraphasia) or by meaning (semantic paraphasia). The response word may be phonemic jargon (nonword) or semantic jargon (dictionary word but totally unconnected). Some patients may describe the word in a roundabout way (circumlocution). Cues or help can be given. A phonemic cue constitutes uttering the first one or two phonemes or sounds of the word or producing its rhythm. A semantic cue involves giving a hint about the synonyms or attributes of that word. In case of persistent failure, the examiner can suggest a wrong answer and ask if it is correct or not, or offer the correct answer and observe if the patient accepts it or not. In total disruption of semantics, the patient fails. The naming of objects can be done category-wise, like action verbs, colors, geometric figures, numbers, letters, body parts, etc. Interestingly, sometimes naming deficits may be restricted to narrow, idiosyncratic semantic categories, for example, living versus nonliving, verbs or nouns, furniture items, eatables, and so on.

READING

At first test the ability to recognize, match and discriminate the graphic symbols of alphabets. Then ask the patient to read aloud words, nonwords, phrases, or paragraphs without paying attention to the meaning. A mixed list of words and nonwords is given for sorting. Reading comprehension involves picture or word—object matching, and carrying out some written commands, like "touch your hair," "make a fist," etc. A somewhat difficult task is to fill in the blanks in progressively longer sentences from among a choice of detractors. Large paragraphs (unseen passages) are given to read, and written questions are asked based on it. The effect of complexity and regularity of spelling is judged for scripts such as the Roman or Arabic but not Devnagri because of transparent grapheme-to-phoneme conversion in the later.

WRITING

If motor dexterity of the writing hand is fair, the patient may be able to copy from written stimuli, write to dictation, and serially write automatized sequences (name, address, numbers, alphabet, weekdays, months, etc.). Patients with nonfluent aphasia will have reduced output, laborious start, pauses, and agrammatism in the output. The mechanics of writing and calligraphy will be distorted. Fluent aphasics may write legibly but the written output will exhibit similar deficits of emptiness, paraphasias, jargon, circumlocution, etc. Picture and object naming, and describing the events going on in a sketch are further tests of written expression. Usually, the oral and written expression reveals comparable degrees of proficiency or deficit. Rarely, strategically situated discrete lesions may dissociate the two performances. More commonly, it is the psychogenic disorders (conversion reaction, malingering) that lead to a glaring disparity of the patient being mute yet able to express normally on writing or vice versa.

RELATED HIGHER MENTAL FUNCTIONS

Aphasia is not an exclusively language related problem. Many other functions are simultaneously affected: working memory, short-term memory, recent memory, attention, executive skills, sensory perception, motor dexterity, apraxia, agnosia, and spatial orientation.[9] Aphasic deficits may be seen as impairments to working memory. A central executive system operates at the level of phonological store to momentarily generate articulatory loop or "inner speech" before a string of sounds may be perceived or uttered in a meaningful manner. If a patient has problems in holding items in working memory, he will have problems in sentence processing. Attention is essential to focus on communication with the partner's speech, particularly when surrounded by competing

TABLE 11.8: **Various forms of aphasia and their clinicoanatomical correlations**

Type of aphasia	Clinical	Anatomy
Broca's aphasia	Sparse, halting speech, often misarticulated, frequently missing function words, and bound morphemes. Disturbance in speech planning and production mechanism	Primary posterior aspects of the third frontal convolution and adjacent inferior aspects of the precentral gyrus. Prerolandic branch of middle cerebral artery. A lesion restricted to classical Broca's area causes a mild reversible nonfluent aphasia. More severe and well-known type of classical Broca's aphasia requires a much larger lesion surrounding regions other than Broca's area
Wernicke's aphasia	Poor reading and auditory comprehension, fluent speech with phonemic, morphological and semantic paraphasias. Disturbance of permanent representations of the sound structures of words	Posterior half of the first temporal gyrus and possibly adjacent cortex. Posterior temporal branch of left middle cerebral artery
Global aphasia	Disruption of all language processing components and severe diminution or loss of all language	Large portion of the perisylvian association cortex. Combined lesions involving Broca's and Wernicke's area. Infarction due to occlusion of stem of left middle cerebral artery (MCA) or internal carotid artery
Conduction aphasia	Repetition is severely impaired out of proportion to verbal expression, fluency and comprehension, literal paraphasic errors are common with frequent attempts at self-correction	A disconnection between Wernicke's and Broca's area due to arcuate fasiculus, a white matter tract in deep temporal lobe. Also due to lesion in superior temporal or inferior parietal region
Transcortical motor	Similar to Broca's aphasia with hesitant, telegraphic speech, normal comprehension, and surprisingly good repetition	Deep white matter in frontal lobe, anterior and superior to Broca's area or near supplementary motor area. Anterior cerebral artery territory
Transcortical sensory	Similar to Wernicke's aphasia with fluent paraphasic speech, poor auditory, and reading comprehension but surprisingly good repetition	Left temporo-occipital watershed infarction between MCA and PCA (pure alexia without agraphia) territories
Anomic	Disturbance of the concepts of the words or the sound patterns of words or both. Most aspects of speech normal except naming	Least localizable of all aphasic symptoms. Inferior parietal lobe or connection between parietal lobe and temporal lobe. Arterial territory: angular branch of left MCA
Alexia without agraphia	Patients can write but cannot read even their own writing. Other aspects of speech are normal except naming, especially for colors	Medial occipital lobe on left dominant side along with splenium of corpus callosum. Within posterior cerebral artery territory. It is a disconnection between intact right visual cortex and left hemisphere language centers

stimuli. Arousal is a basic, physiological level of attention. Vigilance is attention sustained over long periods of time and is critical to hold a conversation. The anterior cingulate gyrus is mainly concerned with supervisory attentional system. Speech automations that are frequent in nonfluent aphasia are related to nonlinguistic factors like attention and pragmatic context.

SYNDROMES, THEIR RELEVANCE, AND NEWER METHODS OF ASSESSMENT

Since, the 19th century, aphasiologists have tried to correlate brain areas with abilities of speaking, understanding, reading, and writing and with traditional syndromes (Table 11.8).

The distinction depends on the presence or absence of a constellation of speech behavioral aspects. The syndromes may be artifactual or arbitrary being dictated by angioanatomical territories and the vulnerability of certain regions to pathological insults.

Syndromic diagnosis also depends upon host factors like handedness and bilingualism. Rapid changes in aphasia profile occur during the initial weeks following stroke due to resolution of edema and diaschisis and restoration of blood flow.

Syndromic classification has been useful as a shorthand summary of a patient's language disorder. However, syndromes have lost their theoretical relevance and they should be replaced by newer classifications based on neurolinguistics and cognitive neuropsychology.[10]

TABLE 11.9: **Cognitive neuropsychological model of language based relationship between the tasks, component, and deficit**

The tasks	The system	If damaged
Discrimination of auditory minimum pair nonwords (same or different)	Auditory phonological analysis	Poor performance in deciding whether two short sequence of sounds (nonwords differing minimally with respect to any one phoneme) spoken by examiner are same or different
Discrimination of written minimum pairs or nonwords (same or different)	Visual orthographic analysis	Poor performance in deciding whether two short sequence of letters (nonwords differing minimally respect to only one graphic symbol) written by examiner are same or different
Lexicality decision for spoken word. (Is it a word or nonword?)	Phonological input lexicon	Failure to recognize that a novel phoneme (sound sequence) is a word or nonword
Lexicality decision for written word (Is it a word or nonword?)	Orthographic input lexicon	Failure to recognize that a novel string of graphic symbols or letters is a word or nonword
Confrontation naming of a picture or object	Semantic system	Semantic errors with comparable deficits in comprehension as well as production in both modalities of oral and written
Reading aloud • Regular words • Irregular words (for English in Roman, not for Hindi in Devnagri)	Phonological output lexicon	Delay and failure in word retrieval, circumlocution, semantic errors, word fragments, frequency effect
Writing to dictation • Regular words • Irregular words	Orthographic output lexicon	Poor spelling for irregular words regularization of exception words. Frequency effect
Repetition of words and nonwords	Phonological output buffer	Equally poor repetition of words and nonwords with significantly worse performance for longer words
Writing to dictation of words and nonwords	Orthographic output buffer	Equally poor writing of words and nonwords in significantly worse performance for longer words
Repetition, reading aloud, and writing to dictation of words and nonwords	Conversion procedures from phoneme to grapheme and grapheme to phoneme	Difficulty more with nonwords
Cross script conversion: Roman to Devnagri and Devnagri to Roman	As above. May also need phonological and orthographic output buffers and probably output lexicon but not semantics	

TABLE 11.10: **Neurolinguistic types of errors and their localizing value**

Error type	Locus of damage	Examples
Semantic	• Semantic system • Phonological output lexicon	Table–chair Five–Fifteen
Phonological		
In general	• Phonological output buffer • Phonological output lexicon	*Chidiya* (Bird)–*Chiriya*
If present only during repetition	Phonological input to output conversion mechanism	
If present only during reading	Grapheme to phoneme conversion mechanism	
Morphological	• Phonological output lexicon • Orthographic output lexicon	*Chain* (patience)–*Bechain* (impatience) *Chhutti* (holiday)–*Chhuttiyan* (holidays) *Shiksha* (education)–*Shaikshanik* (educational) *Dikhana* (to show)–*Dikhava* (showmanship)

Traditional methods of assessment of aphasia described above are still valid and useful, but tectonic conceptual shift has occurred since 1980s in the way the patients are studied. The reference model is no longer the anatomy but the functional structure of normal cognitive functioning. Breakdown of language at linguistic levels of phonology, morphology, lexicon, semantics, syntax, and pragmatics is given due consideration. Many testing protocols straddling across and beyond the traditional aphasia syndrome and based on cognitive analysis have been developed.[11] Table 11.9 summarizes the relationship between assessment tasks, components of language model and the deficit due to disruption of these components. Table 11.10 depicts a classification of errors and their localizing value. Neuroimaging techniques like high-resolution structural mapping, functional MRI, PET and tractography have shaken the dogmas about cerebral lateralization and so-called speech areas. The role of genetics (FOXP2 gene, William's syndrome) shifts the focus from macro to molecular levels in a nonfocal context.

An analogy can be given with epilepsy. The classification of seizures has been revised. More emphasis is on seizure semiology rather than pigeon-holing subjects into straight-jacket of classification. Something similar to video monitoring has happened in aphasiology. Data from single patients have become the basis for cognitive neuropsychological research and therapy.[12,13]

One must concede limitations of cognitive analysis. It is not applicable to all patients, particularly severe cases. It is generally useful for those who have several preserved channels of language through which they can be examined. They need an extensive array of probe tests and are useful mainly for disorders at one-word level, more so in reading and writing, and not much for syntax.

When one argues that the classical aphasia syndromes are passé that does not necessarily mean that we must be ready with some perfect or better alternative. We need not regret living through the phase of transition. We must go for description instead of labeling, use labels as a stem and expand upon them, while waiting for some consensus scheme from a panel of experts.

DIFFERENTIAL DIAGNOSES

Not to Miss the Diagnosis of Aphasia When Present

A diagnosis of aphasia may be missed when the clinical deficit is mild and slowly evolving. Observations like pauses, hesitancy, misarticulation, wrong words, word finding difficulty, and the need to repeat the question

TABLE 11.11: Classification of dyslexia/alexia

Performance	Type of dyslexia		
	Deep dyslexia	Surface dyslexia	Phonological dyslexia
Nonword reading	✗	✓	✗
Regularity effects in reading aloud	✗	✓	✗
Imageability effects in reading aloud	✓	✗	✓ (possibly)
Grammatical class effects in reading aloud	✓	✗	✓ (possibly)
Semantic errors in reading aloud	✓	✗	✗

are helpful. The patient points out that he talks in a way which is hard for people to follow yet thinks that he is talking perfectly well. The patient has trouble when tired or anxious, or when listening to many people with a background of noise.

That the apparent impairment of hearing is in fact due to receptive aphasia can be ascertained by the observation that the patient will be able to listen and respond to nonverbal sounds, including music. Anomia in a patient with aphasia can be differentiated from *amnesia*. Intact memory can be inferred by indirect behavioral observations. *Alexia* or impairment of reading comprehension is a common part of aphasia (Table 11.11), and patients may seek ophthalmological consultation thinking that something is wrong with their *vision*. The visual acuity, however, will be normal for nonlinguistic images.

Jargon speech may look like delirium or psychiatric disorder, including psychosis.

Not to Make a False Positive Diagnosis of Aphasia, When not Present

Developmental disorders of speech are not aphasia. Many children with brain damage learn speaking, reading and related skills late or incompletely or not at all. They are not aphasic.

A developmental suppression of the motor fluency of speech is very common. Stuttering or stammering is not a part of the aphasia rubric. An early damage to the function of hearing influences the development of speech, and an extreme example is *congenital deaf-mutism*.

Pure dysarthria hampers the pronunciation and intelligibility of speech, but language, vocabulary, grammar, reading, writing, and auditory comprehension are intact. In severe cases, hardly any sound emanates from the articulatory apparatus and results in *anarthria*. Disorders of phonation occur due to diseases of the larynx, vocal cord, and respiratory weakness.

In all the above conditions, the cortical areas concerned with cerebral organization of linguistic functions are intact. Written expression is normal, while in aphasia, written and verbal deficits almost always run parallel to each other. Auditory and/or reading comprehension is also normal while in patients with aphasia these are often abnormal.

Regression of normal acquired speech and communicative ability and other cognitive functions occurs in a group of pervasive disorders in children such as autism, Asperger's syndrome, and Rett's syndrome. Landau–Kleffner syndrome in children is also a disorder of acquired aphasia and epilepsy.

Patients with conversion reaction may become mute, speak in whispers or in a bizarre, abnormal manner. Rarely, some patients may behave as if they are not able to listen or comprehend any speech. This should raise the possibility of malingering or Munchausen's syndrome. Verbal and written modes of communication are usually not affected together in conversion reaction. A close observation of behavior over a period of time may confirm the diagnosis. A more complete diagnosis of conversion reaction will also need exploration of the underlying psychological stress.

The speech in schizophrenia may be sparse or excessive, bizarre, and absurd. Flight of ideas, pressure of speech, and evasive, tangential answers may create an impression of logorrheic speech or Wernicke aphasia with defects in auditory comprehension. However, grammar and semantic logic are largely retained.

One of the important prerequisites for a definition of aphasia is a state of normal alertness or sensorium, and normal intellectual or cognitive functions. It does not mean that the two cannot coexist, but it is difficult to decide about their relative contribution. Patients who are in acute confusional state may be labeled as aphasic due to delayed and incorrect responses. Irrelevant muttering may be mistaken as fluent jargon or vice versa. Patients with amnesia, dementia, and Korsakoff's psychosis may involuntarily fill in the gaps in their memory and be diagnosed as suffering from anomic or Wernicke's aphasia.

A patient may fail to comply with a verbal command due to motor apraxia and not because of a defect in auditory comprehension. Visual or tactile agnosia may be responsible for a naming defect rather than aphasia.

The differentiation relies on more comprehensive and repeated examination and on considering the over-all picture. Various methods of testing include (i) auditory comprehension that bypasses motor praxis, (ii) gnosis (recognition) that involves much more than naming (i.e. describing the use of an object, making same-different judgment from among foils), and (iii) memory, which goes beyond language function or bypasses language function. Such elaborate testing methods require the services of an experienced neuropsychologist.

Total loss of speech or *"mutism"* is a clinical situation caused by a wide variety of disorders, aphasia being only one of them. Congenital deaf-mutism is easily identified since early childhood. Patients with severe Broca's and global aphasia may be mute initially or many days to weeks. Anarthria and aphonia (laryngeal) may resemble muteness. Frontal lobe dysfunctions are known to cause akinetic mutism. Psychogenic syndromes (conversion or dissociative states, catatonia) can also render a person totally speechless for a variable period of time.

NEUROIMAGING

Clinicoanatomical correlations are best studied when there is a single well-delineated lesion (infarct) in the brain. However, sometimes interesting and useful insights are provided by instances when a second lesion in an atypical location leads to an atypical clinical profile. The patient may have had a lesion in a classical area without clinical deficits, betraying the fact that unconventional parts of the brain had compensated the function.

A substantial proportion of cases show misfits, such as nonfluent aphasias with retrorolandic or posteriorly placed lesions, fluent aphasias with prerolandic or anterior lesions, an instance of the lesion being present in an unexpected area, discrepancies between lesion size/volume and clinical severity of and recovery from aphasia. The most probable explanation is interindividual variations in the anatomical substrate for language functions in the brain. Left handedness, younger age, female sex, and multilingualism are associated with more bilateral representation and anomalous organization of the speech function.

Magnetic resonance imaging has spatial resolution and is better for three-dimensional volumetric analysis. Subtle but significant variations in volume of a particular gyrus or white matter tract, which may not be visually discernible, may underline host-specific vulnerabilities and clinicoanatomical mismatches. Areas of maximum lesion overlap in group studies are depicted through image templates. Areas of structural damage usually have abnormal function but the converse may not be true. There may be brain regions with abnormal function, which look normal on CT/MRI.

Functional neuroimaging (fMRI, PET, SPECT) techniques are now providing evidence for neural modules or networks (not areas or centers) concerned with cognitive functions, such as speech. A concept of interacting, interconnected but widely distributed neural networks has emerged. Experimental *in vivo* studies are performed in normal and brain-damaged subjects. Well-defined linguistic tasks are given while imaging results are compared before, during, and after the task. It is now possible to characterize the patterns of connection between a damaged region and the undamaged areas that show depressed metabolism on functional neuroimaging.[14]

Neuroimaging assists the research on aphasia recovery by biological processes like reperfusion, disappearance of edema and diaschisis, neurotransmitter changes, and finally neuroplasticity. Structural imaging changes like increased gray matter density as a result of therapy also serve as evidence for its efficacy. Understanding how aphasia treatment influences the brain may improve the selection of the specific treatment approach.

However, there are limitations of functional imaging. The areas around the acute infarct may have compromised function due to low perfusion, which may actually not turn into an infarct. Such areas may not show a BOLD (Blood Oxygen Level Dependent) effect in fMRI, yet contribute to clinical deficit; even in chronic stages. Additional information is needed by CT perfusion, MR dynamic contrast perfusion, arterial spin labeling, MR angio or CT angio, and impairment of vascular reactivity to CO_2 challenge or breath-holding. The relationship of BOLD response to diaschisis is also uncertain and problematic.

Increased activation in a brain region during recovery, with or without therapy, does not necessarily mean it to be a positive or useful phenomenon. Not uncommonly, the increased activation in a nearby or remote region may be counterproductive or maladaptive rather than facilitatory or compensatory.

CONCLUSION

The main purpose of the whole edifice of clinical and imaging approach to aphasia, along with its changing theoretical underpinnings, is to guide the neurologist and speech therapist in better planning of rehabilitation and newer therapies based on advances in neurobiology (pharmacotherapy, cell therapy, reperfusion, magnetic and direct current stimulation of brain). But technology apart, physician is first and foremost a counselor and therapist. The physicians should repeatedly reinforce

many everyday tips to caregivers/family members of persons with aphasia. A well-informed neurologist, who has devoted ample time in clinical evaluation of aphasia, automatically becomes a little bit of the speech therapist himself. The neurologist must also evaluate psychosocial status and quality of life of the patients[15] and workout realistic and meaningful, short-term and long-term goals in consultation with patients, caregivers, and a speech therapist.[16]

The evidence base for efficacy of speech therapy is difficult to come by because of the peculiar nature of the problem, yet the evidence is there, justifying the time and effort for clinical assessment of aphasia not only by a speech therapist but also by a neurologist.[17]

REFERENCES

1. Engelter ST, Gostynski M, Papa S, et al. Epidemiology of aphasia attributable to first ischemic stroke: incidence, severity, fluency, etiology and thrombolysis. Stroke. 2006;37:1379-84.
2. Geschwind N. Disconnexion syndromes in animal and man. II. Brain. 1965;88:585-644.
3. Bhatnagar SC, Jain SK, Bihari M, et al. Aphasia type and aging in Hindi-speaking stroke patients. Brain Lang. 2002;83:353-61.
4. Chow TW, Alobaidy AA. Incorporating new diagnostic schemes, genetics and proteinopathy into the evaluation of frontotemporal degeneration. Continuum. 2013;19(2):438-56.
5. Marian V, Blumenfeld HK, Kaushanskaya M. The language experience and proficiency questionnaire (LEAP-Q): Assessing language profiles in Bilinguals and Multilinguals. J Speech Lang Hear Res. 2007;50:940-67.
6. Veale JF, Edinburgh handedness inventory—short form: a revised version based on confirmatory factor analysis. Laterality. 2013;18.
7. Karanth P. Multilingual/multi-literate/multicultural studies of aphasia—the Rosetta stone of neurolinguistics in the new millennium. Brain Lang. 2000;71:113-5.
8. Spreen O, Risser AH. Assessment of aphasia. Oxford: Oxford University Press; 2003.
9. Code C. The Characteristics of Aphasia. Lawrence Erlbaum Associates; 1989.
10. Ardila A. A proposed reinterpretation and reclassification of aphasic syndromes. Aphasiology. 2010;24:3:363-94.
11. Kay J, Lesser R, Coltheart M. Psycholinguistic assessment of language processing in aphasia (PALPA): an introduction. Aphasiology. 1996;10:159-80.
12. Whitworth A, Webster J, Howard D. A cognitive neuropsychological approach to assessment and intervention in aphasia. A Clinician's Guide. Hove and New York: Psychology Press; 2005.
13. Hillis AE. Aphasia: progress in the last quarter of a century. Neurology. 2007;69-200.
14. Lee A, Kannan V, Hillis AE. The contribution of neuroimaging to the study of language and aphasia. Neuropsychol Rev. 2006;16:171-83.
15. Hillari K, Byng S, Lamping DL, et al. Stroke and Aphasia Quality of life scale-39 (SAQOL-39). Evaluation of acceptability, reliability and validity. Stroke. 2003;34:1944–50.
16. Basso A. Aphasia and its therapy. New York: Oxford University Press; 2003. p. 262.
17. Kelly H, Brady MC, Enderby P. Speech and language therapy for aphasia following stroke. Cochrane Database Syst Rev. 2010;5:CD000425.

Chapter 12

Clinical Evaluation of Apraxia and Agnosia

Sireesha Yareeda, Archana Bethala, Suvarna Alladi

INTRODUCTION

Apraxia is classically defined as a "disorder of skilled movement not caused by weakness, akinesia, deafferentiation, abnormal tone or posture, movement disorders (such as tremor or chorea), intellectual deterioration, poor comprehension, or uncooperativeness."[1] However, to further simplify and apply the definition at the bedside, the following operational definition of apraxia has been proposed. It is the "failure to produce the correct movement in response to a verbal command, failure to imitate correctly a movement performed by the examiner, failure to perform a movement correctly in response to a seen object, or a failure to handle an object correctly."[2]

Based upon the above definition, the three main domains that form the principal defects of apraxia can be formulated. These essentially constitute the steps in evaluation of apraxia and include defects in (1) pantomiming an action in response to verbal command, (2) imitation of gestures, and (3) manipulation of tools and objects.[3] Apraxia predominantly involves manual tasks, i.e., the upper limbs but can also involve the legs, face, and the trunk. Even the axial muscles might be affected, but are less obvious because the tasks like bending the trunk or flexing the neck are less complex and have a greater degree of freedom than the fine distal hand movements. According to Liepmann, a pioneer in the concept of apraxia, patients cannot transform the image of intended action into appropriate motor command, and hence, apraxia is the disturbance at the interface between the cognition and the motor control.[4]

NEURAL SUBSTRATES FOR PRAXIS

An understanding of neural substrates for apraxia is essential in order to recognize the presence of apraxia in a patient, to localize pathology, to identify underlying etiology, and also to plan rehabilitative strategies. Praxis functions are distributed across several distinct anatomofunctional neural systems that work together and mainly involve the parietofrontal systems controlling reaching/grasping processes and the frontostriatal system controlling sequential motor acts.[5]

Studies in primates have identified segregated circuits that operate in parallel and suggest that sensorimotor transformation processes underlie praxis. The posterior parietal cortex plays a key role and consists of several functionally distinct areas. The superior parietal lobule has been found to be involved in somatosensory transformation of reaching movements, and the inferior parietal lobule (IPL), which is separated from the superior parietal lobule by the intraparietal sulcus is mainly involved with visuomotor transformation of grasping movements.[6] The superior parietal lobule guides tasks such as reaching, a proximal movement, thereby guiding to aim the movement toward a particular target or to move away from a target of no interest. It uses visual and somatosensory information for movement organization and projects predominantly to the dorsal premotor cortices and supplementary motor areas of the frontal cortex.[7] Studies in macaque monkeys reveal that the dorsal premotor cortex plays a role in trajectory planning and the supplementary motor area is involved in the postural adjustments that precede voluntary

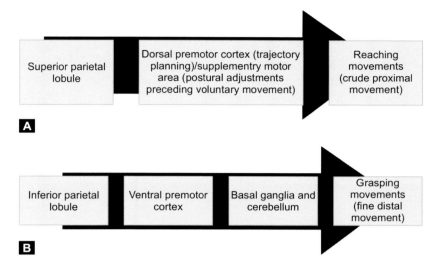

Figs 12.1A and B: (A) Dorsal parietofrontal network system for reaching; **(B)** Ventral parietofrontal network system and the frontostriatal system for grasping.

movements.[6] Similarly, the IPL is connected with the ventral premotor cortex and its connections with basal ganglia and cerebellum and is devoted to grasping and hand manipulation, which are distal actions (Figs 12.1A and B).

Functional brain imaging studies in humans also support the neurophysiological mechanisms of reaching and grasping, and substantiate the role of parietofrontal and subcortical structures in praxis. Lesion studies in patients further provide evidence for the underlying role of parietofrontal circuits in the process of praxis. Patients with lesions in parietal regions report apraxia of limb movements, in subjects with lesions in anterior lateral intraparietal sulcus demonstrating problems with grasping suggestive of a unimodal visuomotor deficit and those with left superior parietal lesions showing abnormal reaching movements. Patients with frontal lobe lesions involving mainly the premotor cortex were found to cause coordination impairment in reaching movements, abnormal sequencing, and deficits in conditioned learning.

Both right and left hemispheric lesions can cause apraxia in patients. In one study, 50% of patients with left hemispheric damage and <10% with right hemispheric damage were found to have apraxia.[8] Left-sided lesions affect the imitation of both single gestures or sequences, while patients with right-sided lesions can imitate single gestures normally but cannot imitate gesture sequences.[8] The other dissociation is that patients with left-sided lesions have difficulty with imitation of hand and foot posture while that of distal finger movements can be normal or minimally affected in contrary to right-sided lesions.[3]

TYPES OF APRAXIA

Apraxia is a defect in both spatial and temporal processing of a sequence of a motor act and consists of two important components, the conceptual system and the production system (Fig. 12.2).[5] Patients with ideational apraxia cannot sequence a multistep act to attain the target goal of action, whereas those with conceptual apraxia commit content errors with problems in manipulating with objects (object misknowledge).[9] The defects in the productive

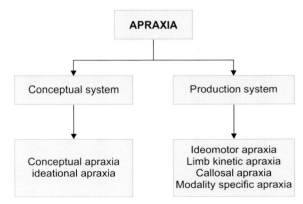

Fig. 12.2: Components of apraxia.

system are ideomotor and limb kinetic apraxia. Patients with ideomotor apraxia have temporal and spatial errors (Table 12.1), more so when performing with a tool, or performing transitive gestures. Limb kinetic apraxia is slowness, coarseness, or fragmentation of the movement that is seen predominantly in pyramidal weakness, but disproportionate to it, i.e., it cannot be explained by the pyramidal weakness alone.[10]

Ideational or Conceptual Apraxia

Ideational or conceptual apraxia occurs due to the defect in the conceptual system of the bimodal system of apraxia. The term ideational apraxia refers to the failure to sequence a series of acts leading to an action goal, and conceptual apraxia refers to loss of different types of tool object knowledge.[11] Patients with ideational apraxia make

TABLE 12.1: **Types of praxis errors**

	Description	Example
Temporal errors		
Sequencing errors	Sequence of steps to complete an action are disturbed with addition, deletion, transposition of a movement element	While mailing a letter, attempting to seal the envelope before inserting the letter into the envelope
Timing errors	The timing or speed of an action is disturbed. Movements are abnormally fast, slow, or irregular	Very fast application of soap over hands before washing away, on pantomiming to washing hands
Occurrence errors	Multiplication of single cycle or reduction of repetitive cycles to a single event	While unlocking the door, repeatedly rotating the key without releasing the lock
Spatial errors		
Amplitude errors	Increase, decrease, or irregularity of amplitude	Increase in the amplitude on pantomiming application of toothpaste over brush
Internal configuration errors	Discrepancy between the finger hand position to the target tool	While holding a glass of water, the subject may grasp his fist too tight with no space to accommodate the glass
External configuration errors	Errors in placing the object in space	While brushing teeth, the subject may hold the brush away from the mouth without gauging the distance necessary to accommodate the imagined object
Body part as object errors	Substituting finger, hand, or arm as the pretend object	Attempt to puff index finger in an attempt to smoke a cigarette
Movement errors	Discrepancy between the movement characteristic of the action	While driving a screw, the subject has to twist at the elbow, but instead of stabilizing the shoulder and wrist and twisting the elbow, the subject twists the shoulder or elbow and fixes the wrist and the intended action cannot be accomplished
Content errors		
Perservative errors	Repetition of all or part of previously produced pantomime	Following being asked how to brush, when the examiner asks to pantomime shaving, he continues to pantomime brushing
Related errors	Errors are related to the task	Playing guitar on asking the subject to pantomime playing veena
Non-related errors	Errors are unrelated to the content	On asking the subject to pantomime playing cricket, the subject pantomimes shaving
Concretization errors	Errors in using object that are not used for the task	On asking to pantomime sawing a log of wood, the subject pretends to saw his or her own leg
No response	Subject does not respond	On asking the subject to pantomime an action (e.g., to wave bye), the subject does not respond/becomes quiet
Unrecognizable response	Response of the subject cannot be recognized or classified	On asking the subject to pantomime an action (e.g., to comb hair) the subject's response is unidentifiable

errors in temporal and spatial sequencing of an act and fail to achieve an action goal. Omissions and confusions in sequencing a multistep task are noted.[12] Patients with conceptual apraxia (agnosia of utilization) have content errors in performing actions such as in tool selection errors or tool object knowledge.[10] They have preserved tool naming, which essentially rules out object agnosia. For instance, when asked to pantomime combing hair, the patient uses a toothbrush, as he has problems associating tools and objects with their corresponding action. He also loses the ability to associate a set of tools with his corresponding actions; for example, when a partially driven nail is shown to him, he could tend to use a scissors rather than a hammer from a tool kit to drive it further. Thus, these patients lose the mechanical knowledge or action semantics, i.e., the mechanical advantage offered by tools in day-to-day life.[5] The most frequent errors are those of omission (neglect to spread paste on the toothbrush before brushing), misuse (use a fork to drink soup), and misallocation (use a pen upside down to write).[8] Other errors include transpositions, additions, perseverations, and substitutions Table 12.1. However, this strict diversification into ideational and conceptual apraxia is not considered to be very purposeful, since errors in sequencing a task are often found to be associated with loss of mechanical knowledge. Ideational apraxia is uncommonly encountered in isolation; however, coexisting aphasia may frequently mask its presentation. Patients with lesions in the left parietotemporal, parietal, frontotemporal, frontal and basal ganglia have been described with this form of apraxia.

Ideomotor Apraxia

Ideomotor apraxia is a disturbance in programming the timing, sequencing and spatial organization of gestural movements.[11] Here the identification of the gesture and the discrimination of the gesture are intact (unlike the apraxia of the conceptual system) and thus is an error of the production system. Transitive pantomimes are more affected than intransitive ones, and acting with real objects is better performed than pantomiming their use. Actions improve with imitation rather than with acting to verbal commands, i.e., pantomime.[1,8] This is because acting with objects provides tactile and kinesthetic cues and helps the patient in performing the movement in a more natural context.[13] This is responsible for the so-called voluntary automatic dissociation, where they can perform their daily activities while being disproportionately disabled during examination.

Ideomotor apraxia usually results from lesions of the parietal association area, and less likely from lesions of the premotor and supplementary motor areas and the white matter bundles that connect the latter to subcortical structures. Heilman et al. and Rothi et al. suggested two forms of ideomotor apraxia: the posterior variant (parietal variant) where the movement formulae or the motor engrams of the IPL are lost and the anterior variant (disconnection variant) where the motor engrams are preserved.[14,15] Thus, patient with posterior variant cannot recognize gestures as the motor engrams are lost, while the anterior variant with ideomotor apraxia can identify the gestures well.

Callosal Apraxia

Patients with lesions involving either the genu or body of the corpus callosum have unilateral apraxia of the nondominant limb, termed as callosal apraxia. These patients are not able to pantomime to verbal commands with their left hand but could improve on imitation and object use.[2]

Limb Kinetic Apraxia/Innervatory Apraxia

In limb kinetic apraxia, the defect is proportional to the innervatory complexity and thereby affects the distal manipulative finger movements.[9] The movements become clumsy and the smoothness of the skill attained through years of practice is lost. For instance, the subject is unable to manipulate a scissors and shows complete failure to knot a thread. The deficit is consistent and does not exhibit the so-called voluntary automatic dissociation.

Orobuccal Apraxia

These patients cannot pretend or imitate facial movements such as blowing out a match or sucking through a straw, but they usually perform normally when presented with a real match or straw. The criteria for buccofacial apraxia include (1) the patient is not paralyzed for voluntary movements and (2) the patient has deficits specific to pretending and or imitating movements with the face,[16] and is served by the circuit originating from the insular or left inferior frontal cortex concerned with complex learned movements.

Several forms of dissociation are observed in apraxias. The term modality specific apraxia is used when there is dissociation between two sensory modalities. For example in verbal dissociation apraxia, there is a dissociation between language areas and movement formulae in IPL. However, the input can reach through other modalities like visual imitation or tactile inputs in the form of holding the object. The reverse is seen in visuoimitative apraxia or visual dissociation apraxia. These patients can pantomime to verbal commands or perform flawlessly under other modalities but cannot imitate an act by inputs from the visual modality.

EVALUATION OF LIMB PRAXIS

A systematic approach to the evaluation of apraxia is essential in order to recognize the presence of apraxia, to identify the type of apraxia and the nature of errors that occur, with an aim to establish the underlying disease process and neural mechanisms. A detailed evaluation is also required to institute appropriate rehabilitation strategies. Clinical evaluation using simple steps, adopting formal apraxia assessment batteries and the use of kinematics study have all been used to evaluate apraxia.

A wide range of movements are tested to evaluate apraxia. Figure 12.3 demonstrate the various steps involved in the comprehensive assessment of praxic functions. To test praxis production system, transitive gestures that involve the use of a real object and intransitive gestures that do not involve the use of objects are used. Gestures tested could be meaningful, i.e., representational and habitual, such as waving good bye, or thumbs up or meaningless, which are nonrepresentational and new to the patient such as wiggling one's fingers, or touching one's nose. Instructions to perform these gestures could be verbal (pantomime) or visual (imitative). In the case of transitive gestures, real objects could be used to test praxis. To test the praxis conceptual system, tasks that involve multiple tests such as preparing a letter for mailing are used. Further, ability of patient to select an appropriate tool to complete a task, such as a hammer for a nail and gesture recognition tasks that assess the capacity to comprehend gestures, by naming gestures performed by examiner, or match gestures performed by the examiner with the object or picture of the tool.[8,17] Limb kinetic movements can be tested by finger tapping, alternate touching each fingertip with thumb, or picking up a coin without sliding.

Among apraxia assessment batteries, the Florida Apraxia Battery-Extended and Revised Sydney (FABERS) score established inter-rater reliability for the qualitative pantomime expression scoring system, and provided

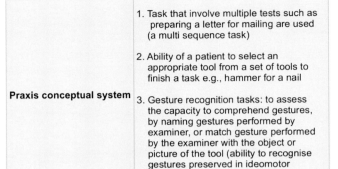

Praxis conceptual system

1. Task that involve multiple tests such as preparing a letter for mailing are used (a multi sequence task)
2. Ability of a patient to select an appropriate tool from a set of tools to finish a task e.g., hammer for a nail
3. Gesture recognition tasks: to assess the capacity to comprehend gestures, by naming gestures performed by examiner, or match gesture performed by the examiner with the object or picture of the tool (ability to recognise gestures preserved in ideomotor apraxia-anterior variant)

First test with the dominant hand and then the non dominant hand
Limb kinetic movements can be tested by finger tapping alternate touching each finger tip with thumb or picking up a coin without sliding

A

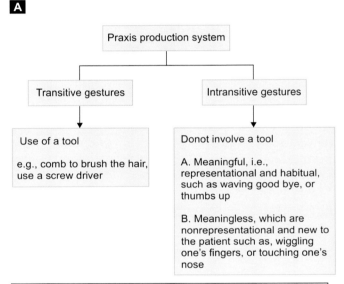

Praxis production system

Transitive gestures   Intransitive gestures

Use of a tool

e.g., comb to brush the hair, use a screw driver

Donot involve a tool

A. Meaningful, i.e., representational and habitual, such as waving good bye, or thumbs up

B. Meaningless, which are nonrepresentational and new to the patient such as, wiggling one's fingers, or touching one's nose

These instructions can be verbal (pantomime) or visual (imitative)

B

Figs 12.3A and B: (A) Steps involved in the evaluation of the praxis conceptual system; **(B)** Steps involved in the evaluation of the praxis production system.

control comparison scores for healthy elderly controls across the battery. It allows comparison across different FABERS scores within an individual, identifying their strengths and weaknesses in different aspects of praxis systems. It is mainly used as a valuable research tool.[18]

ETIOLOGICAL CONSIDERATIONS

Several diseases may present with apraxia. In clinical practice, corticobasal degeneration (CBD) and stroke are most common. The other diseases that manifest apraxia include movement disorders like progressive supranuclear palsy (PSP) atypical variants of Alzheimer's disease, frontotemporal dementia syndromes, motoneuron disease with dementia and Creutzfeldt–Jakob disease (Table 12.2). It is the anatomical location of the pathology rather than the nature of the pathology that determines the occurrence of apraxia.

APRAXIA IN CORTICOBASAL DEGENERATION

Corticobasal degeneration is an asymmetric akinetic-rigid syndrome, with majority of affected individuals demonstrating ideomotor apraxia, while few have orofacial apraxia. Forty percent of patients present with apraxia at disease onset, and 72% develop apraxia later in the course of disease.[19] Patients with CBD present with ideomotor apraxia, though they can have a combination of ideomotor and limb kinetic apraxia. Patients are found to have bilateral deficits with preserved asymmetry (Case study 1). Corticobasal degeneration is

TABLE 12.2: **Etiology of apraxia**

Vascular	Stroke
Degenerative	• Corticobasal degeneration • Alzheimer's disease • Posterior cortical atrophy • Primary progressive aphasia • Creutzfeldt–Jacob disease • Huntington's disease
Structural	• Tumors • Lymphoma • AV malformations
Trauma	Diffuse axonal injury
Demyelination	• Multiple sclerosis • Acute demyelinating encephalomyelitis
Infective	• Tuberculoma • Cysticercosis • Brain abscess • Fungal mass

---

CASE STUDY 1

Corticobasal Degeneration

A 67-year-old advocate presented with a history of difficulty in using his right hand and word finding difficulties since 2 years. He initially complained of clumsiness of his right hand with difficulty in handling common household objects, and 6 months later, he noticed progressive difficulty in using his right hand for eating and dressing. These problems started off very gradually, but were getting worse with time. Since 1 year, he developed stiffness of the right arm, and was noticed to be holding it in an awkward position while walking. He also noticed that he had difficulty in preparing for complex arguments while discussing legal cases, along with a mild word finding difficulty. There was no history of memory, visuospatial, or behavioral disturbances. There was no history suggestive of tremors or gait disturbances.

On cognitive assessment, he was oriented to time and place with normal attention span. Recent and remote episodic memories were normal; fluencies were reduced. He performed normally on visuoperceptual tasks and executive function tests. He had slow and monotonous speech, mild slowing of both horizontal and vertical saccades and mild generalized bradykinesia, along with rigidity of right upper limb without evidence of cortical sensory loss.

On apraxia testing, he could not pantomime to verbal commands in terms of both transitive and intransitive actions. He failed to recognize gestures and lost the sequence of action when given a multisequence task with temporal and spatial errors. He could not associate the tools with their corresponding action when showing the pictures of action. MRI brain showed asymmetric frontoparietal atrophy affecting the motor and sensory cortex, and 18 FDG-PET CT scan showed asymmetric hypoactivity in the frontal and parietal regions and the thalamus, predominantly on the left side (Fig. 12.4). Patient was diagnosed to have CBD based on his clinical and imaging features.

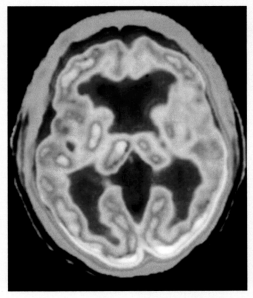

Fig. 12.4: PET-CT scan showing asymmetric hypoactivity in the frontal and parietal regions and thalamus, predominantly in the left side in corticobasal degeneration.

characterized by involvement of the frontoparietal and frontostriatal networks that underlie praxis. Patients with CBD can sometimes function normally with relatively preserved activities of daily living by the aid of tactile cues by manipulating the actual object or visual cues by the target of action. It is proposed that the lack of sensory inputs due to cortical sensory loss could also impede motor functioning and this could be mitigated by providing visual information.[20] Patients with posterior cortical atrophy have evidence of complex visual disorder on examination, visuo-spatial and visuo-perceptual disturbances and apraxia with mild memory disturbances (Case study 2).[21]

APRAXIA IN STROKE

Apraxia occurs in 50–80% of patients with left hemispheric stroke and can persist as a chronic deficit in 40–50%. In majority of the patients with left hemispheric lesions, the presence of coexisting aphasia masks the apraxia that can be mistaken as a comprehension deficit. Similarly, the coexisting right hemiparesis masks the right limb apraxia. Sometimes the normal nondominant hand clumsiness masks the presence of left-limb apraxia. Patients with stroke who have distal impairment have involvement of the contralateral limb alone (Case study 3), unlike in CBD, and the type of apraxia is innervatory apraxia or limb kinetic apraxia.

AGNOSIA

Agnosia is the term used to refer to a disorder of recognition. Sigmund Freud originally used the term agnosia in 1891 to denote disturbances in the ability to recognize and name objects in one sensory modality in the presence of intact primary sensation. Milner and Teuber in 1968, subsequently defined agnosia as a "normal percept stripped of its meaning."[22]

Agnosia is clinically diagnosed when there is (1) failure to recognize an object, (2) normal perception of the object, excluding an primary sensory disorder, (3) ability to name the object once it is recognized, excluding anomia as the principal deficit, and (4) absence of a generalized dementia. Agnosias are classified based on the specific sensory modality affected—visual, auditory, or tactile—or based on one class of items within a sensory modality, such as color agnosia, or prosopagnosia (agnosia for faces). For example, a patient with visual agnosia may fail to identify a bell by sight but readily identifies it by touch or by the sound of its ring.

VISUAL AGNOSIA

Visual agnosia is the inability to recognize or identify objects visually, despite intact visual function, and despite knowing the object previously.[23,24] Patients can neither name the object, nor produce any information about it. In

---

CASE STUDY 2

Posterior Cortical Atrophy

A 58-year-old lady presented with complaints of visuospatial and memory disturbances of 2 years duration. She had difficulties in stepping up and down the stairs, problems in driving, especially while reversing and judging distances. She had problems in cooking and was not orienting vessels properly over the stove nor placing telephone receiver properly over the cradle. In addition, she had dressing difficulties and memory disturbances. Previously alert and fast in calculations, she was unable to handle money correctly. Her language functions were relatively preserved and she had no behavioral changes.

On examination, her mini-mental state examination (MMSE) score was 13/30 and Addenbrooke's Cognitive Examination-Revised (ACE-R) score was 62/100. She had predominant visuospatial deficits, with construction difficulty and was unable to read fragmented letters. She could count dots only in one block out of four of the ACE-R presented to her. She had problems in recall of words and a newly learnt address. Her remote memory was relatively preserved and she had no behavioral disturbances. On testing for apraxia, she could not pantomime to verbal commands nor imitate gestures with both hands, with a lot of errors of omission and substitutions. She could not recognize the gestures either, and she got confused with the sequence of actions in a complicated task, for example, when she was asked to show how she would mail a letter. She was slightly better when the tool of action was given to her. She did not show any evidence of neglect. Her MRI showed evidence of bilateral parietal and temporal atrophy and 18 FDG-PET scan showed evidence of bilateral parietal, occipital, and temporal hypometabolism (Figs 12.5) consistent with the diagnosis of posterior cortical atrophy, a variant of Alzheimer's disease.

Continued

Continued

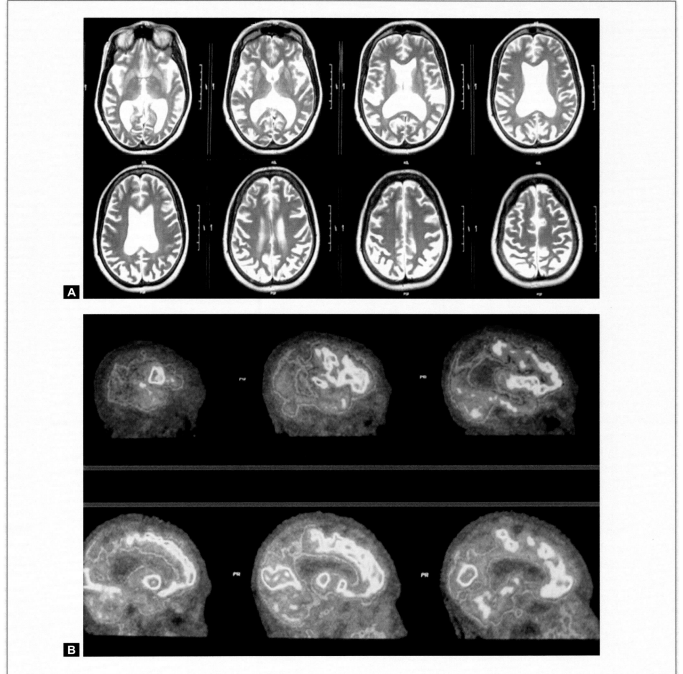

Figs 12.5A and B: (A) MRI of brain showing symmetrical atrophy in posterior cortical region; **(B)** PET-CT scan of brain showing hypometabolism in bilateral parieto-occipital regions.

CASE STUDY 3

Stroke with Apraxia

A 69-year-old gentleman who was a known hypertensive since 15 years, presented with sudden onset mild weakness of right upper limb and lower limb. He had pronator drift of the right upper limb that improved. There was no weakness of hand grip. On clinical examination, power of the intrinsic muscles of the hand was also normal. Gradually, the attendants started noticing that he had clumsiness in using both his hands. He had difficulty in holding objects, attempting to hold them awkwardly. He was unable to grasp a glass of water and attempted to place his palm incongruous to the shape of the glass, and was unable to manipulate the fingers for a grip. He could not hold a toothbrush nor a comb, asking for the help. He had no speech problems, visual or memory disturbances. His cognitive assessment revealed normal attention, memory, language, visuospatial, and executive functions.

On testing for apraxia, he could not pantomime to verbal commands for both transitive and intransitive actions with the right hand. He could not imitate the victory sign nor a salute. His gestural knowledge appeared intact and he could identify all the actions shown as pictures to him. He could describe verbally, all the events in a sequential action like ploughing the field and sowing seeds, but was clumsy and hesitant while demonstrating the actions. He could not count his fingers nor flip a coin, and this did not improve on giving him a real object (coin). CT brain revealed left and posterior parietal infarcts consistent with the diagnosis of stroke with apraxia (Fig. 12.6).

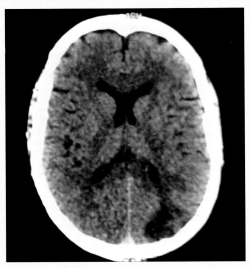

Fig. 12.6: CT scan of brain showing infarcts in left parieto-occipital region.

some cases, it is thought to be a perceptual dysfunction, while in others it seems to be a problem associating what is seen with what is known from the past.

Visual agnosias are classified further into apperceptive and associative agnosia.[25] This distinction is based on two criteria: (1) whether patients can copy drawings and (2) whether they can match simple shapes. Failure on either of these tasks would point to an apperceptive defect. In apperceptive visual agnosia, a defect is thought to be at high level perception and is encountered usually with bilateral occipitotemporal infarction. In associative visual agnosia, high-level perception is preserved but the percept is unable to associate semantic information and is generally associated with lesions located in the anterior left temporal lobe.

Object perception defects involve several types of apperceptive visual agnosia (shape or visual form or integrative agnosias). Integrative visual agnosia can be detected by testing with Escher drawings, in which patient may not appreciate the falsity of objects clubbed together. These patients usually have bilateral peristriate occipital infarcts or posterior cortical atrophy. Associative visual agnosia is divided into semantic access agnosia, the inability to access intact memories (or stored representations) of objects, and semantic agnosia,

in which those memory representations have been destroyed.[26,27] The distinction can be made by probing verbally what a patient remembers about objects. Another classification for associative visual agnosia is based on whether patient can describe the appearance of the object (structural description) or can pantomime its use (semantic knowledge of function, habitat). Related to this concept is the distinction between living and nonliving things. Recognition of living things is more severely affected compared to the nonliving things because they are remembered by their function not by their structure.[28] Associative agnosia and semantic access deficits may be more prominent with left occipital damage that involves the parahippocampal, fusiform, and lingual gyri (Brodmann areas 18, 19, and 37).

Achromatopsia refers to a loss of the ability to perceive colors, described by the subject as watching black-and-white television. It results from lesions affecting the medial occipitotemporal region (fusiform gyri). Color agnosia refers to a loss of semantic knowledge of colors. Patients cannot identify colors, or color line drawings appropriately or tell whether drawings have been colored by others correctly. In shape agnosia or visual form agnosia, patients have trouble seeing shapes because of a defect in perceiving curvature, surface, and volume.[29,30] Selective impairment of motion perception is associated with damage to areas of extrastriate visual cortex, usually the dorsal stream involvement and these patients have difficulties in judging the speed and direction of cars. Simultanagnosia is the inability to comprehend a complex scene in its entirety—that is, only one component of the scene is perceived at a time. Topographagnosia is a disorder in which a person gets lost in familiar surroundings that can be due to deficits in visual association cortices.

ASSESSMENT OF VISUAL AGNOSIA

Bedside tests include recognizing and naming the objects, pointing to objects shown and the ability to provide semantic information about unnamed items, drawing object on command and copying a drawing. Patient can be asked to see an object and mime its use. Further testing is done by overlapping line drawings, partially degraded or fragmented images, judgment of line orientation, face analysis, and matching from different angles. Other tests include recognizing and naming colors separately, telling color of familiar objects, grouping objects according to their color.

AUDITORY AGNOSIA

Auditory agnosia refers to defective recognition of auditory stimuli in the context of normal hearing. Patient is unable to understand the meaning of sounds despite hearing the sounds. Most cortical auditory deficits require bilateral cerebral lesions, involving the temporal lobes, especially the primary auditory cortices in the Heschl gyri. Auditory agnosias are classified into pure word deafness, pure auditory nonverbal agnosia, phonagnosia, and pure amusia.[31] Pure word deafness involves an inability to comprehend spoken words, with preserved ability to hear and recognize nonverbal sounds and usually occurs while recovering from cortical deafness. Auditory nonverbal agnosia refers to patients who have lost the ability to identify meaningful nonverbal sounds but have preserved pure tone hearing and language comprehension. Phonagnosia is analogous to prosopagnosia in the visual modality. Amusia is a music-specific auditory agnosia usually due to right temporal lobe involvement.[32]

TACTILE AGNOSIA

Tactile agnosia is an inability to recognize the object by touch, but the patient is able to do so when accessed through other modalities such as vision in presence of normal primary sensation. It usually results from unilateral parietal cortical lesion. Apperceptive tactile agnosia is difficult to distinguish from astereognosis. Tactile aphasia is an inability to name a palpated object despite intact recognition of the object and intact naming when the object is presented in another sensory modality.

AGNOSIAS IN NEUROLOGICAL DISEASES

Several neurological disorders present with agnosias. Agnosias frequently result from bilateral or diffuse lesions such as hypoxic encephalopathy, multiple strokes, major head injuries and neurodegenerative disorders like dementias. Stroke involving bilateral occipitotemporal areas as a result of basilar artery occlusion, as in Balint's syndrome leads to simultagnosia. Involvement of right parietal cortex in middle cerebral artery territory infarcts results in apperceptive visual agnosia. Most cases of associative visual agnosia have involved the fusiform or occipitotemporal gyri bilaterally.

Agnosias are also prevalent in degenerative disorders, often in early stage of the illness when general cognitive abilities are relatively preserved. Posterior cortical atrophy (a variant of Alzheimer's disease) presents with a progressive decline in complex visual processing and relative sparing of other cognitive domains. It is associated with occipitoparietal atrophy and hypometabolism on positron emission tomography (PET) scans. Patients with this syndrome show a high rate of alexia without oral language difficulty (80%), Balint's syndrome (68%), and apperceptive visual agnosia (44%).[33]

Progressive prosopagnosia is a degenerative disorder presenting with progressive impairment in the recognition of faces, and occurs as a part of the frontotemporal dementias.[34,35] There is prominent atrophy in the right temporal lobe. Schizophrenia is usually associated with associative visual agnosia[36] and a specific impairment to memorizing faces. This deficit is highly correlated with a reduction in the volume of the fusiform gyrus.

REFERENCES

1. Heilman KM, Rothi LJG. Apraxia. In: Heilman KM, Valenstein E (Eds). Clinical Neuropsychology. New York: Oxford University Press; 1985. pp. 131-50.
2. Geschwind N, Damasio AR. Apraxia. In: Vinken PJ, Bruyn GW, K Lawans HL (Eds). Handbook of Clinical Neurology. Amsterdam: Elsevier; 1985. pp. 423-32.
3. Goldenberg G. Matching and imitation of hand and finger postures in patients with damage in the left or right hemispheres. Neuropsychologia. 1999;37:559-66.

4. Liepmann H. Apraxie. Ergebn ges Med. 1920;1:516-43.

5. Leiguarda RC, Marsden CD. Limb apraxias: higher order disorder of sensor motor integration. Brain. 2000;123:860-79.

6. Rizzolatti G, Luppino G, Matelli M. The organisation of the cortical motor system: new concepts. Electroencephalogr Clin Neurophysiol. 1998;106: 283-96.

7. Kalaska JF, Scott SH, Cisek P, et al. Cortical control of reaching movements. Curr Opin Neurobiol. 1997;7:849-59.

8. De Renzi E. Apraxia. In: Boller F, Grafman J (Eds). Handbook of Neuropsychology, Vol. 2. Amsterdam: Elsevier; 1989. pp. 245-63.

9. Kleist K. Kortikale (innervatorische) Apraxie. J Psychiat Neurol. 1907;28: 46-112.

10. Mendez MF, Po heng Tsai. Limb apraxia and related disorders. In: Daroff RB, Fenichel GM, Jankovic J, Mazziotta JC (Eds). Bradley's Neurology in Clinical Practice. Philadelphia: Elsevier; 2012. pp.118-23.

11. Rothi LJG, Ochipa C, Heilman KM. A cognitive neuropsychological model of limb praxis. Cognit Neuropsychol. 1991;8:443-58.

12. Poeck K, Lehmkuhl G. Das Syndrom der ideatorischen Apraxie und seine Lokalisation. Nervenarzt. 1980;51:217-25.

13. Frank JS, Earl M. Coordination of posture and movement. Phys Ther. 1990;70:855-63.

14. Heilman KM, Rothi LJ, Valenstein E. Two forms of ideomotor apraxia. Neurology. 1982;32:342-46.

15. Rothi LJ, Heilman KM, Watson RT. Pantomime comprehension and ideomotor apraxia. J Neurol Neurosurg Psychiatry. 1985;48:207-10.

16. Woolley JD. Buccofacial apraxia and the expression of emotion. Ann NY Acad Sci. 2003;1000:395-401.

17. Rothi LJ, Heilman KM. Apraxia: the neuropsychology of action. Hove (UK): Psychology Press; 1997. pp. 7-18.

18. Power E, Code C, Croot K, Sheard C, et al. Florida Apraxia Battery-Extended and Revised Sydney (FABERS): design, description, and a healthy control sample. J Clin Exp Neuropsychol. 2010;32:1-18.

19. Murray R, Neumann M, Forman MS, et al. Cognitive and motor assessment in autopsy-proven corticobasal degeneration. Neurology. 2007;68:1274-83.

20. Jacobs DH, Adair JC, Macauley B, et al. Apraxia in corticobasal degeneration. Brain Cogn. 1999;40:336-54.

21. Alladi S, Xuereb J, Bak T,et al. Focal cortical presentations of Alzheimer's disease. Brain. 2007;130;2636-45.

22. Teuber HL. Alteration of perception and memory in man. In: Weiskrantz L (Ed). Analysis of Behavioral Change. New York: Harper and Row; 1968.

23. Farah MJ. Visual Agnosia: Disorders of visual recognition and what they tell us about normal vision. Cambridge, MA: MIT Press; 1990.

24. Riddoch M, Humphreys G. Visual agnosia. Neurol Clin. 2003;21:501-20.

25. Lissauer H. Ein fall von seelenblindheit nebst einem beitrag zur theorie derselben. Arch fur Psychiatrie. 1890;21:222-70.

26. Farah MJ. Visual agnosia: once more, with theory. Cogn Neuropsychol. 1988;5:337-46.

27. Riddoch M, Humphreys G. A case of integrative agnosia. Brain. 1987;110: 1431-62.

28. Warrington EK, Shallice T. Category specific semantic impairments. Brain. 1984;107:829-54.

29. Miceli G, Fouch E, Capasso R, et al. The dissociation of color from form and function knowledge. Nat Neurosci. 2001;4:662-7.

30. Humphreys GW, Riddoch MJ. To see but not to see: a case study of visual agnosia. New Jersey: Lawrence Erlbaum;1987.

31. Zatorre RJ, Evans AC, Meyer E, et al. Lateralization of phonetic and pitch discrimination in speech processing. Science. 1992;256:846-9.

32. Mazzucchi A, Marchini C, Budai R, et al. A case of receptive amusia with prominent timbre perception defect. J Neurol Neurosurg Psychiatry. 1982; 45:644-7.

33. Mendez MF, Ghajarania M, Perryman KM. Posterior cortical atrophy: clinical characteristics and differences compared to Alzheimer's disease. Dement Geriatr Cogn Disord. 2002;14:33-40.

34. Evans JJ, Heggs AJ, Auton N, et al. Progressive prosopagnosia associated with selective right temporal lobe atrophy. A new syndrome? Brain. 1995; 118:1-13.

35. Hodges JR. Frontotemporal dementia (Pick's disease): clinical features and assessment. Neurology. 2001;56:S6-10.

36. Gabrovska VS, Laws KR, Sinclair J, et al. Visual object processing in schizophrenia: evidence for an associative agnosic deficit. Schizophr Res. 2003;59:277-86.

Chapter 13

Dementia: Clinical Approach

Suvarna Alladi, Pavan K Cherukuri, Divyaraj Gollahalli

INTRODUCTION

A number of neurological disorders affect cognition and behavior and manifest as dementia syndromes. The prevalence of dementia increases from 5% among 71 to 79-year-olds to 36.1% in those 90 years and older.[1] Further, it is estimated that most people with dementia live in developing countries.[2] This rapid increase in the societal burden of dementia is reflected in the rising numbers encountered in clinical practice. The phenomenon of demographic transition in India that has resulted in increased life expectancy, as well as urbanization and lifestyle factors are thought to underlie the increasing numbers of dementia patients.[3–5]

A range of neurological disorders cause cognitive decline and dementia and different dementia syndromes present differently to the clinician. A rational approach to diagnosis requires the identification of a pattern of cognitive deficits using appropriate tools to localize the pathology and the efficient use of investigations to determine the underlying etiology. Cognitive and behavioral disturbances are a cause of distress to patients and their families, but are often under-recognized during clinical evaluation and management. A specific and early diagnosis of dementia and its functional impact on the patient and her/his family is vital for planning and instituting treatment.

DEFINITION OF DEMENTIA

Dementia refers to impairment of multiple cognitive domains (attention, memory, executive functioning, language, visuospatial domains, etc.) that is sufficient to interfere with social and occupational functioning. Other mental functioning like mood, personality, judgment, and social behavior can also be affected. The disorder can be progressive or static, permanent, or reversible.[6] According to Diagnostic and Statistical Manual of Mental Disorders IV (DSM-IV), dementia syndromes are characterized by the development of multiple cognitive deficits (including memory impairment) that are due to the direct physiological effects of a general medical condition, to the persisting effects of a substance, or to multiple etiologies (e.g., combined effects of cerebrovascular disease and Alzheimer's disease). The essential features for the diagnosis of dementia include memory impairment and any one cognitive disturbance such as aphasia, apraxia, agnosia, or disturbance in executive functioning. More recently, in the Diagnostic and Statistical Manual of Mental Disorders 5 (DSM-5), the diagnosis of dementia is subsumed under the entity major neurocognitive disorder. DSM-5 also recognizes a less severe level of cognitive impairment, mild neurocognitive disorder, which is a new disorder that permits the diagnosis of less disabling syndromes that may nonetheless be the focus of concern and treatment.

CLINICAL APPROACH TO DEMENTIA

The aims of clinical evaluation of dementia are to detect the presence of dementia as early as possible, to determine the specific cause of dementia, to establish its severity, to identify potentially reversible causes, and to treat all other causes with the intention to optimize functioning of the patient and alleviate burden of the caregivers.

HISTORY TAKING IN DEMENTIA

Patients present to the clinic with complaints of forgetting events, conversations, names of familiar people, forgetting routes, repeatedly saying the same thing or asking the same questions, misplacing objects, delusions, hallucinations, personality changes, and behavioral disturbances. Evaluation begins by taking the demographic details and history from the caregiver and the patient separately. Information from a reliable caregiver is important as often an accurate history cannot be obtained from the subject, given the nature of the disease. The history and examination should be conducted in a quiet place without any distractions and adequate time needs to be devoted. The onset, symptoms, and duration of the symptoms are noted which help the clinician diagnose the type of dementia.

Memory loss manifests as forgetting appointments, difficulty in recalling recent events or conversations. Dementia can manifest as visuospatial disturbances or language abnormalities too. Patients with language disturbances have difficulty in speaking and forget the name of common, well-known objects, use inappropriate words, and repeat words and catch phrases. Patients can get disorientated in less familiar places, not know the time of the day or the date, and misidentify family and friends.

Behavioral disturbances and personality changes are common. Symptoms like wandering, disinhibition, and agitation make it very difficult for the caregiver to handle the patient. Patients may show personality changes in some forms of dementia such as frontotemporal dementia (FTD) that manifest as overfamiliarity with strangers, saying embarrassing things, becoming less caring, or more aggressive. Neuropsychiatric symptoms often co-occur with dementia. Paranoid ideation, hallucinations mostly visual and delusional thinking can occur in dementia. Mood disturbances such as depression and euphoria without reason can also be seen. Sleep and appetite disturbances, anxiety and irritability are other common features. History taking involves eliciting symptoms in various domains that will aid in the diagnosis of dementia (Box 13.1).

COGNITIVE ASSESSMENT IN DEMENTIA

A good cognitive evaluation is based on history from the patient and a reliable informant, response of patient to conversational clues and formal cognitive testing. Since, time is always an issue in busy clinics, a clear focus is required early in the evaluation. Diagnosis of cognitive

Box 13.1: Domain screening in dementia

The following are details from some of the domains that will aid in the diagnosis of dementia.

Memory
1. Does one have difficulty remembering recent events (e.g., attending a wedding and meeting guests)?
2. Is one repeating the same thing again and again?
3. Does one misplace things and keeps searching for them?

Language
1. Does one have difficulty in naming?
2. Can one read/write/speak in sentences?
3. Does one understand what is being said to them?
4. Does one substitute wrong words?

Orientation
1. Does one know what time, date, month, and year it is?
2. Does one know which place, city, and state one is in?

Visuospatial
1. Does one misplace objects and search for them?
2. Does one lose their way?

Calculation
1. Does one handle money appropriately (get change back correctly)?

Agnosia
1. Does one have difficulty in recognizing people or objects?

Apraxia
1. Does one find it difficult to use one or both hands?
2. Can one do "namaskaaram," combing, cutting?

Neglect
1. Does one respond correctly to people and objects on both sides?
2. Is one unaware of the sensory stimuli on any one side of the body?
3. Can one copy both sides of the pictures?

Social cognition
1. Does one show concern for other people?
2. Does one can take other people's perspective while taking decisions?
3. Does one behave appropriately at social gatherings?
4. Can one differentiate between sarcasm and appreciation?
5. Can one understand the emotional state of others?

Basic activities of daily living
1. Does one need help with eating, dressing, bathing, hygiene, brushing, etc.?
2. Instrumental activities of daily living
3. Is one still able to function independently in one's job, shopping, business, and financial affairs, make/receive a telephone call, volunteer, and social groups?
4. Does one can stay safely at home?

TABLE 13.1: **Basic clinic assessment and neuropsychological tests for each cognitive domain**

Cognitive feature	Means of assessment	Neuropsychological test
Attention	Digit span forward	Digit span test
Memory		
Working memory	• Digit span backward	• Digit span test
Episodic memory	• Delayed recall of a newly learned material	• Auditory verbal learning test
Semantic memory	• Naming, category fluency	• Cambridge semantic battery
Orientation	Time, location, autobiographical data	Temporal orientation test
Language	• Naming • Fluency (e.g., animals and grocery items) • Repetition (sentences of varying length) • Comprehension (yes-or-no questions; performing multistep tasks) • Reading aloud • Sentence writing (spontaneous, to dictation)	• Boston naming test • Category fluency test • Sentence repetition • Token test
Visuospatial	• Figure copying (two- and three-dimensional figures) • Visual scene analysis (describe whole and individual parts)	Complex figure test
Neglect	• Line bisection (place "X" in center of a line) • Clock drawing (draw clock face with hands set to "10 after 11")	Line bisection test
Praxis	Have patient demonstrate saluting a flag, hammering a nail, demonstrating namaskaram, combing	Florida apraxia screening test–revised
Abstract thinking	Similarities (rose/lotus, poem/statue); proverb interpretation	• Similarity test • Proverb test
Sequencing	• Graphomotor sequencing (have patient draw a simple alternating pattern) • Luria gestures (sequentially alternating fist, side, palm)	Letter number sequencing (WAIS-IV)
Visuoperceptual	Perception of stimulus on field Recognizing fragmented objects/letters	Visual object and space perception test

disorders and identifying pattern of cognitive deficits require availability of user-friendly cognitive tests that can be used in the clinic that are appropriate for local use (Table 13.1). Typically, detection of cognitive impairment rests on comparison of performance with "normal cutoffs" derived from tests on age, gender, and education-matched controls. Availability of cognitive tests that are adapted and validated for use in each of the local context, the different languages spoken by patients in most urban settings, heterogeneity in educational status and cultures, and variability in social setting are some of the issues that have to be taken into account while evaluating patients for the presence of cognitive impairment, and determining its severity. Several standard cognitive screening instruments and neuropsychological test batteries have been successfully adapted and are available for use in the Indian population.[7-11] While assessing illiterates, cognitive tests need to be adapted for illiteracy to diagnose dementia in this large subgroup and education stratified scores need to be used for meaningful comparisons.[8,12]

A brief global cognitive screening scale has to be done in all cases. In the Indian context, the Mini-Mental State Examination (MMSE), the Addenbrooke's Cognitive Examination, and its revised versions are used in clinical practice.[7,8] Hindi Mental State Examination is also used for illiterate population.[12] Montreal Cognitive Assessment (MoCA) is another cognitive test that can be easily used in a busy neurology clinics.[13] Subsequent to this, each cognitive domain is assessed individually. Detailed neuropsychological tests for attention, verbal and visual memory, praxis, language, executive and visuospatial functioning can selectively be used for further evaluation. In selected cases where FTD is suspected, social cognition tests that assess theory of mind, emotion recognition, and empathy can be used. This will guide the physician in differential diagnosis of dementia.[14]

FUNCTIONAL ACTIVITIES

The diagnosis of dementia rests on establishing the subject's impairment in performing activities of daily living. If the subject is still working, there may be difficulties in job performance. There may also be changes in social functioning involving maintaining social relationships and engaging in hobbies. Difficulty can be seen in performing instrumental activities and later activities of daily living. Therefore, a prior level of functioning before onset of illness needs to be assessed. This will help identify the debilitating effects of the disease. Disability assessment for dementia is a measure of functional disability that assesses basic, instrumental and leisure activities, initiation, planning and organization, and effective performance.[15] It is administered through an interview with the caregiver and higher scores represent less disability in activities of daily living. Clinical Dementia Rating (CDR) is a widely used scale to assess the severity of dementia.[16] Caregiver burden, depression, anxiety, and stress also has to be assessed for a comprehensive evaluation of the patient and caregiver unit and also to plan management. This can be done with the help of questionnaires such as Depression Anxiety Stress Scale.[17]

INVESTIGATIVE APPROACH TO DEMENTIA

One of the main aims of investigating patients with dementia is to identify the underlying cause of dementia. The treating doctor must be cautious to avoid missing a reversible or a treatable cause. The American Academy of Neurology recommends the routine measurement of thyroid function, a vitamin B12 level, and a neuroimaging study [computed tomography (CT) or magnetic resonance imaging (MRI)][18] besides the identification of the typical clinical syndrome. The exclusion of reversible and secondary causes of dementia is done by conducting the following tests: complete blood cell count, electrolytes, glucose, blood urea nitrogen, liver function tests, and creatinine. In selected patients, cerebrospinal analysis may be useful in the diagnosis. Cerebrospinal fluid (CSF) studies are indicated in suspected central nervous system infection, reactive serum syphilis serology, when metastatic cancer is suspected, in subjects aged <55 years, in rapidly progressive or unusual dementia syndromes, in immunosuppression, in suspected CNS vasculitis, and in hydrocephalus. Cerebrospinal fluid opening pressure, cell count, and protein and glucose concentrations are normal in neurodegenerative dementias. Other CSF tests that could be considered in diagnostically challenging cases where a diagnosis of Alzheimer's disease dementia (AD dementia) is possible yet not certain include CSF β-amyloid and tau or phospshorylated tau that are currently performed only in research settings. Low CSF β-amyloid (Aβ1-42) coupled with elevated tau or phosphotau increases the likelihood that the patient has AD-type pathology.

Neuroimaging studies such as MRI and CT scan are useful in evaluating patients with dementia.[18] Magnetic resonance imaging is more sensitive than CT scan, and neuroimaging studies help to rule out primary and metastatic neoplasms, infarction, detect subdural hematomas, normal pressure hydrocephalus, or diffuse white matter disease. The degree of atrophy or volume loss on MRI correlates somewhat with the rate and degree of cognitive impairment and the amount of pathological changes at the autopsy. AD dementia is associated with hippocampal atrophy in addition to posterior-predominant cortical atrophy. Focal frontal and/anterior temporal atrophy suggests FTD. Dementia with Lewy bodies (DLB) often features less prominent atrophy, with greater involvement of amygdala than hippocampus. On positron emission tomography (PET) scan, decrease in glucose metabolism can predict dementia in early stages. Single-photon emission computed tomography (SPECT) and PET scanning show temporal and parietal hypoperfusion or hypometabolism in AD dementia and frontotemporal deficits in FTD. Autoimmune encephalitis can be diagnosed by performing autoimmune antibody tests using laboratory-standardized assays that measure anti-Hu, anti-Yo, anti-NMDA (N-methyl-D-aspartate), and anti-VGKC (voltage gated potassium channels) antibodies.

Other investigations that are useful in special conditions are electroencephalogram (EEG), parathyroid hormone estimation, tests for adrenal function, urine for heavy metals, and in selected cases genetic studies and brain biopsy. Electroencephalogram is helpful in certain conditions, e.g., Creutzfeldt–Jakob disease (CJD) (repetitive bursts of diffuse high-amplitude sharp waves, or "periodic complexes") or an underlying nonconvulsive seizure disorder (epileptiform discharges). Brain biopsy, including meninges is done only in certain conditions, e.g., to diagnose vasculitis, potentially treatable neoplasms, or unusual infections. Genetic studies are indicated in familial dementia syndromes but are not widely available and should be done only with the support of genetic counseling.

CLINICAL SUBTYPES OF DEMENTIA

Alzheimer's disease dementia (AD dementia) constitutes the largest proportion of dementias in clinical practice. Other degenerative dementias such as frontotemporal dementia (FTD) syndromes and DLB are also frequently diagnosed[19,20] (Table 13.2). The increasing burden of cardiovascular risk factors such as hypertension, diabetes, obesity, smoking, alcoholism, and stroke have resulted in large numbers of patients with vascular dementia (VaD).[21] In several cases, the etiology may be mixed, with AD and other neurodegenerative dementias and cerebrovascular disease co-occurring in the same patient.

Other neurological diseases such as head injuries, viral encephalitis, chronic infections, multiple sclerosis, and epilepsy are also associated with impairment of intellectual function and behavioral disturbances. A significant proportion of patients with brain tumors also have cognitive decline.[22] Metabolic disturbances also cause cognitive impairment and can present as dementia to the practitioner. Normal pressure hydrocephalus is a cause of dementia that requires careful investigation for proper management. Recently, autoimmune encephalitis is increasingly being recognized as an important cause of cognitive decline in clinical practice. The relative proportions of these different dementia subtypes in a clinic population are variable and are likely to be impacted by several factors. In a general hospital setting, cerebrovascular diseases, neuroinfections, metabolic disorders, and head injuries constitute the important causes, while in specialist clinics, degenerative disorders make up the larger proportion of cases[23] (Table 13.3 and Fig. 13.1).

Challenges that arise in the clinical diagnosis of dementia in resource-poor countries include a low awareness, limited availability of neuropsychological tests that have not been adapted for local needs and limited health care services and personnel specialized for dementia diagnosis and care. Accurate and uniform diagnosis of dementia and its subtypes is required to estimate magnitude and burden of disease, to recognize disease early, treat patients depending on the underlying cause and identify possible protective and risk factors for dementia.

AD Dementia

More common in elderly after 60 years of age, AD dementia has become the most common neurodegenerative disorder and one of the most common diseases of the aging population.[24] AD dementia is a progressive disorder of recent episodic memory, language, visuospatial function, and executive function associated with high frequency of neurobehavioral abnormalities at some point in the course. Memory impairment is the most prominent problem and is noticed as one of the earliest deficits. Episodic memory, particularly for recent events is impaired. Recent episodic memory can be assessed by delayed recall in the context of sufficiently preserved attention and concentration. In AD dementia, semantic memory is also impaired fairly early in the disease. A decline in visuospatial skills is also a common symptom. Most of the AD dementia patients exhibit a wide range of neuropsychiatric symptoms during the course of disease. Mood (depressed, euphoric), vegetative status (eating, sleeping), changes in personality (apathetic, disinhibited), and alterations in perception (hallucinations) or thought (delusions) are the major areas to be probed in the course of diagnostic assessment. Till late in the disease, there are no significant motor problems. In a few instances, AD dementia can present atypically as a nonamnestic condition, as a progressive aphasia, with prominent visuospatial disturbances and apraxia as posterior cortical atrophy, as a frontal variant or a corticobasal syndrome.[25] While most cases of AD dementia are sporadic, family history of AD dementia is a risk factor for AD dementia and Apo E genotype is thought to be involved in the pathogenesis of sporadic AD dementia. Familial AD dementia on the other hand is associated with a strong family history of dementia and includes early-onset autosomal dominant and late-onset familial AD dementia. Early-onset autosomal dominant genetic history is associated with presenilin 1 (PS1) which is located on chromosome 14 and late onset AD dementia is associated with mutations in one of three genes: the amyloid precursor protein (APP), and the PS1 and PS2 genes. PS2 is located on chromosome number 1, and the gene for APP is located on chromosome number 21 which codes for amyloid production in AD dementia.

Magnetic resonance imaging (MRI) brain can be normal or can show diffuse cortical atrophy in AD dementia. More specific findings include atrophy of hippocampus[26] and involvement of entorhinal cortex and limbic structures. The degree of volume loss correlates with the severity of cognitive impairment. On 18-fluoro-deoxyglucose PET scan, decrease in glucose metabolism is present initially in the temporal and parieto-occipital regions bilaterally followed by frontal association areas. More recently amyloid imaging of the brain is being used in research for improving diagnostic accuracy of AD dementia.

TABLE 13.2: **Types of dementia**

Disease	Alzheimer's dementia	Frontotemporal dementia—behavioral variant	Frontotemporal dementia—progressive nonfluent aphasia	Frontotemporal dementia—semantic dementia	Dementia with Lewy bodies	Creutzfeldt-Jakob disease
First symptom	Memory loss (episodic memory)	Poor judgment, behavioral disturbances, apathy, speech disturbances	Expressive aphasia with word finding difficulty, agrammatism and phonemic paraphasias	Fluent dysphasia with impairment of semantic verbal memory	Visual hallucinations, REM disorder, brittle proneness to delirium, psychomotor drug sensitivity, parkinsonism	Movement disorder/dementia
Psychiatric	Normal initially, agitation, aggression, and hallucinations later	Apathy, disinhibition, euphoria, depression	Apathy	Ritualistic behavior	Visual hallucinations, delusions, depression, sleep disorder	Depression, anxiety
Neurological examination	Normal initially	Frontal, executive dysfunction, memory and visuospatial functions spared relatively	Extrapyramidal features	Obsessions and compulsions	Drawing, frontal executive function is involved, memory is spared	Myoclonus, rigidity, parkinsonism
Pathology	Amyloid plaques, neurofibrillary tangles	Tau inclusions, Pick bodies, neurofibrillary tangles	Variable, tau pathology, and TDP-43 positive pathology	Ubiquitin-positive, TDP-43-positive, tau-negative inclusions	Lewy bodies (α-synuclein inclusions)	Spongiform changes, gliosis
Imaging	Entorhinal cortex and hippocampal atrophy initially, and later diffuse brain atrophy	Frontotemporal and insular atrophy	Predominantly left frontotemporal atrophy	Predominantly left anterior and inferior temporal lobe atrophy	Posterior parietal atrophy	Cortical ribboning and basal ganglia hyperintensities in DWI-MRI

TABLE 13.3: **Clinical features of dementias with probable diagnosis**

Clinical features	Probable diagnosis
Dementia with myelopathy and peripheral neuropathy	Vitamin B12 deficiency
Dry cool skin, hair loss, bradycardia and dementia	Hypothyroidism
Dementia with neuropathy	Vitamin deficiency, heavy metal intoxication, thyroid dysfunction, Lyme disease, vasculitis
Subacute onset amnesia and psychosis	Autoimmune encephalitis
High-risk sexual behavior or IV drug abuse	Syphilis, HIV
Recurrent head trauma	Chronic subdural hematoma, dementia pugilistica , NPH
Unexplained falls, axial rigidity, vertical gaze defects	Progressive supranuclear palsy
Asymmetric akinesia, rigidity, dystonia, myoclonus, alien limb executive dysfunction, apraxia	Corticobasal degeneration
Sudden onset focal weakness, apathy, emotional lability, incontinence, with cortical or subcortical infarctions, confluent white matter disease	Vascular dementia

HIV, human immunodeficiency virus; NPH, normal-pressure hydrocephalus.

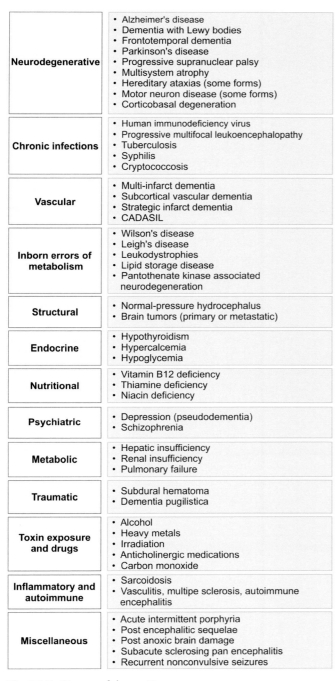

Neurodegenerative	• Alzheimer's disease • Dementia with Lewy bodies • Frontotemporal dementia • Parkinson's disease • Progressive supranuclear palsy • Multisystem atrophy • Hereditary ataxias (some forms) • Motor neuron disease (some forms) • Corticobasal degeneration
Chronic infections	• Human immunodeficiency virus • Progressive multifocal leukoencephalopathy • Tuberculosis • Syphilis • Cryptococcosis
Vascular	• Multi-infarct dementia • Subcortical vascular dementia • Strategic infarct dementia • CADASIL
Inborn errors of metabolism	• Wilson's disease • Leigh's disease • Leukodystrophies • Lipid storage disease • Pantothenate kinase associated neurodegeneration
Structural	• Normal-pressure hydrocephalus • Brain tumors (primary or metastatic)
Endocrine	• Hypothyroidism • Hypercalcemia • Hypoglycemia
Nutritional	• Vitamin B12 deficiency • Thiamine deficiency • Niacin deficiency
Psychiatric	• Depression (pseudodementia) • Schizophrenia
Metabolic	• Hepatic insufficiency • Renal insufficiency • Pulmonary failure
Traumatic	• Subdural hematoma • Dementia pugilistica
Toxin exposure and drugs	• Alcohol • Heavy metals • Irradiation • Anticholinergic medications • Carbon monoxide
Inflammatory and autoimmune	• Sarcoidosis • Vasculitis, multipe sclerosis, autoimmune encephalitis
Miscellaneous	• Acute intermittent porphyria • Post encephalitic sequelae • Post anoxic brain damage • Subacute sclerosing pan encephalitis • Recurrent nonconvulsive seizures

Fig. 13.1: Causes of dementia.

The important neuropathological hallmark for AD dementia are neurofibrillary tangles (NFT) and neuritic plaques that are more than expected for patients' age and are typically located in the pyramidal neurons of the neocortex, hippocampus, and amygdala. Granulovacuolar

degeneration and amyloid accumulation are also present in most of the patients. These changes occur normally in aging brain and it is the number and concentration that plays an important role in the diagnosis. The NFTs are composed of silver-staining neuronal cytoplasmic fibrils composed of abnormally phosphorylated tau protein and neuritic plaques are spherical silver-staining structures located outside the neuron. Amyloid plaques[27] are usually more located in the cerebral cortex and hippocampus but also occur in the corpus striatum, amygdala, and thalamus. The accumulation of $A\beta$ in cerebral arterioles is termed as amyloid angiopathy and is frequently found in the brains of patients with AD dementia.

Criteria intended to serve as a guide for the diagnosis of probable, possible, and definite Alzheimer's disease were first proposed in 1984.[28] More recently, the National Institute of Aging (NIA) and the Alzheimer's association (AA) reviewed the biomarker, epidemiological, and neuropsychological evidence in relation to AD, and proposed conceptual frameworks as well as operational research criteria. The major reason for including biomarker evidence to the criteria is to increase diagnostic certainty (Appendix 4.1).[29]

Frontotemporal Dementia

The clinical syndrome of frontal lobe degeneration is with onset typically between the ages of 50 and 60 years featuring insidious personality change, disinhibition, and subsequent gradual loss of speech output. The FTD spectrum is a clinically and pathologically inhomogeneous group. Originally, Lund-Manchester criteria were used to diagnose FTD. Others provided research diagnostic criteria for the clinical syndromes associated with frontotemporal lobar degeneration (Box 13.2).[30]

Frontal variant frontotemporal dementia (fvFTD) also called as behavioral variant frontotemporal dementia (bvFTD) manifests as disinhibition, apathy, social isolation, impaired judgment, lack of empathy, obsessions, and compulsions. Abstract thinking, decision making, and planning are impaired. Despite relatively well-preserved general language skills, patients with bvFTD have particular problems with verb processing with characteristic sparing of visual memory.[31] In 2011, an international consortium developed revised guidelines for the diagnosis of bvFTD based on recent literature and collective experience (Appendix 4.2).[32]

Patients with a language variant of FTD include either progressive nonfluent aphasia (PNFA) or semantic dementia (SD). Progressive nonfluent aphasia shows early prominent language impairment with dysfluent, effortful, and agrammatical language output in the context of preserved language comprehension until late in the disease course. Speech output requires manifest effort and is nonfluent and hesitant with phonemic and semantic errors. Word finding and repetition are impaired, and spelling is poor. Semantic dementia is characterized by prominent loss of semantic knowledge. Therefore, in SD while the language output in fluent, well–articulated, and grammatically correct, it shows impoverished content and semantic supraordinate paraphasias (e.g., naming a lion an "animal" or a flower a "plant"). Further patients with SD frequently substitute many nouns with "it" or "thing" and this can cause difficulty in understanding the message the patient is trying to convey. Semantic dementia is characterized by a unique type of dyslexia called surface dyslexia where irregular words are written and read with spelling to sound correspondence. These patients show frontal behaviors similar to those seen in FTD (Appendix 4.3) (Box 13.3).

The MRI in bvFTD frequently shows frontal and temporal cortical atrophy, which is asymmetrical or sometimes symmetrical, in particular involving anterior cingulate and frontoinsular regions. Nonfluent aphasia usually presents with left perisylvian atrophy, particularly in the inferior-frontal cortex, frontal opercular, and dorsal insular regions, while SD tends to be associated with more anterior and inferior temporal lobe involvement.[35] The PET or SPECT imaging reveals profound hypoperfusion/

hypometabolism in the affected areas that also shows atrophy on MRI.

FTD is characterized by both genetic and pathological heterogeneity. An autosomal dominant inheritance has been found in 10–27% of all FTD patients. About 30–50% of bvFTD patients have a positive family history, whereas PNFA and SD patients are less frequently associated with a family history. The most common mutations identified with FTD are in microtubule-associated protein tau (MAPT) and progranulin (GRN) genes accounting for nearly 50% of mutations. In rarer instances, genetic mutations in valosin containing protein (VCP), charged multivesicular body protein 2B (CHMP2B), TAR-DNA binding protein (TARDP), and fused in sarcoma (FUS) genes have been described. Familial FTD-MND has been linked to chromosome 9 (Box 13.4).[35]

Apart from the classically described FTD syndrome, Pick's disease, other tauopathies include progressive supranuclear palsy, corticobasal degeneration, and argyrophilic grain disease. The FTD-TDP subtypes include SD, FTD-MND, GRN mutations, and VCP mutations. Some correlations between genetic and pathologic changes have been observed. Patients with FTD-tau are associated with MAPT mutations generally and different types of tau inclusions (Pick bodies, neurofibrillary tangles, and pretangles) in the frontal and temporal cortex, hippocampus, subcortical nuclei and sometimes in brainstem, cerebellum, and spinal cord.[36] The FTD-TDP patients have ubiquitin-positive inclusions that have TDP-43 protein as major constituent.[37] Semantic dementia is associated with dystrophic neuritis, FTD-MND with neuronal cytoplasmic inclusions, GRN mutations with cytoplasmic inclusions, dystrophic neuritis, neuronal intranuclear inclusions, and VCP mutations with numerous intraneuronal inclusions and fewer cytoplasmic intrusions and dystrophic neurites. A small number of patients with ubiquitin-positive, TDP-43 negative pathology show FUS antibody reactivity.[38]

Dementia with Lewy Bodies

The DLB is found in approximately 20% of late-onset dementias (alone or in combination with AD dementia). The mean age of onset is 75 years, with a range of 50–80 years. There is a slight male predominance.[39] Fluctuating cognition is observed in upto 90% of the patients. Psychotic symptoms (delusions and hallucinations) are present in up to 75% of DLB patients. Visual hallucinations are the most frequent symptoms. They are detailed, brightly colored, three-dimensional images of people and animals. Delusions also occur commonly and the most common themes are delusional misidentification, followed by paranoid beliefs (theft, conspiracy, harassment, abandonment, infidelity). Nondelusional suspiciousness and paranoia are also frequent. Extrapyramidal features and neuroleptic sensitivity are commonly associated.

The MRI brain imaging shows disproportionate atrophy of the temporal lobes but not to the degree seen in AD dementia. 18-Fluoro-deoxyglucose positron emission tomography (FDG-PET) shows bilateral temporoparietal hypometabolism as seen in AD dementia and in addition it also shows hypometabolism of bilateral occipital lobes and there is mild degree of hypometabolism in frontal lobes. The hypometabolism in the primary visual cortex in DLBD explains the presence of visual hallucinations.[40] Presence of Lewy bodies in limbic (e.g., hippocampus and amygdala), paralimbic (e.g., anterior cingulate),[39] and neocortical regions is the neuropathological hallmark of DLB. Lewy bodies are concentric hyaline cytoplasmic inclusions that are found in the cortex of patients with DLBD. Lewy bodies stain with periodic acid–Schiff (PAS) and ubiquitin. They can also be identified with antibodies to the presynaptic protein and α-synuclein.[41] α-Synuclein is the major filamentous component of LBs and Lewy neuritis although ubiquitin and tau proteins are also present.

The consensus criteria for the clinical diagnosis of probable and possible DLB were first established in 1996. However, the Dementia with Lewy Bodies Consortium revised criteria for the clinical and pathologic diagnosis of DLB in 2005, incorporating new information about the core clinical features and suggesting improved methods to assess them (Appendix 4.4).[42]

Vascular Dementia

Stroke and cerebrovascular disease is a common cause of dementia in India due to the increased prevalence of atherosclerosis and cardiovascular risk factors. VaD is not a single entity, but represents a complex dementia subtype that occurs as a result of interaction between vascular risk factors, such as hypertension, diabetes, obesity, dyslipidemia, and brain parenchymal changes such as macro and microinfarcts, hemorrhages, white matter changes and brain atrophy occurring in an aging brain. VaD is a group of syndromes that represent a clinicoradiologic and pathological spectrum (Box 13.5).

Emotional lability, gait disturbances, and urinary incontinence are clinical clues toward this diagnosis. Cognitive examination reveals frontal/executive dysfunction, cognitive slowing, and can spare memory. Neurological examination demonstrates motor slowing, pyramidal signs, focal deficits and sometimes examination can be normal. A slowly progressive disorder without clinically obvious cerebrovascular accidents is not uncommon in subcortical VaD. Neuropsychiatric examination shows apathy, delusions, depression, and anxiety. The clinical diagnosis of VaD is still very complex because of the heterogeneity in pathophysiology, clinical presentation, and imaging. Research criteria for the diagnosis of VaD[43] were perhaps first provided in 1993 (Appendix 4.5). Milder forms of the disease exist and term vascular cognitive impairment (VCI) is used to encompass the entire spectrum of the disorder. The National Institute for NINDS and the Canadian Stroke Network developed common standards in clinical diagnosis, epidemiology, brain imaging, neuropathology, experimental models, genetics, and clinical trials to recommend minimum, common, clinical, and research standards for the description and study of VCI.

Mild Cognitive Impairment

Recognizing that the development of dementia is a long process, which extends over several years with gradual accumulation of pathology and slow decline in cognitive functions from normal to very subtle and then significant deficits, the concept of mild cognitive impairment (MCI) has been proposed to identify an early but abnormal state of cognitive impairment. The MCI is regarded to be a cognitive continuum between normal aging and early Alzheimer's disease.[44] Individuals with MCI have complaints of poor memory, have normal activities of daily living, have abnormal memory and other cognitive functions for age, and do not meet the criteria for dementia but are at increased risk. This entity is considered to be useful in identifying subjects with mild memory complaints who are at a high risk of developing AD dementia.[45-47] MCI represents the gray zone between normal cognitive aging and early dementia.[48]

Increasing urbanization, change in lifestyles and a shift from joint family system to nuclear families is reducing the "sociocultural protection" of elderly with cognitive problems. This trend is demonstrated by the finding that a significant proportion of people seeking help in specialist clinics present with mild memory complaints.[49] Various criteria defining MCI using clinical features and neuropsychological profile have been proposed over the past decade.[50-52] Petersen's criteria are most widely used and depend on clinical and neuropsychological features in defining MCI and its subtypes.[44] The criteria for MCI have been recently revised by the National Institute on Aging and the Alzheimer's Association (NIA-AA) and recommend the use of imaging and CSF biomarkers to improve the diagnostic confidence in identifying subjects with mild cognitive complaints whose underlying pathophysiological process could be AD dementia. The FDG-PET brain imaging, SPECT perfusion imaging and assessment of MRI temporal lobe volumes by visual rating, amyloid imaging, voxel-based measures, and CSF amyloid and tau biomarkers are being studied in dementia and MCI. Currently, these biomarkers are advocated for use for research and once validated could potentially find their place in clinical practice to improve the diagnostic accuracy of dementia and MCI.

ILLUSTRATIVE CASE STUDIES

Behavioral Variant of Frontotemporal Dementia

A 56-year-old gentleman presented with a 4-year history of behavioral disturbances. He was noticed to have become tactless, easily distractible and impersistent in his work at a bank. He developed a habit of hoarding stationary items such as pins and paper weights. He had verbal stereotypies and a new found preference for sweets. There was a family history of similar disease in his brother, mother, and grandmother.

On examination, he was alert but easily distracted. The MMSE was 24/30. Cognitive function assessment revealed impairment of attention (digit forward 4, digit backward span 3). He was oriented to time and place. He had preserved memory (RAVLT 12/15 Immediate recall and 10/15 delayed recall scores) and visuospatial functions on Rey-Osterrieth Figure Test. Language assessment was normal except for mild reduction in fluencies (animals 11/minute, p letter fluencies 10/minute). His performance on Trail-Making Test B (7 minutes 20 seconds with frequent errors) was impaired. He had no other neurological signs. Magnetic resonance imaging brain showed asymmetric frontotemporal atrophy and SPECT brain showed bilateral (right more than left) frontotemporal hypoperfusion (Fig. 13.2). Clinical diagnosis based on history, cognitive, and behavioral profile and imaging was suggestive of familial behavioral variant FTD.

Progressive Nonfluent Aphasia

A 68-years-old gentleman, a retired geologist, presented with the sole complaint of difficulty in speaking of a year's duration. His speech had become slow and halting. Sentences were short with frequent pauses between words. He repeated the same word two or three times and sometimes mispronounced them. He did not have problems understanding speech and did not substitute wrong words. He had no difficulty in remembering events or appointments and had no problems finding his way around. No behavioral problems were noted. There was no family history of a similar illness in his father.[4]

On examination, he was conscious, alert, and cheerful. The MMSE was 21/30 and the ACE-R was 67/100. Neuropsychological assessment revealed normal digit span (digit forward 6 and digit backward 4) and impaired serial subtraction. On language evaluation, comprehension, reading, and writing were preserved. Repetition and naming were impaired with phonological errors. Verbal fluency was reduced, with a significant degree of perseveration. Western aphasia battery revealed a profile of expressive nonfluent aphasia. Assessment of verbal episodic memory was interfered with by language impairment. Visual memory was fairly well preserved on Rey-Osterrieth Complex Figure Test. Performance on the semantic battery showed phonological errors while naming of objects in the categories of animals, birds, fruits, vegetables, household items, vehicles and tools, and normal category sorting, with accurate pointing was seen. Frontal executive function as assessed by Trail-Making Test B was normal. He had no apraxia and rest of the neurological examination was normal. Magnetic resonance imaging brain showed left frontotemporal atrophy. Clinical and imaging findings were consistent with a diagnosis of PNFA variant of FTD.

Continued

Continued

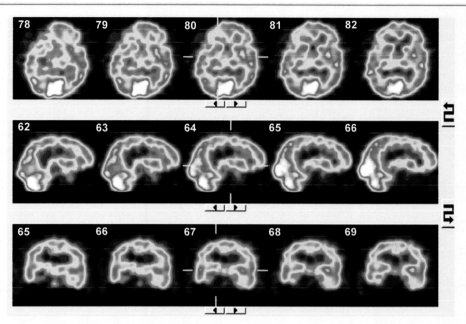

bvFTD, behavioral variant frontotemporal dementia; SPECT, single-photon emission computed tomography.

Fig. 13.2: SPECT scan of brain in a patient with bvFTD showing bilateral (right > left) frontotemporal hypometabolism.

Semantic Dementia

A 55-years-old lady presented with difficulties in naming objects and behavioral problems for 4 years. The lady was a highly functional housewife. Since, 4 years her relatives noticed changes in behavior characterized by ritualistic behavior with obsessive tendencies. Her daughter noticed that she used to talk "nonstop" but only about few restricted topics. She was also noticed to have profound difficulty in naming persons and objects.

Detailed neuropsychological testing and language evaluations were carried out. The MMSE was 14/30 and the ACE-R was 24/100. Patient had a profound impairment of language involving deficits in word fluencies and confrontation naming with moderate impairment of comprehension and preserved repetition. While orientation and visuospatial functions were fairly well preserved there was an inability to learn new verbal material. Episodic memory was evaluated in the patient by conducting an interview. She was able to describe her routine of the previous day clearly, as also recent events in her life. She was also able to recount autobiographical details, suggesting that her episodic memory was relatively preserved.

Language assessed by Western aphasia battery revealed an aphasia quotient of 54.2 that was suggestive of sensory aphasia. She had fluent speech with marked inability to name, preserved repetition, and impairment of single word comprehension. On assessing semantic memory using the modified Cambridge Semantic Battery, she had profound impairment of semantic knowledge across various categories including animals, birds, vegetables, household items, vehicles, and tools.

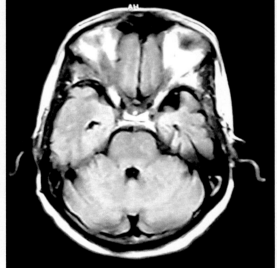

Fig. 13.3: MRI brain of patient with semantic dementia showing left anterior and inferior temporal atrophy.

Magnetic resonance imaging revealed left anterior and temporal lobe atrophy (Fig. 13.3). Clinical observations, neuropsychological evaluations, language evaluations, and neurodiagnostic findings on MRI were consistent with a diagnosis of SD.

Continued

Continued

Vascular Dementia

A 62-years-old farmer presented to the hospital with sudden onset of memory loss of 2 years duration. His relatives noticed that he was not able to remember names of close relatives, and recent conversations and events. He had mild clumsiness of his right hand while performing activities. The patient gradually improved, and became independent for activities of daily living, but with mild residual memory complaints. Six months later, he suddenly developed left sided facial weakness. His family members revealed that his memory disturbances had begun increasing again. He had become dull and disinterested in events happening around him and was interacting less with people. There were outbursts of anger, irritability, low mood with frequent crying spells. There was history of occasional urinary incontinence. Patient was hypertensive since 10 years and diabetic since 3 years on irregular treatment. He had no history of cardiac disease, smoking, or chronic alcoholism. On examination, patient was apathetic with delayed responses. On neurological examination, he had mild right facial weakness and right-sided ataxic hemiparesis.

Cognitive examination MMSE scores of 22/30 and ACE-R scores: 57/100. Impairment in attention and executive functioning was noted on the performance of Color Trails and Digit Span tests. The CDR score was 2 showing moderate level of dementia. Neuropsychiatric inventory scores show that the patient has moderate levels of depression, anxiety and apathy, with an increase in severity levels. Conventional neuropsychological testing revealed moderate levels of deficits in attention, memory, executive functions and relatively spared language and visuospatial functions. Behavioral evaluation was done with Frontal Systems Behavior Scale (FrSBe). Patient was found to have increased apathy and executive dysfunction.

The MRI of brain showed infarcts in bilateral basal ganglionic regions and cerebral deep white matter. There was also evidence of grade II periventricular hyperintensities (Figs. 13.4). Intracranial MR angiogram showed bilateral stenosis (>50%) of middle cerebral arteries and diffuse intracranial atherosclerosis in other cerebral vessels ECG showed evidence of left ventricular hypertrophy. Lipid profile was normal. Neck vessel Doppler showed 40% stenosis of left internal carotid artery and 35% stenosis of right internal carotid artery. Patient was diagnosed to have subcortical vascular dementia.

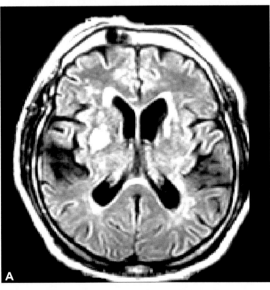 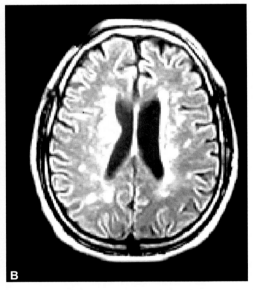

Figs 13.4A and B: MRI images of patient with vascular dementia, showing subcortical basal ganglionic and white matter infarcts and periventricular hyperintensities.

CONCLUSION

Dementia syndromes are many, and varied in clinical presentations. The evolution of symptoms as indicated by history and pattern of cognitive deficits identified on clinical and cognitive examination are essential to subtype dementia. A combination of simple clinic based tests, more extensive neuropsychological tests, assessment of functional impairment, and neurologic examination for motor and sensory deficits coupled with appropriate investigations help the clinician arrive at a proper diagnosis. Since, the clinical profile reflects location of pathology rather than a specific etiology, an accurate pathological diagnosis may not always be possible. In the future, the use of biomarkers may aid in arriving at a more certain diagnosis, with implications for instituting appropriate treatment and for prognosis.

REFERENCES

1. Plassman BL, Langa KM, Fisher GG, et al. Prevalence of dementia in the United States: aging, demographics, and memory study. Neuroepidemiology. 2007;29:125-32.
2. Kalaria RN, Maestre GE, Arizaga R, et al. Alzheimer's disease and vascular dementia in developing countries: prevalence, management, and risk factors. Lancet Neurol. 2008;7:812-26.
3. Yusuf S, Reddy S, Ounpuu S, et al. Global burden of cardiovascular diseases: Part I: general considerations, the epidemiologic transition, risk factors, and impact of urbanization. Circulation. 2001;104:2746-53.
4. Skoog I, Lernfelt B, Landahl S, et al. 15-year longitudinal study of blood pressure and dementia. Lancet. 1996;347:1141-5.
5. Shaji KS, Jotheeswaran AT, Girish N, (Ed). The Dementia India Report: prevalence, impact, costs and services for dementia. New Delhi: ARDSI; 2010.
6. Saddock BJ, Saddock VA. Delirium, dementia, and amnestic and other cognitive disorders. In: Grebb JA, Pataki CS, Sussman N (Eds). Kaplan and Saddock's Synopsis of Psychiatry Behavioral Sciences/Clinical Psychiatry, 10th edition. Philadelphia: Lippincott Williams and Wilkins; 2007. p. 329.
7. Folstein MF, Folstein SE, McHugh PR. "Minimental state." A practical method for grading the cognitive state of patients for the clinician. J Psychiatr Res. 1975;12:189-98.
8. Mathuranath PS, Hodges JR, Mathew R, et al. Adaptation of the ACE for a Malayalam speaking population in southern India. Int J Geriatr Psychiatry. 2004;19:1188-94.
9. Das SK, Bose P, Biswas A, et al. An epidemiologic study of mild cognitive impairment in Kolkata, India. Neurology. 2007;68:2019-26.
10. Rao SL, Subbakrishna DK, Gopukumar K. NIMHANS Neuropsychology Battery- 2004 Manual, 1st edition. Bangalore: NIMHANS publications; 2004. pp. 6-201.
11. Pershad D, Verma SK. Handbook of PGI Battery of Brain Dysfunction (PGI-BBD). Agra: National Psychological Corporation; 1990.
12. Ganguli M, Ratcliff G, Chandra V, et al. A Hindi version of MMSE: the development of a cognitive screening instrument for a largely illiterate rural elderly population in India. Int J Geriatr Psychiatry. 1995;10:367-77.
13. Nasreddine ZS, Phillips NA, Bédirian V, et al. The montreal cognitive assessment, MoCA: a brief screening tool for mild cognitive impairment. J Am Geriatr Soc. 2005;53:695-9.
14. Kipps CM, Hodges JR. Cognitive assessment for clinicians. J Neurol Neurosurg Psychiatry. 2005;76:22-30.
15. Gelinas I, Gauthier L, McIntyre M, et al. Development of a functional measure for persons with Alzheimer's disease: the disability assessment for dementia. Am J Occup Ther. 1999;53:471-81.
16. Morris JC. The clinical dementia rating (CDR): current version and scoring rules. Neurology. 1993;43:2412-4.
17. Lovibond PF, Lovibond SH. The structure of negative emotional states: comparison of the Depression Anxiety Stress Scales (DASS) with the Beck Depression and Anxiety Inventories. Behav Res Ther. 1995;33:335-43.
18. Knopman DS, DeKosky ST, Cummings JL, et al. Practice parameter: diagnosis of dementia (an evidence-based review). Report of the quality standards subcommittee of the American academy of neurology. Neurology. 2001;56:1143-53.
19. Srikanth S, Nagaraja AV, Ratnavalli E. Neuropsychiatric symptoms in dementia-frequency, relationship to dementia severity and comparison in Alzheimer's disease, vascular dementia and frontotemporal dementia. J Neurolsci. 2005;236:43-8.
20. Krishnan S, Mathuranath PS, Sarma S, et al. Neuropsychological functions in progressive supranuclear palsy, multiple system atrophy and Parkinson's disease. Neurol India. 2006;54:268-72.
21. Plassman BL, Langa KM, Fisher GG, et al. Prevalence of cognitive impairment without dementia in the United States. Ann Intern Med. 2008;148:427-34.
22. Tucha O, Smely C, Preier M, et al. Cognitive deficits before treatment among patients with brain tumors. Neurosurgery. 2000;47:324-33.
23. Alladi S, Mekala S, Chadalawada SK, et al. Subtypes of dementia: a study from a memory clinic in India. Dement Geriatr Cogn Disord. 2011;32:38.
24. Alzheimer's Association; Thies W, Bleiler L. 2011 Alzheimer's disease facts and figures. Alzheimers Dement. 2011;2:208-44.
25. Alladi S, Xuereb J, Bak T, et al. Focal cortical presentations of Alzheimer's disease. Brain. 2007;130:2636-45.
26. Apostolova LG, Dutton RA, Dinov ID, et al. Conversion of mild cognitive impairment to Alzheimer disease predicted by hippocampal atrophy maps. Arch Neurol. 2007;64:1360-1.
27. Mathis CA, Lopresti BJ, Klunk WE. Impact of amyloid imaging on drug development in Alzheimer's disease. Nucl Med Biol. 2007;34:809-22.
28. McKhann G, Drachman D, Folstein M, et al. Clinical diagnosis of Alzheimer's disease: report of the NINCDS-ADRDA Work Group under the auspices of Department of Health and Human Services Task Force on Alzheimer's disease. Neurology. 1984;34:939-44.
29. McKhann GM, Knopman DS, Chertkow H, et al. The diagnosis of dementia due to Alzheimer's disease: Recommendations from the National Institute on Aging-Alzheimer's Association Workgroups on Diagnostic Guidelines for Alzheimer's Disease. Alzheimer Dement. 2011;7:263-9.
30. Neary D, Snowden JS, Gustafson L, et al. Frontotemporal lobar degeneration. A consensus on clinical diagnostic criteria. Neurology. 1998;51:1546-54.
31. Hodges JR, Miller B. The neuropsychology of frontal variant frontotemporal dementia and semantic dementia. Introduction to the special topic papers: Part II. Neurocase. 2001;7:113-21.
32. Rascovsky K, Hodges JR, Knopman D, et al. Sensitivity of revised diagnostic criteria for the behavioral variant of frontotemporal dementia. Brain. 2011;134:2456-77.
33. Apostolova LG, DeKosky ST, Cummings JL. Dementias. In: Daroff RB, Fenichel GM, Jankovic J, Mazziotta JC (Eds). Bradley's Neurology in Clinical Practice. Philadelphia: Elsevier; 2012. pp. 1534-82.
34. Grono-Tempini ML, Hillis AE, Wintraub S, et al. Classification of primary progressive aphasia and its variant. Neurology. 2011;76:1006-14.
35. Seelaar H, Rohrer JD, Pijnenburg YAL, et al. Clinical, genetic and pathological heterogeneity of frontotemporal dementia: a review. J Neurol Neurosurg Psychiatry. 2011;82:476-86.
36. Van Swieten J, Spillantini MG. Hereditary frontotemporal dementia caused by Tau gene mutations. Brain Pathol. 2007;17:63-73.
37. Neumann M, Sampathu DM, Kwong LK, et al. Ubiquitinated TDP-43 in frontotemporal lobar degeneration and amyotrophic lateral sclerosis. Science. 2006;314:130-3.
38. Josephs KA, Lin WL, Ahmed Z, et al. Frontotemporal lobar degeneration with ubiquitin-positive, but TDP-43-negative inclusions. Acta Neuropathol. 2008;116:159-67.
39. Gesser F, Wenning GK, Poewe W, et al. How to diagnose dementia with Lewy bodies: state of art. Mov Disord. 2005;20:11-20.

40. Beyer MK, Javin CC, Larsen JP, et al. A magnetic resonance imaging study of patients with Parkinson's disease with mild cognitive impairment and dementia using voxel-based morphometry. J Neurol Neurosurg Psychiatry. 2007;78:254-9.
41. Jellinger KA, Wenning GK, Seppi K. Predictors of survival in dementia with Lewy bodies and Parkinson dementia. Neurodegener Dis. 2007;4:428-30.
42. McKeith IG, Dickson DW, Lowe J, et al. Diagnosis and management of dementia with Lewy bodies. Third report of the DLB consortium. Neurology. 2005;65:1863-72.
43. Roman GC, Tatemchi TK, Erkinjuntti T, et al. Vascular dementia: diagnostic criteria for research studies. Neurology. 1993;43:250-60.
44. Petersen RC. Mild cognitive impairment as a diagnostic entity. J Intern Med. 2004;256:183-94.
45. Grudman M, Petersen RC, Ferris SH, et al. Mild cognitive impairment can be distinguished from Alzheimer disease and normal aging for clinical trials. Arch Neurol. 2004;61:59-66.
46. Manly JJ, Tang MX, Schupf N, et al. Frequency and course of mild cognitive impairment in a multiethnic community. Ann Neurol. 2008;63:494-506.
47. Prestia A, Caroli A, van der Fleir WM, et al. Prediction of dementia in MCI patients based on core diagnostic markers for Alzheimer disease. Neurology. 2013;80:1048-56.
48. Geda YE, Petersen RC. Mild cognitive impairment. In: Weiner MF, Lipton AM (Eds). Clinical Manual of Alzheimer Disease and Other Dementias. Virginia: American Psychiatric Publishing; 2012. p. 159.
49. Alladi S, Shailaja M, Mridula KR, et al. Mild Cognitive Impairment: clinical and imaging profile in a memory clinic setting in India. Dement Geriatr Cogn Disord. 2014;37:113-24.
50. Petersen RC, Smith GE, Waring SC, et al. Aging, memory, and mild cognitive impairment. Int Psychogeriatr. 1997;9:65-9.
51. Winblad B, Palmer K, Kivipelto M, et al. Mild cognitive impairment-beyond controversies, towards a consensus: report of the International working group on mild cognitive impairment. J Intern Med. 2004;256:240-6.
52. Portet F, Ousset PJ, Visser PJ, et al. Mild cognitive impairment (MCI) in medical practice: a critical review of the concept and new diagnostic procedure. Report of the MCI working group of the European consortium on Alzheimer's disease. J Neurol Psychiatry. 2006;77:714-8.

Chapter 14

Approach to Disturbances of Smell and Taste

Sahil Mehta

INTRODUCTION

The sense of smell and taste is the least understood of all the sensory systems. It is the most neglected part of neurological examination due to the sparse training in medical colleges and neurology residency programs on this subject.[1]

The importance of sense of smell and taste lies in appreciating the flavor and palatability of foods and protection against toxins, polluted air, smoke, and spoiled food products. Physiologically, smell and taste aid in digestion by triggering gastrointestinal secretions.[2] The olfactory system is necessary for odor recognition and food flavors. The taste system comprising of receptors on the tongue, palate, and pharynx is necessary for identifying five types of taste sensation: sweet, sour, bitter, salt, and umami [Japanese word for savory or broth taste, represented by monosodium glutamate (MSG)].

The sensory portion of the trigeminal nerve recognizes texture, temperature, and spiciness of food.[1]

About 2% of the individuals less than 65 years of age have smell and taste dysfunction and this proportion increases to 50% in people aged 65–80 years and up to 75% beyond 80 years. Smell and taste dysfunction can have a significant impact on quality of life. Deficits of these senses can result in weight loss, malnutrition, impaired immunity, and worsening of medical illness.[3,4] Patients commonly confuse symptoms of flavor loss, which results from smell disturbance, with taste dysfunction. Olfactory disturbances are hallmark features of preclinical or presymptomatic Alzheimer's or Parkinson's disease.

The evaluation of patients with abnormalities of taste or smell requires a multidisciplinary approach, including a neurologist, an otolaryngologist and a primary care physician (Table 14.1).

TABLE 14.1: **Definitions**

Disorders of smell	Disorders of taste
Normosmia: Normal smell function	Normogeusia: Normal taste function
Hyposmia: Diminished smell function	Hypogeusia: Diminished taste function to one or more specific tastants
Anosmia: Complete loss of smell	Ageusia: Absent taste function
Parosmia: Aberrant odor perception either without an odorant stimulus (phantosmia) or with an odorant stimulus (troposmia)	Dysgeusia: Persistent sweet, sour, salty, bitter, or metallic taste
Dysosmia: Distortion of smell sensation	Aliageusia: Unpleasant taste of food or drink that is usually pleasant
Hyperosmia: Enhanced odorant sensitivity	Phantogeusia: Unpleasant taste produced indigenously due to a gustatory hallucination

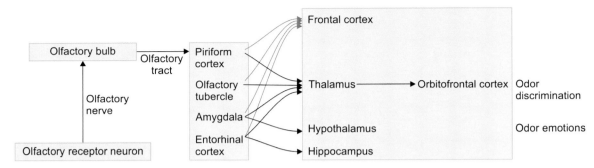

Fig. 14.1: Simplified diagrammatic representation of the olfactory pathway.

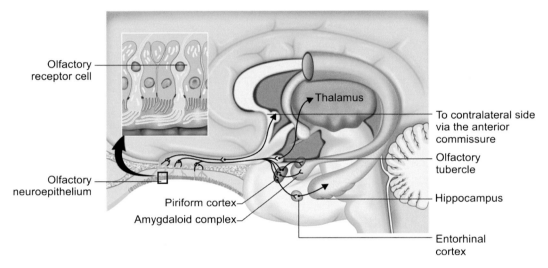

Fig. 14.2: The olfactory pathway.

DISTURBANCES OF OLFACTION

Anatomy and Physiology

The olfactory epithelium is located in the roof of the nasal cavity and is comprised of 6 million receptor cells. This olfactory cleft is open for both ortho and retronasal flow where odors can reach via sniffing through the nostrils or via the nasopharynx by passing retronasally into the nose while eating or drinking.[5]

About 1,000 olfactory receptors are coded in the human genome, although only 380 of these are functionally expressed in the epithelium.[6,7] These receptors are not highly specific to a single odorant; rather single odorants evidently bind to different receptor types. Olfactory receptor neurons send their axons that project through the cribriform plate to the glomeruli in the olfactory bulb at the base of the frontal lobes (Figs 14.1 and 14.2). Activation of different receptor types causes different excitation patterns in the bulb explaining the basis of quality coding of the odors. The orbitofrontal cortex plays a major role in the conscious perception of odors; other important structures include the piriform cortex, amygdala, hippocampus, thalamus, nucleus accumbens, and the cerebellum.[8]

Possible Causes of Smell Disturbance

Olfactory disturbance can be due to trauma, viral infections, mechanical obstruction or inflammatory damage, ageing, neurodegenerative disorders etc. (Box 14.1, Tables 14.2 and 14.3).

Box 14.1: Causes of olfactory disturbance

1. Trauma: Possibly due to severance of the fila olfactoria or due to contusions in the orbitofrontal cortex
2. Viral infections that damage the olfactory receptor neurons
3. Nasal causes such as sinusitis or nasal polyp causing mechanical obstruction or inflammatory damage to the olfactory epithelium
4. Smell disorders associated with aging
5. Neurological disorders like Parkinson's disease, Alzheimer's disease, etc. Olfactory disturbances are present in over 95% of patients with idiopathic Parkinson's disease and precede the motor symptoms by many years

TABLE 14.2: Causes of olfactory disturbances classified on the basis of their relative frequency

Common causes	Less common causes	Uncommon causes
Nasal and sinus disease (allergic or vasomotor rhinitis, chronic sinusitis, nasal polyps)	Medications	Neoplasms or brain tumor (olfactory groove or cribriform plate meningioma, frontal lobe tumor, temporal lobe tumor, pituitary tumor)
Upper respiratory infection	Cocaine abuse (intranasal)	Psychiatric conditions (malingering, schizophrenia, depression)
Head trauma	Toxic chemical exposure (benzene, carbon disulfide, ethylacetate, paint solvents)	Endocrine disorders (adrenocortical insufficiency, Cushing's syndrome, diabetes mellitus, hypo-thyroidism, Turner's syndrome, pregnancy)
Cigarette smoking	Industrial agent exposure (ashes, cadmium, chalk, lead, nickel)	Epilepsy (olfactory aura)
Neurodegenerative disease (Alzheimer's disease, Parkinson's disease, multiple sclerosis)	Nutritional factors (vitamin A, B6, B12 deficiency, zinc and copper deficiency, malnutrition, chronic renal failure, liver disease, cancer, AIDS)	Migraine headache
Age	Radiation treatment of head and neck	Cerebrovascular accident
	Congenital conditions (congenital anosmia, Kallmann's syndrome)	Sjogren's syndrome, systemic lupus erythematosus

TABLE 14.3: Medications which alter smell and taste

Selected medications that alter smell and taste

Antibiotics
- Ampicillin
- Azithromycin
- Ciprofloxacin
- Clarithromycin
- Metronidazole
- Ofloxacin

Antihistamines and decongestants
- Chlorpheniramine
- Pseudoephedrine
- Loratadine

Anti-inflammatory agents
- Colchicine
- Dexamethasone
- Gold
- Penicillamine

Antimanic drug
- Lithium

Lipid lowering agents
- Fluvastatin
- Lovastatin
- Pravastatin

Anticonvulsants
- Carbamazepine
- Phenytoin

Antihypertensives and cardiac medications
- Acetazolamide
- Amiloride
- Captopril
- Diltiazem
- Enalapril
- Hydrochlorothiazide
- Nifedipine
- Propranolol
- Spironolactone

Antineoplastics
- Cisplatin
- Doxorubicin
- Methotrexate
- Vincristine

Antiparkinsonian agents
- Levodopa

Antipsychotics
- Clozapine
- Trifluoperazine

Antidepressants
- Amitriptyline
- Desipramine
- Nortriptyline
- Imipramine

Antithyroid agents
- Methimazole
- Propylthiouracil

Muscle relaxants
- Baclofen
- Dantrolene

APPROACH TO A PATIENT WITH SMELL DISTURBANCE

The first step involves taking a detailed history including the nature of eating, drinking, and smoking habits, any past history of head injury, surgery, medications, and a history of upper respiratory infection or nasal complaints like rhinorrhea or nasal obstruction.[5] Questions must be asked relevant to a history of diabetes, hypothyroidism, connective tissue diseases, vitamin deficiencies, or any history of allergies.

A thorough ENT, dental, and general physical examination is important to evaluate for various local and systemic causes responsible for smell loss. The nasal cavity and sinuses should be examined for any masses, inflammation, or obstruction. A complete neurological examination of the cranial nerves, cerebellum, and sensory and motor function may be required. MRI brain may be done to rule out the cerebral causes of smell disorders like tumors, stroke, and head injury or to look for congenital aplasia of the olfactory bulbs. Blood tests may be helpful to identify diabetes, infection, heavy metal exposure, vitamin B6 and B12 deficiency, thyroid, liver, and kidney disease (Table 14.4).

Tests of Olfaction[9]

The University of Pennsylvania Smell Identification Test (UPSIT)

This is a commercially available commonly used standardized scratch and sniff test. It consists of 40 microencapsulated odorants. The test scores range from 0 to 40, where scores from 34 to 40 indicate normosmia, 26 to 30 indicate moderate hyposmia, and 6 to 18 indicate anosmia. A score of 0 to 5 indicates a malingerer. Scoring is useful in longitudinal serial examinations to determine if a patient's performance is constant or worsening over time.[10]

TABLE 14.4: **Approach to a patient with smell loss**

History	
Sudden loss of function	• Head trauma
	• Cerebrovascular accident
	• Acute upper respiratory infection
	• Psychiatric condition
Intermittent loss of function	Inflammatory processes (allergy, infection, chemical exposure)
Gradual loss of function	Nasal polyps, chronic upper respiratory infection, presbysomia
Difficulty passing air through nose	Obstruction secondary to polyps, inflammation or fracture
Physical examination	
Rhinorrhea	Rhinitis (allergy, infection), head trauma (fracture of cribriform plate)
Intranasal mass lesion	Polyps, neoplasm
Oral or perioral skin infection	Viral infection
White plaque on tongue	Candidiasis, HIV, leukoplakia
Facial palsy	Bell's palsy
Memory impairment	Alzheimer's disease
Motor findings (bradykinesia, cogwheel rigidity, tremor, ataxia, weakness)	Parkinson's disease, multiple sclerosis
Laboratory tests	
Anemia	Cancer, malnutrition
Altered red cell indices	Vitamin deficiencies (B12)
Leucocytosis	Infection
Deranged renal function tests	Kidney disease
Hyperglycemia	Diabetes mellitus
Deranged liver function tests	Viral hepatitis, Liver disease
Elevated prothrombin time	Liver disease, malnutrition
Altered thyroid function tests	Thyroid disease
Elevated ESR	Sjogren's syndrome, SLE
Elevated eosinophil count and IgE level	Allergy

IgE, immunoglobulin E; ESR, erythrocyte sedimentation rate; HIV, human immunodeficiency virus; SLE, systemic lupus erythematosus.

The Sniffin Sticks

This is a reusable screening test and involves smelling 12 odors. Shortened versions with three or five odor probes are also available.[11] The odors are distributed in pen like devices. On removal of the cap, the odor is released. The pen is held for 3 seconds about 2 cm under both the nostrils. The patients are asked to identify the odor from a list of four choices. [10]

The Threshold Olfactory Test

This test has two components. Firstly, it finds out the threshold at which the patient is able to detect an odorant, and secondly his ability to distinguish between various odorants. The odorants most frequently used are butanol or phenylethyl alcohol because of their minimal trigeminal components. The aim is to find the weakest concentration of butanol that the patient can detect. The test starts with the weakest concentration and proceeds to progressively stronger concentrations until the patient can detect the smell. The test is continued until the patient either gives five consecutive incorrect answers or consistently shows no ability to detect the butanol. The test takes around 20 minutes.

Next, the odor identification component tests the patient's ability to identify eight different smells. Each nostril is tested separately (Box 14.2).

Assessment of the Trigeminal Nerve

The trigeminal nerve endings in the nasal epithelium are important in detecting tactile pressure, pain, and temperature sensations. Trigeminal nerve function is assessed by the ability to detect pungent odors such as mustard oil, capsicum, and onion.

Psychophysical Test of Retronasal Olfaction

This involves placing a so-called Schmeckpulver (taste powder) in the mouth (20 different powdered forms from various foods and spices) and the patient is asked to identify the taste from a list of four choices.

Olfactory Event-Related Potentials

It is an objective method of testing the smell. The olfactometer must allow presentation of chemical stimuli of defined duration, concentration, and stimulus rise time. The presence of an olfactory event potential is suggestive of the ability to smell. It is primarily of importance for medicolegal purposes.[12]

THE SENSE OF TASTE

Anatomy and Physiology

Taste buds present in the tongue papillae consist of gustatory receptor cells and have a half-life of about 15 days.[13] These receptor cells are present on the base of the taste buds and are innervated by afferent neurons. The transduction of acid stimuli occurs by blocking of the potassium channels in the membrane of taste receptors. A potential independent sodium channel is involved in the transduction process for salty stimuli, while the transduction of sweet and bitter stimuli is associated with specific membrane receptors coupled to second messenger systems.[14]

Taste sensations are transported via four cranial nerves (Box 14.3).

The brainstem, thalamus, and the anterior insula are involved in the processing of taste information by the central nervous system.

Etiology of Taste Disorders

Only about 5% of the patients actually suffer from taste disorders. The majority have smell disorders due to altered odor perception (Box 14.4; Table 14.5).[15]

Box 14.2: Cutoff scores for the threshold olfactory test

- 0–1.75 indicates anosmia
- 2–3.75 indicates hyposmia
- 4–4.75 indicates moderate hyposmia
- 5–5.75 indicates mild hyposmia
- 6–7 indicates normosmia

Box 14.3: Cranial nerves that transport taste sensations

1. The sensory branch of nervus intermedius (facial nerve) innervates the taste receptors on the anterior two-thirds of the tongue (chorda tympani) and the palate (superficial petrosal nerve)
2. The glossopharyngeal nerve innervates taste receptors on the posterior third of the tongue
3. The vagus nerve innervates the taste receptors in the oropharynx and the pharyngeal portion of the epiglottis
4. The trigeminal nerve is responsible for temperature and texture of food

Box 14.4: Etiology of taste disorders

The main causes of taste disorders include:

- Head trauma with lesions in thalamus, brainstem, and temporal lobes which are important for processing taste stimuli. A fracture of the temporal bone or mandible can lead to damage to the facial nerve (the glossopharyngeal and the vagus nerves are relatively well-protected deep in the neck)[16]
- Upper respiratory tract infections
- Exposure to toxic substances and medications
- Iatrogenic causes (dental treatment or exposure to radiation)[17]
- Glossodynia or burning-mouth syndrome

  It is associated with hypogeusia with bitter or metallic taste. It is seen most commonly in postmenopausal females. Results with hormone replacement therapy are usually disappointing with spontaneous remission in only 50% of the cases[18]

TABLE 14.5: **Selected possible causes of taste disturbance**

Common causes	Less common causes
Oral and perioral infections	Nutritional factors (vitamin B3, B12 deficiency, zinc and copper deficiency, chronic renal failure, liver disease, AIDS)
Bell's Palsy	Tumors (oral cavity cancer, skull base neoplasm)
Medications	Head trauma
Oral appliances (dentures, tooth prosthetics)	Toxic chemical exposure (benzene, benzol, carbon disulfide, paint solvents)
Dental procedures (tooth extraction, root canal)	Industrial agent exposure (chromium, lead, copper)
Age	Radiation treatment of head and neck
Uncommon causes	
Psychiatric conditions (depression, anorexia nervosa)	Sjogren's syndrome
Epilepsy (gustatory aura)	Multiple sclerosis
Migraine	Endocrine disorders (adrenocortical insufficiency, Cushing's syndrome, diabetes mellitus, hypothyroidism, Kallmann's syndrome)

APPROACH TO A PATIENT WITH TASTE DISTURBANCES

Enquire about smoking and dietary habits. Ask about dental hygiene, dry mouth, and ability to taste. Focused examination of oral cavity, ears, and chorda tympani should be done.

Taste Testing

Taste versus Flavor

The first task is to differentiate between loss of taste and impairment of flavor. Flavor involves taste, smell, texture, and temperature. About 75% of the flavor sensation is produced by odorants. So, patients with taste loss complaints require smell testing.

Whole Mouth Taste Test[19]

This test assesses the patient's ability to detect, identify, and evaluate the intensity of different concentrations of sweet, sour, salty, and bitter taste solutions. Small amounts of the flavored solution are kept for few seconds in the mouth (sip and spit method).[20] Sugar (sweet), citric acid (sour), sodium chloride (salty), and quinine (bitter) are normally used as the test stimuli.

Spatial Taste Test

It is used to assess localized areas of impairment. A cotton swab dipped in a special taste solution is placed in different areas of the mouth. The patient is asked to swallow a part of each taste solution and assess the taste quality and intensity.

Box 14.5: Key points in the evaluation of smell and taste disorders

- Olfactory dysfunction is more common than taste dysfunction
- Three most common causes of loss of smell are nasal and sinus disease, upper respiratory infection, and head trauma
- Enquire about the use of tobacco, intranasal cocaine, or alcoholism
- Medications can interfere with smell and taste and should be reviewed in all patients
- Quantitative sensory evaluation, neurological, and otorhinolaryngological examination with appropriate brain and nasosinus imaging aid in evaluation of patients with olfactory or gustatory complaints
- Management of chemosensory disorders is condition specific
- Reassurance is the most important aspect of treatment

Flavor Discrimination Test

It is used to evaluate both taste and smell sensations. Four different solutions with different degrees of sweetness are used. The patient is asked to taste the solutions in random order.

Electrogustometry[21]

Weak electric currents are delivered to various taste bud fields in the mouth cavity. The sensation is similar to that if one licks the poles of a battery.

Somatosensory Testing

This test measures contact detection and spatial acuity thresholds. The contact detection threshold is tested with Stemmes-Weinstein monofilaments, which exert a force proportional to their gauge when applied to a peripheral nerve field. Different areas of the mouth are tested likewise.

Taste Strips

In this, a threshold is recorded by presenting stimuli in the form of tastant saturated filter paper or taste strips of different concentrations. The patient is asked to identify the flavor/taste.

Three-Drop Test

In this test, three drops of liquid are presented to the patient. One of the drops is the taste stimulus, and the other two drops are of pure water. The threshold is defined as the concentration at which the patient identifies the taste correctly three times in a row.

CONCLUSION

Smell and taste examination is usually neglected in the clinical examination. The key points in the evaluation of smell and taste disorders are summarized in Box 14.5.

REFERENCES

1. Devere R. Smell and taste in clinical neurology: five new things. Neurol Clin Prac. 2012;2:208-14.
2. Bromley SM. Smell and taste disorders: a primary care approach. Am Fam Physician. 2000;61(2):427-36.
3. Mattes RD, Cowart BJ. Dietary assessment of patients with chemosensory disorders. J Am Diet Assoc. 1994;94:50-6.
4. Schiffman SS, Wedral E. Contribution of taste and smell losses to the wasting syndrome. Age Nutr. 1996;7:106-20.
5. Hummel T, Landis BN, Hüttenbrink KB. Smell and taste disorders. GMS Curr Top Otorhinolaryngol Head Neck Surg. 2011;10:Doc04.
6. Buck L, Axel R. A novel multigene family may encode odorant receptors: a molecular basis for odor recognition. Cell. 1991;65:175-87.
7. Firestein S. How the olfactory system makes sense of scents. Nature. 2001;413:211-8.
8. Gottfried JA. Smell: central nervous processing. Adv Otorhinolaryngol. 2006;63:44-69.
9. Mann NM. Management of smell and taste problems. Cleve Clin J Med. 2002;69(4):329-36.
10. Hawkes CH, Doty RL. Neurology of olfaction. Cambridge: Cambridge Publishers; 2009.
11. Hummel T, Pfetzing U, Lötsch J. A short olfactory test based on the identification of three odors. J Neurol. 2010;257:1316-21.
12. Lötsch J, Hummel T. The clinical significance of electrophysiological measures of olfactory function. Behav Brain Res. 2006;170:78-83.
13. Beidler LM, Smallman RL. Renewal of cells within taste buds. J Cell Bio. 1965;27:263-72.
14. Chaudhari N, Roper SD. The cell biology of taste. J Cell Biol. 2010;190:285-96.
15. Deems DA, Doty RL, Settle RG, et al. Smell and taste disorders: a study of 750 patients from the University of Pennsylvania smell and taste center. Arch Otorhinolaryngol Head Neck Surg. 1991;117:519-28.
16. Heckmann JG, Lang CJ. Neurological causes of taste disorders. Adv Otorhinolaryngol. 2006;63:255-64.
17. Doty RL, Bromley SM. Effects of drugs on olfaction and taste. Otolaryngol Clin North Am. 2004;37:1229-54.
18. Grushka M, Epstein JB, Gorsky M. Burning mouth syndrome and other oral sensory disorders: a unifying hypothesis. Pain Res Manag. 2003;8:133-5.
19. Gudziol H, Hummel T. Normative values for the assessment of gustatory function using liquid tastants. Acta Otolaryngol. 2007;127:658-61.
20. Delwiche JF, Halpern BP, Lee MY. A comparison of tip of the tongue and sip and spit screening procedures. Food Qual P. 1996;7:293-7.
21. Hummel T, Genow A, Landis BN. Clinical assessment of human gustatory function using event related potentials. J Neurol Neurosurg Psychiatry. 2010;81:459-64.

Chapter 15

Approach to Visual Loss

Prem S Subramanian, Sarita B Dave

INTRODUCTION

The differential diagnosis for a patient with visual loss is broad and includes disease involving every aspect of the visual pathways from the tear film to the occipital lobe. The goal of evaluation of such a patient is to strategically acquire the key elements of the history and physical presentation, generate a precise differential diagnosis, and proceed with a targeted diagnostic evaluation. This chapter discusses the necessary components of the history and examination of a patient with visual loss. The subsequent discussion of visual loss is divided into three categories: transient visual loss, acute stationary visual loss, and progressive visual loss. While, there is some overlap between these categories, the general organization is helpful when approaching a patient.

HISTORY

A patient presenting with visual loss will provide tremendous aid to the clinician by describing three features of his symptoms: monocularity or binocularity, course of visual loss, and associated symptoms.

Monocular or Binocular

Laterality or bilaterality of vision loss is critical for accurate localization of a disease process. Monocular vision loss is most likely due to disease anterior to the optic chiasm; i.e., ipsilateral ocular, orbital, or optic nerve disease. Binocular vision loss may be due to bilateral ocular, orbital, or optic nerve disease, or to a chiasmal or retrochiasmal process. Although a patient may describe his symptoms as monocular, it is further imperative that the clinician clarify if the patient truly has monocular symptoms or if the patient has homonymous symptoms. This can be easily determined by asking the patient to occlude the poorly seeing eye and ensure that the vision in the contralateral eye is unaffected. A patient with homonymous pathology will often attribute their symptoms to the eye on the side of the affected temporal field and often not appreciate the binocularity of their vision loss until examined or specifically asked by the clinician.

Course of Visual Loss

The timing or pace of the vision loss relates to the underlying pathology. Transient vision loss (TVL) occurring over seconds may be due to raised intracranial pressure (ICP) and be triggered by changes in posture, whereas TVL lasting minutes is often due to an ischemic process from emboli. Onset of vision loss over hours to days may be due to ischemia or inflammation. Vision loss progressing over weeks to months may be due to inherited disease, as in Leber's Hereditary Optic Neuropathy, or a toxic cause, though vision loss from methanol and ethylene glycol toxicity is much more rapid. Slowly progressive vision loss over years can be due to compressive pathology, nutritional deficiencies, or inherited disease. Dominant optic atrophy classically causes very slow vision loss of approximately one line of visual acuity per decade.

Just as a patient may confuse monocularity for a homonymous defect, so might a patient complain of sudden vision loss, when in fact the vision loss has been suddenly recognized. This is typically the case for very gradual monocular vision loss occurring over months to years, and can suddenly be appreciated under monocular conditions, for instance while applying eye makeup or having a routine vision examination.

While these patterns of vision loss are typical, they are not definite, and there is considerable overlap between causes of vision loss and the pace of loss.

Associated Symptoms

See Table 15.1 for a list of pertinent associated symptoms and potential diagnoses. Because of the inapparent connection of some symptoms with loss of vision, a patient may not offer this information without direct questioning.

EXAMINATION

The goal of physical examination in a patient with vision loss is to characterize the extent of vision loss, and garner as much localizing information as one can. A thorough and thoughtful examination can narrow the differential to

TABLE 15.1: Associated symptoms and potential diagnoses

Associated symptoms	Differential diagnosis
Headache	• Idiopathic intracranial hypertension • Malignant hypertension • Giant cell arteritis • Intracranial mass • Migraine
Pain with eye movements	• Demyelinating disease • Orbital myositis
Eye redness or prominence	• Orbital mass • Thyroid eye disease • Orbital apex or cavernous sinus syndrome
Diplopia	• Thyroid eye disease • Orbital myositis • Orbital apex or cavernous sinus syndrome
Symptoms of hormonal deficiency (e.g., hair loss, weight gain/loss, palpitations, galactorrhea, sexual dysfunction, etc.)	Sellar mass
Numbness/weakness, ataxia	• Demyelinating disease • Stroke

those processes involving a particular accurately localized anatomical location and provide clues to the underlying etiology.

Visual Acuity

Visual acuity testing should be performed at distance and near when possible. If visual acuity is not 20/20, pinhole acuity should be measured to estimate the best-corrected visual acuity, assuming refraction cannot be readily performed. Distance and near acuity should be approximately equal, and if not, suggests media opacity (corneal or lenticular opacity) if distance acuity is better than near acuity (due to pupil constriction at near), and macular pathology if near acuity is better than distance (near testing projects the image beyond the macular portion of the retina).

Visual acuity worse than 20/400 can be documented using a 200 optotype E and documenting the distance at which its orientation is identified (i.e., "2/200 E" for proper identification at 2 feet). For worse vision loss, ability to defect finger-counting, hand motion, and light projection should be assessed.

Additional information can be obtained by observing for eccentric fixation (suggesting a central scotoma but intact peripheral field), or consistent inability to read letters on the left or right side of the chart (homonymous defect).

Color Vision

Color vision testing can facilitate identification of retinal versus optic nerve disease, or certain types of optic nerve disease. In retinal disease, color vision and visual acuity may be equally affected, whereas in compressive or demyelinating optic neuropathies, color vision is affected out of proportion to visual acuity. Reliable color vision testing requires visual acuity of 20/200 or better, and is most practically tested using pseudoisochromatic plates such as the Ishihara or Hardy-Rand-Rittler tests.

Confrontational Visual Fields

Confrontational visual field testing using finger-counting can detect gross, dense visual field defects and is most helpful in determining if vision loss is diffuse or if it respects horizontal or vertical meridians. Visual field defects respecting the horizontal meridian are typically caused by retinal or optic nerve disease, while those respecting the vertical midline, especially if bilateral, suggest chiasmal or postchiasmal pathology. If a

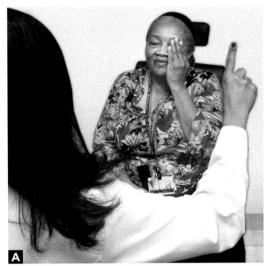 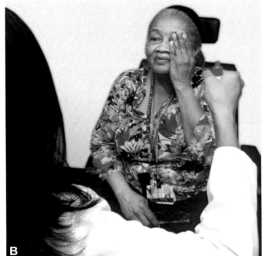

Figs 15.1A and B: Confrontation visual field testing. **(A)** Finger-counting. While fixating on the examiner's nose, the patient states the number of fingers demonstrated in each of four visual field quadrants. **(B)** Red object. The patient states if two red objects demonstrated simultaneously across the vertical midline appear equally red.

homonymous defect is suspected, detection of a spared "temporal crescent" may further localize a lesion to the posterior occipital lobe. Subtle defects can be detected by using simultaneous red objects (see Fig. 15.1 for a depiction of testing techniques).

Formal visual field testing using static and kinetic techniques are beyond the scope of this text, but are more accurate in assessing for visual field defects and are useful in monitoring over time.

Pupil Examination

A strong penlight and dim ambient lighting are essential for accurate pupil examination. Afferent unilateral or asymmetric bilateral disease will create a relative afferent pupillary defect (RAPD) on the affected side or on the more significantly affected side if bilateral. The pupils are best assessed for an RAPD utilizing the swing flashlight test. During testing, the examiner should note the velocity and amplitude of initial constriction to a light response, as well as the subsequent amount and rapidity of dilation. An RAPD typically suggests optic nerve disease, but can be present in contralateral optic tract disease, significant retinal disease, or in dense amblyopia.

Anisocoria, or asymmetry in pupil size, suggests efferent disease (oculomotor nerve palsy, Horner syndrome, tonic pupil, etc.) and will not be discussed in detail in this chapter.

Cranial Nerve Examination

A complete assessment of cranial nerves II through VII should be performed on all patients presenting with vision loss. Subtle cranial nerve palsies from raised ICP and orbital or cavernous sinus infiltration may be detected in a patient who complains solely of vision loss.

Direct Ophthalmoscopy

A direct ophthalmoscope provides a magnified (15X) view of the fundus, and although it does not provide tremendous stereoscopic detail, it allows a clinician to assess for visible signs of optic nerve or retinal disease. The optic nerve should specifically be assessed for hyperemia, pallor, hemorrhages, swelling (often appreciated as blurring of the disc margins), and size of the optic cup. Tortuosity, dilation, or attenuation of retinal vessels may also be observed.

TRANSIENT VISUAL LOSS

When approaching a patient with TVL, it is important to identify whether the vision loss is monocular or binocular, and to determine the duration and pattern of vision loss. This strategy allows targeting clinical testing and management (see Fig. 15.2 for a diagnostic algorithm of transient visual loss).

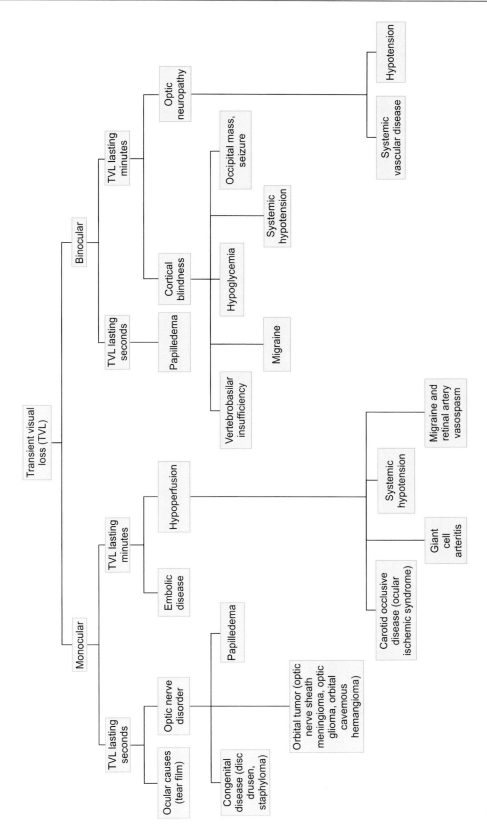

Fig. 15.2: Diagnostic algorithm for transient visual loss.

Monocular

TVL Lasting Seconds

Episodes of monocular TVL lasting seconds can be due to ocular, optic nerve, or orbital disease. Triggering or alleviating factors are often suggestive of the underlying etiology.

Individuals with papilledema may experience TVL due to the effects of raised ICP on the blood flow to the optic nerve.[1] These episodes are often precipitated by a change in posture and typically last <30 seconds. Although anxiety-provoking to a patient, there is no association with poor visual outcome.[2]

Similar TVL may occur in optic nerve sheath meningiomas and congenital abnormalities such as peripapillary staphyloma or optic disc drusen.

A common ocular cause of transient visual loss is tear film irregularity. Individuals may note difficulty with vision after prolonged visual activity (reading or watching television) and will often report improvement with blinking or closing the eyes for a few minutes. This presentation should be distinguished from rarer gaze-evoked (eccentric gaze) or reading-evoked TVL, which have been reported in cases of intraorbital mass (usually optic nerve sheath meningiomas or cavernous hemangiomas), papilledema, and intermittent angle closure.

Individuals with monocular TVL lasting seconds should have a complete ophthalmologic examination, with particular attention paid to the ocular surface, orbit and optic nerve. Findings suggestive of orbital disease (proptosis, limited motility, etc.), or the presence of papilledema should prompt magnetic resonance imaging (MRI) of the brain and orbits with contrast to investigate the possibilities of intraorbital compressive lesion, or intracranial tumor. In a patient with papilledema and normal MRI, a lumbar puncture should subsequently be performed to check for signs of CNS inflammation and infection. This is also a necessary step in diagnosing individuals with idiopathic intracranial hypertension.

Although, embolic disease typically causes TVL lasting minutes (see below), this should also be considered in individuals with brief TVL and an unrevealing examination.

TVL Lasting Minutes

Transient monocular vision loss lasting minutes is far more likely due to vascular disease than those episodes lasting seconds. The Dutch Transient Monocular Blindness Study Group described particular features of TVL associated with the presence of internal carotid artery (ICA) occlusion: altitudinal onset or disappearance of symptoms, precipitation of symptoms by bright light, occurrence of >10 attacks. Onset of vision loss occuring over seconds, and a duration of loss lasting between 1 and 10 minutes were significantly associated with ipsilateral ICA stenosis of 70–99%. Interestingly, patients who could not recall details of the onset, disappearance, or duration of symptoms were likely to have a normal ICA.[3]

In addition to the carotid artery, thromboembolic disease may from the heart or aorta may cause monocular TVL lasting minutes. Fundus examination may reveal emboli within retinal vessels. The most common types of emboli are cholesterol (Hollenhorst plaques), platelet-fibrin, and calcific (see Table 15.2). Presence of emboli should prompt general medication evaluation as well as studies of carotid patency, the heart and great vessels, using ultrasound, MRA or CTA, cardiac monitoring, and echocardiography.[4]

Non-embolic cause of monocular TVL include giant cell arteritis (GCA), hypoperfusion from carotid occlusive disease (ocular ischemic syndrome), collagen vascular disease, and hypercoagulable states. If pain is present, carotid dissection should be considered, especially if an ipsilateral Horner syndrome is also present.

In young patients (<45 years old) with a strong personal or family history of migraine, retinal vasospasm may produce monocular TVL with or without positive visual phenomena. During acute episodes, vasospasm of retinal

TABLE 15.2: **Emboli causing monocular transient vision loss**

Type of embolus	Appearance	Location	Origin
Cholesterol (Hollenhorst plaques)	Refractile yellow or copper colored	At a major bifurcation	• Atheromatous plaques • Carotid artery
Platelet-fibrin	Dull, gray white, elongated, fragmented, mobile	Along course of vessel with distal fragments	• Walls of atherosclerotic arteries • Heart valves
Calcific	Large, chalky white	Over or adjacent to the optic disc, or at a bifurcation	Heart valves

vessels may be observed on ophthalmoscopy. Additional history of premonitory symptoms or migrainous headache is supportive of vasospasm. Vision loss from vasospasm has been reported to progress in a lacunar pattern (gradual onset of scotomas which coalesce over time), rather than in an altitudinal "descending curtain" pattern seen in embolic or atheromatous causes.[5]

Other causes of transient monocular vision loss include impending anterior ischemic optic neuropathy (AION), impending retinal vessel occlusion, and TVL in the setting of optic neuritis (Uthoff's phenomenon).

Evaluation of monocular TVL, in addition to embolic workup described above, may include erythrocyte sedimentation rate (ESR), C-reactive protein (CRP), and platelets if GCA is suspected. Additionally, antiphospholipid antibodies, anticardiolipin antibody, antinuclear antibody, serum protein electrophoresis, prothrombin and partial thromboplastin times, protein C and S, antithrombin III, factor V Leiden, prothrombin, factor VIII, and plasma homocysteine may be included if there is suspicion of connective tissue disorders or hyper-coagulability.[6]

Binocular

TVL Lasting Seconds

Transient visual loss lasting seconds may be monocular or binocular in the setting of increased ICP and papilledema.

TVL Lasting Minutes

The most common cause of binocular TVL is the vision loss due to migraine with aura. The typical visual aura consists of flickering uncolored zig-zag lines in the center of the visual field that gradual expand toward the periphery over up to 30 minutes, typically leaving a scotoma. The scotoma may have a surrounding "fortification spectra". The visual symptoms are often bilateral and homonymous and resolve generally within 60 minutes. Individuals may or may not develop subsequent headache. Patients without prior headache history, those with vision loss or headache always on the same side, those with persistent visual symptoms, and those with accelerating frequency or severity of headache warrant imaging to rule out a space-occupying lesion such as tumor or arteriovenous malformation.

Bilateral TVL may also be due to bilateral occipital lobe ischemia from vertebrobasilar disease. Individuals with vertebrobasillar insufficiency will typically have other symptoms at the time of vision loss, including vertigo, dysarthria, dysphagia, diplopia, weakness, sensory loss, or gait and coordination difficulties. Vision loss may be bilateral or hemianopic.

Bilateral optic neuropathy from GCA or impending bilateral AION may rarely cause bilateral TVL. Other causes, including systemic conditions such as hypo-glycemia, hypotension, and occipital seizures (usually accompanied by unformed positive visual phenomena such as colored lights), should be considered.

Evaluation of someone with binocular TVL may include complete blood count, ESR, CRP, MRI, MRA, and electroencephalogram.

ACUTE STATIONARY VISION LOSS

Monocular

Anterior Ischemic Optic Neuropathy

Anterior ischemic optic neuropathy is the most common acute optic neuropathy in patients over 50 years old. Vision loss is typically painless and monocular and develops over hours to days. Ocular examination reveals visual acuity loss and visual field defects (often altitudinal), an RAPD, and optic disc edema with or without hemorrhages. Late pallor may be appreciated diffusely or in the involved sector.

Anterior ischemic optic neuropathy may be classified as nonarteritic or arteritic (see Fig. 15.3). Differentiation between the two is crucial. In arteritic AION, vision loss is secondary to inflammatory and thrombotic occlusion of the short posterior ciliary arteries which supply the optic nerve head. Immediate steroid therapy is critical, without which the fellow eye may become involved within days to weeks. Conversely, with treatment, 34% may experience visual improvement.[7] If there is suspicion of arteritic AION, ESR, CRP, and CBC should be obtained, steroids should be immediately initiated, and plans should be made for temporal artery biopsy.

In nonarteritic anterior ischemic optic neuropathy (AION), vision loss is attributed to hyperperfusion of the optic nerve head through a combination of a crowded, small optic nerve head, and a drop in systemic blood pressure. Patients may report visual impairment upon awakening possibly due to nocturnal hypertension, or temporally related to the use of antihypertensive medications or phosphodiesterase inhibitors such as sildenafil. Vision loss may be static or may progress either steadily or in stepwise decrements over several weeks.

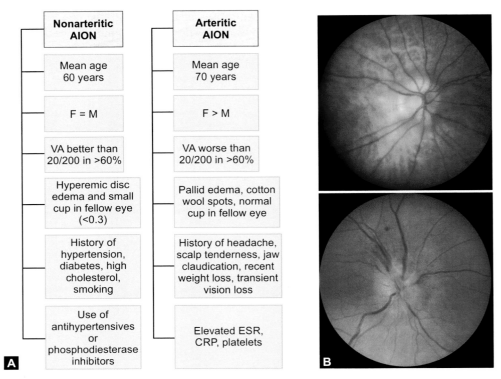

Figs 15.3A and B: (A) Comparison of nonarteritic versus arteritic AION; **(B)** Fundus photographs of nonarteritic (above) and arteritic (below) AION.

Recurrence has been reported to occur in 6% at 2 years, whereas onset in the fellow eye has been reported in 17% at 5 years.[8,9] Patients who present with typical features of AION should have a medical evaluation for underlying risk factors including hypertension, diabetes, and hypercholesterolemia. A hypercoaguable workup may be warranted in atypical cases (patients <45 years, absence of small cup in the fellow eye, bilateral simultaneous NAION, recurrent NAION, personal or family history of recurrent thrombotic events).[10]

Optic Neuritis

Optic neuritis generally refers to any optic neuropathy resulting from idiopathic, inflammatory, infectious, or demyelinating etiology. The terms papillitis or anterior optic neuritis are used if visible disc swelling is present, whereas retrobulbar optic neuritis refers to a normal optic nerve appearance.

Patients with typical demyelinating optic neuropathy present with periorbital ache and painful eye movement (92%), followed or accompanied by monocular vision loss. The pain diminishes and the vision loss reaches a nadir at around 4 days. Color vision is decreased out of proportion to visual acuity. Vision improves substantially by 6 weeks and continues to improve slowly up to 12–18 months. Examination reveals an RAPD and diffuse central visual field loss. In retrobulbar optic neuritis (65%), the disc may appear normal. Imaging will reveal optic nerve enhancement.[11]

Magnetic resonance imaging of the brain is recommended in every case of retrobulbar optic neuritis. The presence of periventricular white matter lesions is the greatest risk factor for progression to MS. The overall rate of conversion to MS is 50% at 15 years, with a 25% risk in patients with zero lesions on MRI and a 72% risk in patients with at least one lesion.[12]

Individuals with atypical features of optic neuritis warrant further testing to rule out infection, systemic inflammation, neuromyelitis optica, or polyneuropathies such as Guillain Barre, Miller Fisher, and chronic inflammatory demyelinating polyradiculoneuropathy (see Box 15.1).

Children with optic neuritis are more likely to have bilateral optic neuritis, papillitis, and an association with recent viral illness or vaccination. Younger children (<10

- Bilateral simultaneous or rapidly sequential optic neuritis in an adult
- Pain and vision loss lasting >30 days
- Exam findings: Retinal vasculitis, lipid maculopathy, marked hemorrhages or cotton wool spots, vitreous cells
- Exquisite steroid sensitivity
- Age >50 years

Differential and evaluation of atypical optic neuritis

- Sarcoidosis: Chest CT, gallium scan, serum ACE levels
- Syphilis: Serum and CSF, VDRL and FTA-ABS
- Lupus and other vasculitides: ESR, ANA, Anti-DNA
- Lyme: IgG and IgM Elisa, Western blot
- Neuromyelitis optica: MRI spine, NMO antibody, CSF pleocytosis

MRI, magnetic resonance imaging; ACE, angiotensin-converting enzyme; NMO, neuromyelitis optica; CSF-VDRL, cerebrospinal fluid-Venereal Disease Research Laboratory; FTA-ABS, fluorescent treponemal antibody-absorption; ANA, antinuclear antibody; ESR, erythrocyte sedimentation rate.

years) with normal brain imaging are more likely to have bilateral disease and are less likely to develop multiple sclerosis.[13]

Neuroretinitis

Neuroretinitis is a clinical syndrome of children and adults characterized by optic disc edema and macular start (lipid exudates). It is a distinct entity from optic neuritis and does not carry an increased risk of demyelinating disease. Individuals with neuroretinitis typically present with unilateral (66%) acute painless loss of vision. One half of individuals will have a history of preceding viral illness. Fundus examination will initially reveal optic disc edema alone, followed 1–2 weeks later by macular star formation.

Neuroretinitis is generally benign and self-limited and has been associated with a wide variety of infectious causes. The most common of these is cat-scratch disease (*Bartonella henselae)*, which accounts for up to two thirds of cases. Although self-limited, treatments with antibiotics are thought to shorten the course of disease. Additional infectious causes of neuroretinitis include syphilis, tuberculosis, Lyme disease, and toxoplasmosis. Extent of workup should be guided by the patient history and examination findings. Generally, testing should include *Bartonella* titers, fluorescent treponemal antibody-absorption (FTA-ABS) test, and chest CT.[14]

Traumatic Optic Neuropathy

Traumatic optic neuropathy is often apparent from patient history and occurs in two forms. The direct form results from injury to the nerve by bone fragments or other foreign bodies, avulsion of the nerve, or compression by intraorbital or intrasheath hemorrhage. The indirect form occurs with head injury often to the frontal or brow region in which the force of the injury is transmitted along the frontal bone to the optic canal where a shear injury occurs. Visual loss is severe and permanent and accompanied by an RAPD. Pallor becomes apparent within 1–2 months.

Neuroimaging is required to assess the extent of the injury and detect any associated injury or fractures. Management of these individuals is directed toward these injuries, as there is no clear benefit of treatment either with surgery or high-dose steroids. In fact, treatment with high-dose steroids is associated with a higher rate of mortality than no treatment.[15]

Binocular

Binocular, acute vision loss is typically associated with a suggestive history or associated symptoms indicative of the underlying etiology.

Posterior AION is an often bilateral condition characterized by severe vision loss. It often follows spinal surgeries or cardiac surgeries and has been associated with significant blood loss and face-down positioning. Radiation optic neuropathy also causes a posterior AION, and is discussed below (see Table 15.3).

Severe hypertensive retinopathy is characterized by narrowing of retinal vessels, hemorrhages, and disc swelling. This is typically bilateral and should be included in the differential of any patient presenting with bilateral disc edema.

Any cerebral vascular event involving the chiasmal or retrochiasmal visual pathways will cause bilateral visual field loss. Temporal and parietal strokes are often associated with other neurologic symptoms, whereas occipital strokes may be characterized by vision loss in isolation.

PROGRESSIVE VISION LOSS

The differential diagnosis for progressive vision loss is extensive. Accompanying symptoms, unilaterality versus bilaterality, and nature of visual field loss are the most helpful features in narrowing the differential. A schematic

TABLE 15.3: Features of radiation optic neuropathy

Focus of irradiation	Paranasal sinuses, skull base, pituitary adenoma, parasellar meningiomas, craniopharyngiomas, frontal and temporal gliomas, intraocular tumors, dysthyroid orbitopathy (in patients with diabetes mellitus)
Mechanism	• Vascular endothelial cell injury • Direct injury to replicating glial tissue • Demyelination, neuronal degeneration, vascular occlusion, and necrosis
Risk factors	• Dose and daily fractionation size • (>50 total Gy, daily fractions >2 Gy) • Increasing age • Pre-existing optic nerve injury (as in compression and vascular compromise from pituitary tumors) • Concurrent chemotherapy
Onset	Average 18 months after radiation therapy (range 3 months to 8 years)
Symptoms	• Episodes of transient vision loss • Acute, painless vision loss in one or both eyes • Progression over weeks to months
Signs	• Altitudinal or central visual field loss • Optic nerve pallor • Optic nerve enhancement on MRI
Differential	• Tumor recurrence, secondary malignancy, arachnoiditis
Treatment	Unsuccessful (hyperbaric oxygen, anti-coagulation, corticosteroids)
Prognosis	• No light perception in 45% • 20/200 or worse in 85%

illustration of one approach to progressive vision loss is shown in Fig. 15.4.

Raised Intracranial Pressure

Individuals with elevated ICP may present with a constellation of symptoms, including headache, pulsatile tinnitus, diplopia, and transient obscurations of vision. While visual field loss occurs to some degree in most cases of elevated ICP, central vision is spared unless the condition is severe or long standing. This is a key feature in distinguishing raised ICP from other optic neuropathies and is critical in determining the urgency of treatment. The differential diagnosis for raised ICP is vast (see Box 15.2).

Box 15.2: Differential diagnosis of raised intracranial pressure

Decreased absorption
• Meningitis
• Subarachnoid hemorrhage

Obstructive hydrocephalus
• Chiari malformation
• Aqueductal stenosis
• Mass lesions (ependymoma, astrocytoma, choroid plexus papilloma, hypothalamic or optic nerve glioma, craniopharyngioma, pituitary adenoma, metastatic tumors)

Obstructed venous outflow
• Venous sinus thrombosis
  ○ Middle ear infection
  ○ Hypercoagulable state
  ○ Systemic lupus erythematosus
• Venous sinus stenosis
• Glomus tumor, bilateral radical neck dissection, superior vena cava syndrome
• Arteriovenous malformation

Endocrine
• Addison disease
• Hypoparathyroidism
• Obesity
• Steroid withdrawal
• Growth hormone use in children

Exogenous factors
• Anabolic steroids
• Hypervitaminosis A
• Lithium
• Tetracycline antibiotics
• Nalidixic acid
• Oral contraceptives

Idiopathic Intracranial Hypertension

Idiopathic intracranial hypertension (IIH) is a syndrome of increased ICP typically occurring in obese women of childbearing age. Diagnostic criteria are shown in Box 15.3. Most individuals with IIH complain of headache (94%), transient visual obscurations (68%), pulsatile tinnitus (58%), and photopsias (54%). Diplopia and visual loss are less common (38% and 30%, respectively). Fundus examination reveals papilledema, the severity of which is associated with the extent of vision loss.[16] Additional findings may include sixth cranial nerve palsy (10–20%)[2] which has been attributed to compression as the nerve enters Dorello's canal.

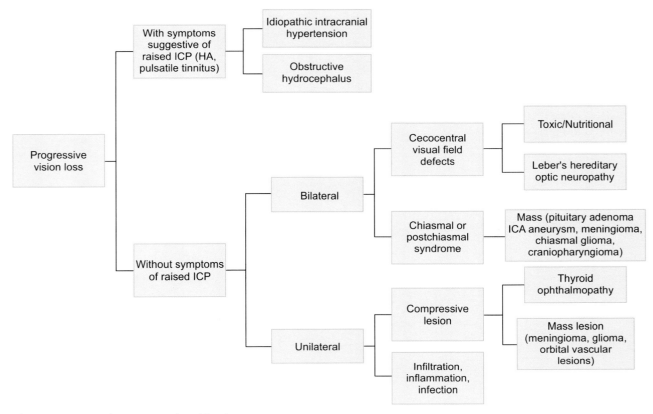

Fig. 15.4: Approach to progressive vision loss.

As mentioned previously, visual acuity remains normal in patients with IIH, unless the condition is chronic or severe, or if optic disc edema extends into the macula. Therefore, visual acuity testing alone is insufficient in detecting vision loss. Individuals with uncontrolled IIH must be followed by an ophthalmologist with formal visual field testing (static or kinetic), and with stereofundus photographs or optical coherence tomography (OCT), if available. Visual field loss other than enlargement of the physiologic blind spot is present in 92–96% of patients on formal testing, one-third of which is mild and unnoticed by the patient. The most common defects include blind spot enlargement, inferonasal defects, arcuate defects, and peripheral constriction. Severe or chronic disease is associated with generalized depression of the entire field, most pronounced peripherally. Central defects alone are so uncommon that their presence should prompt a search for another diagnosis.[17]

A heightened level of caution should be used in treating men with IIH. Men may require more aggressive intervention and are more likely than women to have visual loss.[18] Additionally African American men may be at great risk of vision loss.[19] Obstructive sleep apnea (OSA) has been shown to be a common finding in men with IIH, and studies have demonstrated a relationship between increased ICP during apneic periods and also while awake.[20-22] Therefore, sleep study is recommended in all men and women with a history suggestive of OSA.[23]

Box 15.3: Modified Dandy criteria for IIH

- Signs and symptoms of raised intracranial pressure (ICP)
- Absence of localizing findings on neurologic examination (aside from sixth cranial nerve palsy)
- Raised opening pressure on lumbar puncture (>25 cm water) with otherwise normal cerebrospinal fluid studies and normal imaging (aside from flattening of posterior globes, tortuosity of orbital optic nerve, optic nerve sheath dilation, empty sella)
- Awake and alert patient
- No other identifiable cause of raised ICP

Bilateral Progressive Vision Loss

In the absence of symptoms of raised ICP, the pattern of visual field loss in an individual with progressive bilateral vision loss can be suggestive of the underlying pathology. The differential of bilateral vision loss with central or cecocentral visual defects should include toxic or nutritional optic neuropathy, and hereditary optic

neuropathies. Alternatively, junctional, bitemporal, or homonymous defects suggest a sellar mass.

Toxic Agents and Nutritional Deficiencies

Toxic or nutritional optic neuropathy causes gradual, progressive, bilaterally symmetric, painless vision loss with central or cecocentral scotoma (Fig. 15.5). Pupils may

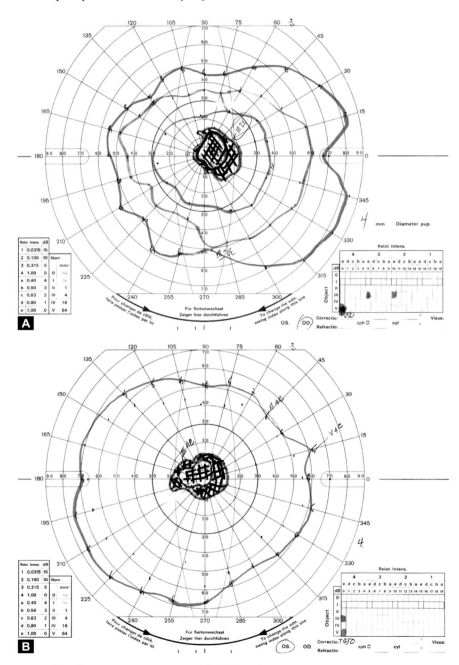

Figs 15.5A and B: Characteristic cecocentral field loss of toxic/nutritional optic neuropathy. The defect extends from the physiologic blind spot to the central field in each eye.

be sluggish, and because of bilaterality, there is no RAPD. Color vision may be diminished. Fundus examination may demonstrate mild or moderate edema, with eventual optic atrophy, particular of the temporal nerve with corresponding loss of the papillomacular bundle.

Methanol and ethylene glycol toxicity are characterized by rapid and severe vision loss with significant disc edema. While ethanol abuse is associated with optic neuropathy, it is more likely due to the associated malnutrition. Amiodarone use has also been associated with bilateral visual loss, and although it has been described in association with NAION, it is characterized by subacute onset of bilateral, diffuse peripheral rather than altitudinal loss, and disc edema, both of which resolve within months of discontinuing the medication. Other medications and toxic substances attributed to toxic optic neuropathy are listed in Box 15.4.[23]

A history of gastric bypass or resection, dietary restriction, alcoholism, pernicious anemia, or long-term veganism should prompt a more detailed history of diet history. If nutritional optic neuropathy is suspected, it is prudent to obtain neuroimaging to rule out other causes unless the diagnosis is certain. All patients suspected of nutritional deficiency should have thiamine (vitamin B1),

> **Box 15.4: Medications and substances associated with toxic optic neuropathy**
>
> - Methanol
> - Ethylene glycol
> - Amiodarone
> - Ethambutol
> - Isoniazid
> - Chloramphenicol
> - Hydroxyquinolones
> - Penicillamine
> - Cisplatin
> - Vincristine
> - Lead
> - Tobacco

vitamin B12, and red blood cell folate levels evaluated. Prognosis is excellent if the underlying condition is corrected prior to the onset of optic nerve pallor.

Radiation optic neuropathy, although likely due to ischemic injury rather than direct toxicity to the nerve, may also cause central visual field loss and should be considered in an individual with history of prior radiation to the brain or orbit. Features of RON are listed in Table 15.3.[24]

Hereditary Optic Neuropathy

Leber's Hereditary Optic Neuropathy

Leber's hereditary optic neuropathy (LHON) is a mitochondrial condition classically affecting men more than women (80–90%). The onset of vision loss typically occurs acutely between age 15 and 35 years (range 1–80 years) and is painless and unilateral. The second eye is affected weeks to months later. Vision loss is severe (<20/200), with central or cecocentral visual field loss and typically stabilizes after 3–4 months. Color vision is severely affected. Uniquely, pupil light responses may be relatively preserved.

On fundus examination, the optic nerve appears hyperemic and elevated with peripapillary retinal nerve fiber layer thickening and telangiectasias (Fig. 15.6). The retinal arterioles may appear tortuous. A similar appearance may be seen in asympomatic relatives. Late findings include nerve pallor and loss of the papillomacular nerve fiber layer bundle.

In the absence of a positive family history, neuroimaging is warranted to rule out treatable causes of vision loss.

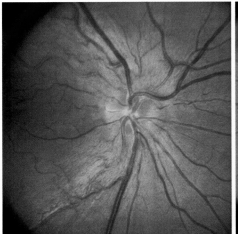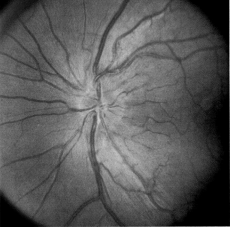

Figs 15.6A and B: Classic disc appearance of LHON. Note hyperemic appearance.

Genetic testing for the underlying mutation carries prognostic value. Of the three most common mutations (11778, 14484, and 3460), the 14484 mutation carries the best prognosis with the highest chance of spontaneous improvement (65%), while the 11778 mutation has the lowest chance (4%).[25]

Dominant Optic Atrophy

Dominant optic atrophy is the most common of the hereditary optic neuropathies. The disease onset occurs insidiously in the first decade of life and progressively declines approximately one line of visual acuity per decade, with most individuals maintaining vision of 20/200 or better. The condition is bilateral and often asymptomatic due to its lack of acute progression. The condition is diagnosed either because of a family member with the condition, failure to pass a routine school vision screening, or at a "routine" eye examination.

Examination is often significant for dyschromatopsia, central, paracentral, or cecocentral scotomas, and optic nerve pallor. In addition to family history, genetic testing for the OPA1 gene may facilitate diagnosis.

Parasellar Lesions

Presence of a bilateral visual defect with either a homonymous, bitemporal, or junctional pattern should prompt suspicion of a parasellar mass (Fig. 15.7). The differential for masses in the parasellar region includes pituitary adenoma, meningioma, craniopharyngioma, internal carotid artery aneurysm, and chiasmal glioma. Though not discussed in detail here, conditions including multiple sclerosis, lymphocytic hypophysitis, sarcoidosis, Wegener's granulomatosis, syphilis, and tuberculosis can also cause mass effect on the chiasm.

These lesions typically cause gradually progressive, bilateral visual loss involvement is asymmetric, or if the optic tract is involved. There may be impaired visual acuity or dyschromatopsia. Fundus examination may be normal or show mild optic disc pallor. Evaluation by an ophthalmologist with formal visual acuity and visual field testing at baseline and following any intervention is critical in establishing progression, success of treatment, or evidence of recurrence.

Pituitary Adenoma

Pituitary adenomas are the most common chiasmal tumors and occur at any adult age. Nonsecreting tumors typically present with visual loss, whereas secreting tumors present with symptoms related to hormonal aberrations. In addition to vision loss, pituitary tumors

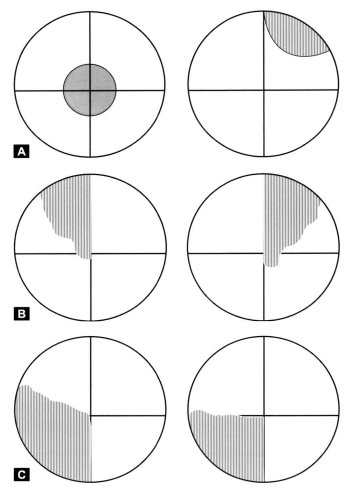

Figs 15.7A–C: Schematic representations of visual field defects indicating of posterior optic nerve, chiasmal, and tract lesions, respectively. **(A)** Junctional scotoma; **(B)** Bitemporal hemianopia; **(C)** Homonymous hemianopia.

may cause a multiple cranial neuropathy if there is extension into the cavernous sinus. Tumors may present during pregnancy due to enlargement of the tumor with compression of the chiasm. Because of their location inferior to the chiasm, they may present with field defects that are denser superiorly.

Pituitary apoplexy is a life-threatening condition caused by acute hemorrhage or infarction of the pituitary tumor. Symptoms include severe headache, abrupt vision loss, diplopia, and decreased level of consciousness. Treatment of pituitary apoplexy with immediate corticosteroids is imperative.

Meningioma

Parasellar meningiomas arise from the tuberculum sella, planum sphenoidale, or clinoids. Particular features of meningioma will be discussed in further detail below. These masses may also present due to growth during pregnancy because of the presence of estrogen and progesterone receptors on tumor cells.

Craniopharyngioma

Craniopharyngiomas more commonly present in childhood. They often arise superior to the chiasm and thus produce inferior visual field defects.

Internal Carotid Artery Aneurysm

Parasellar aneurysm often produces an asymmetric chiasmal syndrome, with the denser defect on the side of the aneurysm.

Chiasmal Glioma

Most common in children, gliomas are discussed in greater detail below.

Unilateral Compressive Lesions

Optic Nerve Sheath Meningioma

Optic nerve sheath meningioma (ONSM) usually occurs in women three times more often than men, with a mean age of onset of 41 years. Individuals present with a slowly progressive loss of visual acuity, poor color vision, and field loss. Pain, double vision, and TVL are less common. The optic nerve may be swollen, usually without hemorrhages or exudates, though there may also be signs of chronic disease such as optic nerve pallor and shunt vessels.

Characteristic imaging findings of ONSMs include an enhancing sheath of tumor surrounding a hypodense optic nerve. On axial imaging, this may appear as the classic "tram-track" sign (Fig. 15.8).[26]

Because the tumor is interposed between the nerve and its extradural blood supply, surgical removal is generally not a treatment option. Untreated, however, these tumors invariably grow and cause progressive vision loss with eventual blindness. Radiation treatment has been shown to be effective in overall disease control (94.3%) and in improvement (54.7%). Patients should be counseled on treatment options and followed long-term with or without treatment.[27]

Optic Nerve Gliomas

Optic nerve gliomas typically become symptomatic in childhood, with 75% presenting in the first decade of

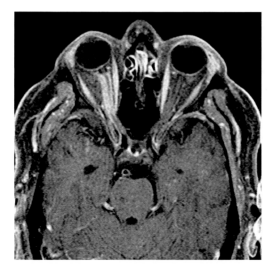

Fig. 15.8: Radiographic appearance of optic nerve sheath meningioma.

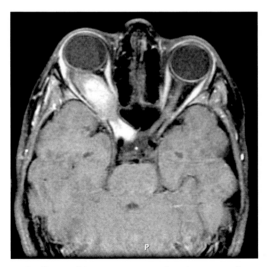

Fig. 15.9: Radiographic appearance of optic nerve glioma.

life and 90% presenting in the second decade.[28] Signs of optic nerve glioma include proptosis, visual loss, optic disc pallor, edema, and strabismus. Patients may present with an asymptomatic optic atrophy. Optic nerve glioma is associated with neurofibromatosis 1 (NF1), with 7.8–21% incidence of glioma in those with NF1, and 10–70% incidence of NF1 in those with glioma.[29]

Neuroimaging reveals a fusiform enlargement of the optic nerve with diffuse or partial enhancement. The dural sheath appears separate from the tumor (Fig. 15.9).

The natural history of optic nerve gliomas is usually benign and observation is indicated. If there is severe vision loss at presentation, evidence of progression, or involvement of the optic chiasm with secondary obstructive hydrocephalus or hypothalamic dysfunction, chemotherapy with carboplatin, and vincristine is accepted.

Thyroid Ophthalmopathy

Severe thyroid ophthalmopathy can cause optic neuropathy in the setting of compression of the optic nerve at the orbital apex. The visual loss is typically slowly progressive and may be unilateral or bilaterally. Visual fields may show central or diffuse depression. Signs of lid retraction and lag, restricted motility, lid and conjunctival edema, and proptosis are supportive of thyroid ophthalmopathy. If an optic neuropathy is present, orbital CT imaging should be obtained to investigate for enlargement of the extraocular muscles, apical crowding, and optic nerve compression. Treatment includes intravenous pulse corticosteroids and surgical decompression.[30]

Inflammation, Infection, and Infiltration

Inflammatory, infectious, and infiltrative processes can all be associated with vision loss, though rare. These conditions may present as vision loss from optic neuropathy, retinal disease, or secondary to orbital or CNS involvement. The differential diagnosis is broad and includes sarcoidosis, connective tissue diseases, Bartonella, Lyme, Syphilis, Tuberculosis, Toxoplasmosis, Herpes viridae (HSV, HZV), lymphoma, leukemia, and carcinomas. A suggestive review of systems may narrow the workup, though thorough laboratory and radiographic evaluation is often needed in most cases.

Ocular

In cases where the cause or anatomic site of vision loss is unclear, ophthalmic examination may be revealing. A comprehensive evaluation by an ophthalmologist will exclude common conditions, such as cataracts, glaucoma, diabetic retinopathy, and age-related macular degeneration. Individuals may present with these conditions acutely, either after abrupt onset or worsening, or after being acutely appreciated. Rarer ophthalmic conditions, such as uveitis and autoimmune retinopathies (cancer-associated and melanoma-associated retinopathy), may also be considered at the time of ophthalmic evaluation, particularly in cases of acute or severe vision loss.

Ophthalmic evaluation with fluorescein angiography, optical coherence tomography, and electroretinography are beyond the scope of this text, but may have critical importance in diagnosing ocular conditions or in isolating the affected anatomic structure.

REFERENCES

1. Sadun A, Currie J, Lessell S. Transient visual obscurations with elevated optic discs. Ann Neurol. 1984;16:484-94.
2. Wall M, George D. Idiopathic intracranial hypertension: a prospective study of 50 patients. Brain. 1991;114:155-80.
3. Donders RC, Dutch TMB Study Group. Clinical features of transient monocular blindness and the likelihood of atherosclerotic lesions of the internal carotid artery. J Neurol Neurosurg Psychiatry. 2001;71:247-9.
4. Miller NR. Embolic causes of transient monocular visual loss. Ophthalmol Clin North Am. 1996;9:359-80.
5. O'Sullivan E, Rossor M, Elston JS. Amaurosis fugax in young people. Br J Ophthalmol. 1995;76:660-2.
6. Biousse V, Trobe JD. Transient monocular visual loss. Am J Ophthalmol. 2005;140:717-21.
7. Liu GT, Glaser JS, Schatz NJ, et al. Visual morbidity in giant cell arteritis. Clinical characteristics and prognosis for vision. Ophthalmology. 1994;101:1779-85.
8. Hayreh SS, Podhajsky PA, Zimmerman B. Ipsilateral recurrence of nonarteritic anterior ischemic optic neuropathy. Am J Ophthalmol. 2001;132:732-42.
9. Beck RW, Hayreh SS, Podhajsky PA, et al. Aspirin therapy in nonarteritic anterior ischemic optic neuropathy. Am J Ophthalmol. 1997;123:212-7.
10. Lee AG. Prothrombotic and vascular risk factors in nonarteritic anterior ischemic optic neuropathy. Ophthalmology. 1999;106:2231.
11. Optic Neuritis Study Group. The clinical profile of optic neuritis. Experience of the optic neuritis treatment trial. Arch Ophthalmol. 1991;19:1673-8.
12. Optic Neuritis Study Group. Multiple sclerosis risk after optic neuritis: final optic neuritis treatment trial follow-up. Arch Neurol. 2008;65:727-32.
13. Waldman AT, Stull LB, Galetta SL, et al. Pediatric optic neuritis and risk of multiple sclerosis: meta-analysis of observational studies. J AAPOS. 2011;15:441-6.
14. Purvin V, Sundaram S, Kawasaki A. Neuroretinitis review of the literature and new observations. J Neuroophthalmol. 2011;31:58-68.
15. Levin LA, Beck RW, Joseph MP, et al. The treatment of traumatic optic neuropathy: the International Optic Nerve Trauma Study. Ophthalmology. 1999;106:1268-77.
16. Wall M, White WN. Asymmetric papilledema in idiopathic intracranial hypertension: prospective interocular comparison of sensory visual function. Invest Ophthalmol Vis Sci. 1998;39:134-42.
17. Digre KB, Corbett JJ. Pseudotumor cerebri in men. Arch Neurol. 1988;45:866-72.
18. Bruce BB, Kedar S, Van Stavern GP, Monaghan D, et al. Idiopathic intracranial hypertension in men. Neurology. 2009;72:304-19.
19. Lee AG, Golnik K, Kardon R, et al. Sleep apnea and intracranial hypertension in men. Ophthalmology. 2002;109:482-5.
20. Sugita Y, Iijima S, Teshima Y, et al. Marked episodic elevation of cerebrospinal fluid pressure during nocturnal sleep in patients with sleep apnea hypersomnia syndrome. Electroencephalogr Clin Neurophysiol. 1985;60:214-9.

21. Jennum P, Borgesen SE. Intracranial pressure and obstructive sleep apnea. Chest. 1989;95:279-83.
22. Wall M. Idiopathic intracranial hypertension. Neurol Clin. 2010;28:593-617.
23. Rizzo JF III, Lessell S. Tobacco amblyopia. Am J Ophthalmol. 1993;116:84-7.
24. Miller NR. Radiation-induced optic neuropathy: still no treatment. Clin Experiment Ophthalmol. 2004;32:2330-5.
25. Riordan-Eva P, Sanders MD, Govan GG, et al. The clinical features of Leber's hereditary optic neuropathy defined by the presence of a pathogenic mitochondrial DNA mutation. Brain. 1995;118:319-37.
26. Dutton JJ. Optic nerve sheath meningiomas. Surv Ophthalmol. 1992;37: 167-83.
27. Miller NR. New concepts in the diagnosis and management of optic nerve sheath meningioma. J Neuroophthalmol. 2006;26:200-8.
28. Dutton JJ. Gliomas of the anterior visual pathway. Surv Ophthalmol. 1994;38:427-52.
29. Listernick R, Louis DN, Packer RJ, et al. Optic pathway gliomas in children with neurofibromatosis type 1: consensus statement from the NF1 Optic Glioma Task Force. Ann Neurol. 1997;41:143-9.
30. Kahaly GJ, Pitz S, Hommel G, et al. Randomized, single blind trial of intravenous versus oral steroid monotherapy in Graves' orbitopathy. J Clin Endocrinol Metab. 2005;90:5234-40.

Chapter 16

Clinical Approach to Pupillary and Eyelid Abnormalities

Wesley Chan, Fiona E Costello

INTRODUCTION

The pupil is an aperture in the iris that allows light to be directed upon the retina. Differences in pupillary light response between the two eyes can help localize lesions affecting the pregeniculate regions of the afferent visual pathway. Because pupil size and movement are mediated by input from the autonomic nervous system, "anisocoria", or intereye asymmetry in pupil size can implicate underlying disorders affecting the sympathetic or parasympathetic supply to the iris musculature. Recognizing efferent pupil abnormalities is often a key step in identifying potentially life-threatening diagnoses that affect autonomic innervation to the eye.

USING THE PUPIL EXAMINATION TO LOCALIZE AFFERENT VISUAL PATHWAY PROBLEMS

In the afferent visual pathway, light enters the pupil and is directed upon the retina. Here, light energy is converted by retinal photoreceptors (rods and cones) into electrical signals that are transmitted from the outer to the inner layers of the retina to reach the retinal ganglion cells.[1] The retinal ganglion cell axons travel in the retinal nerve fiber layer to exit the eye through the optic nerve. From there, afferent visual pathway fibers travel to the optic chiasm that lies just above the sella turcica. Nasal retina fibers from each eye decussate to join axons from the temporal retina of the contralateral eye. This anatomical organization brings together information from the halves of each retina that view the same region of the visual field.[1] Fibers from each eye are then represented in the

right and left optic tracts, which exit the chiasm, en route for the lateral geniculate nuclei located in the thalami. Postsynaptic fibers in the afferent visual pathway leave the lateral geniculate body via the optic radiations, to reach the mesial surface of the occipital lobe in the striate ("calcarine") cortex.[1] Light information that originated in the retina is processed to provide a visual representation of the world we perceive.

In approaching a patient with a suspected afferent visual pathway lesion, it is necessary to take a detailed clinical history to help determine whether the problem represents a lesion of the retina, the optic nerve, or the retrochiasmal visual pathways. In addition, understanding the anatomical organization of the afferent visual pathway is crucial to localizing lesions therein. The pupil examination can facilitate this process, because afferent sensory fibers that mediate pupillary function leave the visual sensory pathway just prior to their synaptic targets in the lateral geniculate nucleus, to reach the pretectal nuclei in the dorsal midbrain.[2,3] Accordingly, a lesion anywhere from the retina to the optic tract can impair the pupillary light reflex, without resulting in anisocoria.[3] Both optic nerves provide input to the pretectal nuclei in the midbrain, which is followed by distribution of equal output to each oculomotor nucleus. This anatomical organization means that pupils appear equal in size in the setting of asymmetric input from a unilateral optic nerve lesion.[3] The hallmark of a unilateral lesion affecting the retina, optic nerves, chiasm, or tract is, therefore, not anisocoria, but the relative afferent pupillary defect (RAPD). Notably, lesions of the lateral geniculate nucleus and retrogeniculate limbs of the afferent visual pathway do not cause the RAPD.[2] Similarly, the RAPD is not observed in cases of refractive error, cataract, or corneal lesions.[2,3]

Detecting a Relative Afferent Pupillary Defect

Prior to checking for the RAPD, it is important to ascertain that the direct and consensual pupillary light responses are normal, meaning that there is no coexisting efferent pupil problem in either eye. With the "Swinging Flashlight Test," the patient is examined in a dimly lit room. In bright lighting conditions (commonly encountered in an emergency room or clinic setting), the ambient light hinders the ability to control the amount of illumination entering each eye separately, making inequality in the pupillary light response difficult to discern. In darkness, both pupils will dilate, whereas in bright light both pupils will constrict equally. Shining the light into either pupil will cause brisk pupil constriction (direct response) in the illuminated pupil, and an equal magnitude of constriction (consensual response) in the pupil of the fellow eye. The light is alternately swung back and forth to illuminate one pupil and then the next, approximately every 1–4 seconds.[3] Both pupils will dilate when light is shone into the eye with the RAPD, whereas both pupils will constrict when light is shone into the normal or relatively unaffected eye.[2,3] When, the disparity in how intensely the light is perceived is great between the two eyes, the RAPD can be detected with a few relatively quick swings of the light. In contrast, when the difference between perceived sensory input is more subtle, the examiner will often have to move the light alternately and with more moderate speed between the two eyes several times to detect the RAPD. Once the presence of the RAPD is established, its severity can be quantified by placing neutral density filters in front of the better or normally functioning pupil. This results in less light entering the "good" eye, which will eventually counter the imbalance in light input causing the RAPD in the "bad" eye. When this balance is attained, the pupillary light reflex will appear symmetric between both eyes and the RAPD size can be measured by noting the filter strength needed to equalize the pupillary responses between the two eyes.[3,4] If one pupil manifests a coexisting efferent problem (pharmacological dilation or iris sphincter damage), it is still possible to test for a RAPD by the "reverse method."[3] Because the pupils react consensually, the reactivity of the pupil without the efferent pathway problem can be used to gauge the relative light intensity perceived by either eye. The detection of the RAPD is a simple, objective clinical test that can be used to localize, and follow many sensory visual pathway problems including inflammatory and compressive lesions of the afferent visual pathway.

USING THE PUPIL EXAMINATION TO LOCALIZE DISORDERS OF THE AUTONOMIC NERVOUS SYSTEM

The resting size and shape of the pupils represents a balance between the parasympathetic and the sympathetic tone to the iris constrictor and dilator muscles, respectively.[2,5] Normally, the autonomic input regulating the efferent pupillomotor signals to both eyes is equal, so that the pupils are the same size or "isocoric" in varying lighting conditions.[6] Anisocoria results when there is an imbalance in the sympathetic or parasympathetic input to the iris musculature between the eyes.

Sympathetic Innervation to the Pupil

Dilation of the pupil occurs through sympathetic innervation, which is mediated via a three-neuron circuit. The first-order neuron (presynaptic) begins in the posterolateral region of the hypothalamus, and runs along the brainstem to the intermediolateral gray matter of the spinal cord (C8-T2) to reach the ciliospinal center of Budge–Waller.[2,3] From there, fibers in the second-order neuron (preganglionic) leave the spinal cord and enter the paravertebral sympathetic chain, where they travel to reach the superior cervical ganglion at the base of the skull.[2,3] Sympathetic fibers in the third-order neuron (postganglionic) ascend along the internal carotid artery to enter the skull and travel with the trigeminal nerve in the cavernous sinus before finally reaching the orbit, and Muller muscle through the superior orbital fissure.[2,3]

Parasympathetic Innervation to the Pupil

Parasympathetic input to the iris constrictor muscles originates in the Edinger–Westphal subnucleus in the rostral portion of the third nerve nuclear complex.[2] The fibers travel via the third cranial nerve to synapse in the ciliary ganglion located behind the globe in the orbit.[2] Notably, pupillomotor fibers are situated superficially and dorsally in the subarachnoid segment of the oculomotor nerve, which renders them vulnerable to compressive lesions such as an aneurysm of the posterior communicating artery.[2]

A Clinical Approach to Anisocoria

In the setting of anisocoria, it is important to note whether the patient has had prior surgery (especially of the head or neck), trauma, migraine, or previous infections. The clinician must also elucidate any relevant occupational exposures to chemicals, drugs, or plants that could influence pupillary dilation or constriction.

The approach to the pupil examination begins with inspection, to determine whether either one of the pupils is irregular in shape.[7] Distortion in pupillary shape is often due to damage of the iris stroma, and can arise as a consequence of prior cataract extraction, surgery (retinal detachment repair), inflammation (postinflammatory synechiae and fibrosis), and iris ischemia. During the process of inspection, the pupils should first be visualized in normal room light, with attention to whether the pupils appear equal, round, and centered within the iris. Irregularities in pupil shape and contour can be detected with slit lamp examination of the anterior segment, with inspection for signs of corneal injury, anterior chamber inflammation, and iris defects.[7]

To test the pupillary light reflex, it is best to examine the patient in a darkened room with a bright focal light source (Box 16.1).[7] This approach will help maximize the amplitude and velocity of the pupillary contraction.[6,8] Testing the light reflex of each pupil involves noting the size of each pupil and the speed of reaction. An abnormal or absent light reflex should prompt the examiner to perform a near reflex test to rule out light-near dissociation. This should be done by having the patient focus on an accommodative target, such as a near card, while watching for symmetric pupillary constriction.[7] The amplitude and velocity of the pupillary contraction from the near reflex is normally equal to or less than the light reflex.[7]

Careful inspection of the lids, ocular motility, and orbital features is another key aspect of the examination that helps discern whether any pupil abnormalities noted are isolated or part of a more complicated clinical syndrome.[7] Generally speaking, intereye pupillary asymmetry exceeding 0.4 mm is considered to represent anisocoria.[6] To localize the anatomical basis of anisocoria,

it should next be determined whether the anisocoria is greatest in darkness or in light (Fig. 16.1).

Anisocoria Greatest in Darkness

If both pupils are normal in shape and the pupillary inequality is greatest in dim light, it indicates a failure of dilation in the smaller pupil, suggesting disruption of the sympathetic pupillary pathway versus physiological anisocoria. Less common causes of this clinical presentation include pharmacological miosis, mechanical anisocoria, and aberrant regeneration of the oculomotor nerve.[6] Approximately 20% of the normal population has mild intereye pupillary asymmetry[9,10] that is physiological in nature (Fig. 16.2). This type of anisocoria in affected individuals is typically <1 mm, and is often the same in dark or bright lighting conditions.[10] This finding can be transient, vary from day to day, and occasionally switch sides. It is characterized by normal pupillary dilation and contraction.[10] In cases of physiological anisocoria, there should be no dilation lag of the smaller pupil since the sympathetic pupillary pathway is intact.

Horner syndrome results from a disruption in the central, preganglionic, or postganglionic arms of the sympathetic pathway. The classic triad is characterized by unilateral miosis (constricted pupil that is slow to dilate in dim light), ptosis (drooping eyelid), and sometimes anhidrosis (lack of sweating on only one side of the face). Other symptoms that may be present include upside-down ptosis (lower eyelid is slightly elevated), conjunctival redness, and flushing on the affected side of the face. The finding of "heterochromic irides" (different colored eyes) in patients with Horner syndrome implicates a congenital origin, with the lighter colored iris being ipsilateral to the sympathetic denervation.[7] Notably, the classic triad of ptosis, miosis, and anhidrosis is often incomplete, and many patients will present with only one salient feature of the Horner syndrome in the clinical setting. Ptosis is absent, for example, in 12–13% of patients, and anhidrosis is rarely reported.[6] Unlike physiological anisocoria, patients with Horner syndrome manifest dilation lag in the affected pupil since there is disrupted sympathetic innervation to the pupillary dilator muscle. Clinically, this means that the anisocoria is typically greatest at about 4–5 seconds after the onset of darkness, with the affected pupil gradually dilating to the same degree as the unaffected pupil at around 20 seconds. While dilation lag is a highly specific test for Horner syndrome, it is not particularly sensitive,[11] being detected in only 50% of affected individuals.[6]

Box 16.1: Clinical pitfalls

A Horner syndrome can be overlooked if patients are only examined in bright lighting conditions, because both pupils will be constricted and intereye pupillary asymmetry will be minimized.

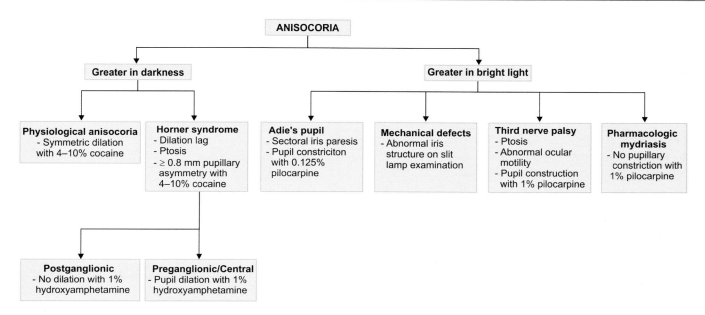

Fig. 16.1: Flowchart of broad differential diagnoses presenting with anisocoria. When anisocoria is noted, the first step should be to determine whether it is greatest in darkness or in bright light. From there, it is possible to discern the potential causes for anisocoria using clues from the patient's history, ocular examination, and pharmacological testing.[10]

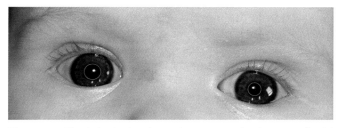

Fig. 16.2: Physiological anisocoria case study. A 4-month-old baby girl is noted by her mother to have episodic anisocoria, with a smaller pupil in the left eye. The anisocoria is most evident in dim lighting when observed, though it frequently disappears. The red circles in this figure border the child's pupils, demonstrating physiological anisocoria with a larger right pupil compared to the left.

Pharmacological Testing for Horner Syndrome

If Horner syndrome is suspected based on the history and physical examination, then pharmacological testing can be performed to confirm the diagnosis (Fig. 16.1).

Cocaine

Cocaine blocks the reuptake of norepinephrine, and therefore acts as an indirect sympathomimetic in the synaptic cleft, causing dilation of the normal pupil.[6] Patients have one to two (4–10% solution strength) cocaine hydrochloride drops instilled in both eyes. The size of the pupils should be measured in room light 40–60 minutes postadministration. A positive cocaine test for the diagnosis of Horner syndrome is inferred if there is at least 0.8 mm intereye asymmetry in pupillary size postcocaine administration.[10,12]

Apraclonidine

Apraclonidine is a α2-adrenergic drug used to lower intraocular pressures, with weak α1 agonist activity. Patients with Horner syndrome have denervation supersensitivity of α1 receptors on the iris dilator muscles of the affected eye,[10] making the pupil dilator more responsive than normal to the weak α1 effect of apraclonidine.[10] Hence, with the administration of one drop (0.5–1%) of topical apraclonidine to both eyes, there is a reversal of anisocoria such that the Horner syndrome pupil becomes larger (and the ipsilateral upper eyelid may elevate) approximately 45 minutes postapraclonidine administration.[6] Apraclonidine testing has frequently replaced cocaine testing in the clinical setting since it is often more readily available.

Hydroxyamphetamine

Hydroxyamphetamine causes the release of norepine-phrine from the presynaptic terminals of an intact third-order neuron. In cases of preganglionic Horner's syndrome, the pupil will dilate posthydroxyamphetamine administration. In cases of postganglionic Horner's syndrome, however, the pupil will not respond to hydroxy-amphetamine stimulation and remain constricted. Thus, the hydroxyamphetamine test is often used to distinguish between preganglionic and postganglionic lesions in patients with Horner syndrome.[13] Testing is generally performed a minimum of 72 hours after cocaine testing, versus 24 hours after apraclonidine testing. Approximately one to two drops of (1%) hydroxyamphetamine can be instilled into both eyes, and pupil size is measured before and 40–60 minutes after administration. It is important to note that norepinephrine vesicle stores can remain for nearly a week postneuronal insult and result in a false preganglionic Horner syndrome diagnosis if the patient is tested at this time point (Box 16.2).[9,13,14]

Horner Syndrome: Localizing the Diagnosis

The differential diagnosis of Horner syndrome is governed by the localization of the order neuron affected (Table 16.1). If a preganglionic lesion (central) is suspected, it is important to look for accompanying brainstem signs. In this case, a cranial magnetic resonance imaging (MRI) scan with angiography can help localize the lesion. In the case of a suspected second-order neuron Horner syndrome, a CT scan of the chest/head/neck (or MRI scan) will help identify lesions that may include a Pancoast tumor of the lung or mediastinal mass (Table 16.1). A painful third-order neuron Horner syndrome also warrants cranial imaging, with specific angiographic views as carotid artery dissection[6] could present in this manner and may be a life-threatening condition (Box 16.3).

Anisocoria Greatest in Bright Light

If the pupillary inequality is greatest in bright light, it often indicates relatively poor constriction of the larger

Box 16.2: Clinical pitfalls

Patients with acute Horner syndrome (<72 hours) may manifest conjunctival redness, tearing, and mild periorbital edema due to loss of vasomotor tone. The diagnosis in this context may be wrongly attributed to conjunctivitis or an ocular infection.

TABLE 16.1: Potential causes of Horner syndrome by area of the affected oculosympathetic innervation

Central	Preganglionic	Postganglionic
• Stroke	• Mediastinal mass	• Carotid artery dissection
• Syringomyelia	• Lung cancer	• Cluster headache
• Prolapsed disc	• Pancoast tumor	• Epipharynx carcinoma
• Spinal cord tumor	• Sympathoblastoma	• Cavernous sinus tumor
	• Goiter	
	• Thyroid malignancy	
	• Lymphoma	
	• Tonsil carcinoma	

Source: Adapted from Walton KA, Buono LM. Horner syndrome. Curr Opin Ophthalmol. 2003;14(6):357-63.

Box 16.3: Clinical pitfalls

Horner syndrome acquired in early childhood may indicate an underlying neuroblastoma arising from the sympathetic chain. Imaging of the chest, neck and abdomen; and urine analysis for catecholamine excretion (6) should be performed on an urgent basis in this clinical context.

pupil, implicating disruption of the parasympathetic innervation to the iris. Causes of this clinical syndrome include mechanical defects, oculomotor nerve palsy, tonic pupil, and pharmacological mydriasis.[6]

In cases of oculomotor nerve palsy, parasympathetic fibers destined for the iris constrictor muscle run peripherally in the oculomotor nerve, where they are vulnerable to compressive effects from adjacent lesions, including posterior communicating artery aneurysms and masses invading the cavernous sinus.[6] In cases of oculomotor nerve disorder, there will often be associated defects of lid position (ptosis) and ocular motility that can help localize the lesion.

Parasympathetic inhibitory agents (anticholinergic substances) and sympathomimetics can cause pupil mydriasis,[6] resulting in anisocoria that is greatest in bright light. Pupils dilated by anticholinergics generally appear quite large (8–9 mm) and do not respond to light or near stimuli.[6] The absence of vermiform movements (segmental sphincter palsy) or pupillary constrictor response to 1–2% (full strength) pilocarpine distinguishes pharmacologically dilated pupils from acutely denervated pupils.[6] Sympathomimetics are adrenergic substances that excessively stimulate the pupillary dilator muscle to cause an enlarged pupil. Because the sphincter muscle is not paralyzed, the affected pupil will typically respond to light.[6] Therefore, the pupil retains a light reflex but has less amplitude compared with the fellow eye, and will constrict to full strength (1–2%) pilocarpine.[6]

Damage to the ciliary ganglion or short ciliary nerves produce a tonic pupil, characterized by poor reaction to light with sectoral palsy of the iris sphincter and a tonic pupillary response to near stimulation (light-near dissociation) in the chronic state. This is a result of aberrant regeneration of accommodative neurons innervating the iris sphincter.[10] Dilute pilocarpine (0.125% or less) will cause a tonic pupil to constrict, whereas a normal pupil will manifest no change in pupil size postadministration. Notably, the finding of cholinergic supersensitivity is also found in mydriatic pupils caused by preganglionic denervation, including oculomotor nerve dysfunction. Adie's pupil refers to a tonic pupil where no local cause for denervation is evident (idiopathic). Young women are most commonly affected.[10] Slit lamp examination typically shows segmental denervation of the iris sphincter, with other segments reacting normally, creating vermiform movements of the iris to light stimulation.[10]

Light-Near Dissociation in Tonic Pupils

After acute denervation of the pupil, the short ciliary nerves regrow to reach the iris. During this process of reinnervation, accommodative fibers reconnect to the ciliary muscle. Aberrant reinnervation of the iris sphincter muscle is characterized by an intact pupilloconstrictor response to the near reflex and a relatively poor response to light.[6] This clinical phenomenon is referred to as "light-near dissociation."

CLINICAL APPROACH TO EYELID ABNORMALITIES

Overview

Normally, the upper eyelid just covers the upper cornea, whereas the lower lid lies below the inferior corneal margin.[2] Eyelid opening is controlled by the levator palpebrae muscle, which is innervated by the oculomotor nerve.[2] Accessory muscles include Muller's muscle, which receives sympathetic innervation, and inserts on the tarsal plate.[2] Eyelid closure occurs when levator action ceases and the orbicularis oculi muscles, innervated by the facial nerve, are activated. Neurological disorders of eyelid function fall broadly into the following categories: abnormal eyelid opening, abnormal eyelid closure, or abnormal eyelid movements.

Localization of eyelid abnormalities is facilitated, first by the examination of the lid position; and secondly, when a lid abnormality is detected, careful inspection for the "company it keeps." Deficits in eyelid function may be an isolated phenomenon or may occur with other cranial nerve deficits. It is, therefore, important to look for associated abnormalities of pupillary function and ocular motility deficits.

Localizing Problems with Eyelid Opening

During the history taking, patients should be asked about any history of trauma, congenital pupil defects, fatigability, variability, pain, and associated symptoms. On examination, the upper eyelid fold is normally located 5–7 mm above the upper eyelid margin.[2] The excursion of the eyelid from maximal downgaze to maximal upgaze can be determined with a millimeter ruler.[2] Levator function is usually 10–12 mm. Movement of 4 mm or less is considered poor levator function, 5–7 mm is fair levator function, and 8 mm or more is considered good levator function.[2] Ptosis refers to eyelid drooping, which can arise from multiple causes including lesions of the oculomotor complex, oculosympathetic lesions, neuromuscular junction abnormalities, myopathies, and mechanical lid abnormalities.[2] Typically, ptosis is seen with lesions of the oculomotor fascicle or nerve, and is associated with pupil mydriasis and ocular motility deficits. In cases of myasthenia gravis, a Cogan's eyelid twitch sign can be seen in association with ptosis. When the patient looks up after assuming a downgaze position for 20–30 seconds, the affected eyelid may twitch before settling into a ptotic position. Patients with chronic progressive external ophthalmoplegia manifest bilateral eyelid ptosis, with reduced eye movements in all fields of gaze. Apraxia of eyelid opening refers to the inability to voluntarily open the eyes in the absence of ptosis or blepharospasm caused by difficulty in overcoming levator inhibition.[2] This interesting clinical finding can be seen in patients with progressive supranuclear palsy, Huntington's disease, Wilson's disease, and after a right hemispheric stroke.[2,15] A ptotic eyelid appearance can be caused by mechanical factors, including disinsertion of the levator tendon, which results in involutional ptosis. Dermatochalasis refers to stretched, redundant eyelid skin that is often observed with age. Patients with aberrant regeneration of the orbicularis oculi after a lower motor neuron facial palsy can get a ptotic appearing eye with facial grimacing, caused by inappropriate eye closure rather than the weakness of eyelid opening.

Localizing Problems with Eyelid Opening

Volitional eye closure is mediated through the orbicularis oculi muscles, which are controlled by the facial nerves.[2] Difficulties with eye closure can arise from cranial nerve VII (facial nerve) dysfunction, neuromuscular junction abnormalities, or muscle pathology. Similarly, eyelid retraction can cause an abnormal eyelid appearance, and reduce the proficiency of eyelid closure. The eyelid position is considered retracted if it exposes a white band of sclera (often referred to as "scleral show") between the lid margin and corneal limbus.[2] This may be caused by overactivity of the levator muscle or overaction of Muller's muscle.[2] Eyelid retraction noted in downgaze is referred to as lid lag, and may be seen in Graves-related eye disease or aberrant regeneration in patients with oculomotor nerve dysfunction. Eyelid retraction, or Collier's sign, also occurs in dorsal midbrain syndrome. In patients with myasthenia gravis, lid retraction may be observed in one eye if there is ptosis in the other according to Hering's law. Manually elevating the ptotic lid can cause the retracted lid in the contralateral eye to assume a normal or even ptotic appearance (Box 16.4).

Identifying Problems Characterized by Abnormal Eyelid Movements

Patients can manifest tics and "habit spasms" that affect eyelid activity.[2] Eyelid myokymia, or a rhythmic twitching of the upper or lower eyelids, is relatively a common phenomenon that can be linked to fatigue and excessive caffeine use. Excessive eyelid closure due to blepharospasm refers to repeat, involuntary, bilateral contractures of the orbicularis oculi.[2] It is most often idiopathic and is considered a focal dystonia.[2]

Box 16.4: Clinical pitfalls

The presence of redundant eyelid skin (dermatochalasis) can sometimes mask underlying lid retraction and create a false impression of ptosis.

CONCLUSION

The pupil and lid examinations can be instrumental in diagnosing important underlying disorders. Like any neurological problem, localizing abnormalities requires a detailed clinical history and thorough examination based on knowledge of the underlying anatomical substrates that govern function.

REFERENCES

1. Prasad S, Galetta SL. Anatomy and physiology of the afferent visual system. Handb Clin Neurol. 2011;102:3-19.
2. Brazis PW, Masdeu JC, Biller J. Localization in Clinical Neurology, 6th edition. Philadelphia: Wolters Kluwer Health/Lippincott Williams & Wilkins; 2011.
3. Wolintz RJ. Isocoric Pupil Dysfunction. CONTINUUM: lifelong learning in neurology. Neuro-ophthalmology. 2009;15(4):213-7.
4. Thompson HS, Corbett JJ, Cox TA. How to measure the relative afferent pupillary defect. Surv Ophthalmol. 1981;26(1):39-42.
5. Kandel ER, Schwartz JH, Jessell TM. Principles of neural science, 4th edition. New York: McGraw-Hill, Health Professions Division; 2000. pp. 527-28, 904-6.
6. Kawasaki A. Anisocoria. CONTINUUM: lifelong learning in neurology. Neuro-ophthalmology. 2009;15(4):218-35.
7. Kawasaki A. Anisocoria. In: Levin LA, Arnold AC (Eds). Neuro-Ophthalmology: The Practical Guide. New York: Thieme; 2005. pp. 156-66.
8. Kawasaki A. Physiology, assessment, and disorders of the pupil. Curr Opin Ophthalmol. 1999;10(6):394-400.
9. Antonio-Santos AA, Santo RN, Eggenberger ER. Pharmacological testing of anisocoria. Expert Opin Pharmacother. 2005;6(12):2007-13.
10. Falardeau J, Kardon R. Anisocoria. In: Givre SJ, Kawasaki A, Mitchell J (Eds). Focal Points: Clinical Modules for Ophthalmologists, 3rd edition. American Academy of Ophthalmology; 2013. pp. 1-10.
11. Wilhelm H. The pupil. Curr Opin Neurol. 2008;21(1):36-42.
12. Kardon RH, Denison CE, Brown CK, et al. Critical evaluation of the cocaine test in the diagnosis of Horner's syndrome. Arch Ophthalmol. 1990;108(3):384-7.
13. Thompson HS, Mensher JH. Adrenergic mydriasis in Horner's syndrome. Hydroxyamphetamine test for diagnosis of postganglionic defects. Am J Ophthalmol. 1971;72(2):472-80.
14. Wilhelm H. Neuro-ophthalmology of pupillary function—practical guidelines. J Neurol. 1998;245(9):573-83.
15. Egan RA. Ptosis ad Lagophthalmos. In: Levin LA, Arnold AC (Eds). Neuro-Ophthalmology: The Practical Guide. New York: Thieme; 2005. pp. 167-80.

Chapter 17

Approach to a Dizzy Patient

Sudhir Kothari

INTRODUCTION

Dizziness is among the most common complaints in medicine, affecting approximately 20–30% of the general population.[1] But it is often inadequately diagnosed and treated, leading to tremendous anguish for the patient. Of note, dizziness is not always due to benign disorders and one may sometimes end up with a problem on missing the diagnosis.

We need to understand first, that patients use the expression, "dizzy" in a rather loose manner in order to describe a number of different sensations. They might often simply expect the examining physician to understand directly what he means when they use the expression, "dizzy." Second, examining physicians themselves often feel intimidated in approaching such patients. Nor can any simple test make it easy for the physician in this situation. In fact, investigations like audiometry or MRI may throw up red herrings, further adding to the confusion. A busy neurologist, being pressed for time, may assume that "dizzy" means vertigo and initiate investigations or worse still suppressive treatment for vertigo! This complacence may lead to missing out sinister causes of dizziness such as vertebrobasilar stroke, brain tumor, or cardiac disorders. Likewise, it would be an embarrassment to miss easily treatable disorders like benign positional paroxysmal vertigo (BPPV) or vertiginous migraine.

We shall outline here a simple approach to dizzy patients, using history to generate some hypotheses and then using a targeted neuro-otological and neurological examination to pinpoint the diagnosis.

Thus, the road to diagnosis remains as follows: History → Hypotheses → Examination → Investigations. Any change or shortcut in this sequence is fraught with peril.

HOW CAN DIFFERENT TYPES OF DIZZINESS BE DISTINGUISHED?

Dizziness is an imprecise complaint that patients often use to describe vertigo, light headedness, near-syncope, syncope, gait instability, generalized weakness, or anxiety. Vertigo, however, is a specific type of dizziness most often caused by a dysfunction of the vestibular system or its central connections. The first step is to use history to try to distinguish the different types of dizziness. This immediately narrows down the diagnostic possibilities. But, in addition to paying attention to this "quality or type of dizziness," one also needs to look at and closely correlate it with the triggers, aggravating factors, the circumstances in which the dizziness occurs as well as the duration of each spell of dizziness.

THE FIRST STEP: CLARIFYING THE TYPE OF DIZZINESS

As a first step, it is useful to ask the patient to describe her/his symptoms, using word other than "dizzy" and try to find out what exactly the patient means by "dizziness". Some patients may even use the expression to describe fatigue, weakness, or anxiety or even difficulty in focusing vision and even actually passing out due to seizures or syncope (Box 17.1).

TYPES OF DIZZINESS

Type 1: Dizziness or True Vertigo

The patient with true vertigo describes his/her dizziness as a clear spinning or rotatory or whirling sensation that is precipitated or aggravated by head movement. There is at least aggravation of the dizziness by sudden head (often with neck) movement, e.g., looking up, or down, or turning to one side, or rolling over in bed, or lying down in bed, getting out of bed. It does not matter whether the feeling of rotation is referred to self or the surroundings. Sometimes patients get a feeling of being tilted or pushed to one side or may get thrown backwards or feel as if they are swaying like in a boat.

True vertigo, makes a vestibular lesion very likely, either peripheral or of its central connections. But, as with all symptoms, it can be inconsistent and unreliable and sometimes even cardiogenic disorders can present with true vertigo. We shall subsequently see how to approach the problem of rotatory vertigo, and distinguish the various peripheral causes from central ones and from each other.

Type 2: Dizziness or Presyncope

Syncope is easy to distinguish from dizziness. But patients who experience a milder form, i.e., presyncope may only feel as if they are going to pass out. The patient may describe a sensation of feeling faint or he may feel darkness before his eyes. This is due to reduced blood flow to the brain. It is essentially a cardiovascular disorder, commonly due to postural hypotension or vasovagal syncope.

Postural hypotension typically happens when the patient stands up after sitting for a long time or gets up from a squatting position.

Vasovagal syncope may be triggered by seeing blood, sudden pain, emotional stress, cough, or micturition. Other causes are low cardiac output or hyperventilation due to a panic attack.

Presyncope almost never occurs in bed, or when lying down, or turning in bed, or turning the head, or looking up or down, unlike in true vertigo.

Type 3: Dizziness or Disequilibrium

Imbalance or disequilibrium is a feeling of loss of balance or feeling unsteady on one's feet. Naturally, it happens when one is walking or gets up. It will be aggravated by walking on uneven ground, while turning in the dark or in the shower. This type of dizziness will not occur while sitting or lying down in the bed. There is no true spinning or rotatory sensation, just a feeling of impending falling down or loss of balance. It will reduce when there are other sensory cues, e.g., visual or tactile.

The causes of loss of balance are myriad and there can be clinical clues. This type of dizziness mandates a careful neurological examination and evaluation of the gait.

Type 4: Dizziness or Psychogenic Dizziness

Psychogenic factors like stress, depression, feelings of insecurity, may lead to a dizzy feeling. The dizziness may be described vaguely as light-headedness or a heavy head, or as tingling and numbness in the head, or inability to think clearly. It is often triggered by stressful situations and not necessarily related to posture or change of position (Tables 17.1 and 17 2).

TABLE 17.1: Types of dizziness

Types of dizziness	Characteristic features
Type 1 Dizziness or True vertigo	• Spinning or tilting feeling • Aggravation by head movement • Vestibular lesion very likely, peripheral, or central
Type 2 Dizziness or Presyncope	• Usually when getting up from sitting position, or prolonged standing • Almost never in bed or just looking up or down • A cardiovascular problem usually • Postural hypotension • Vasovagal syncope • Low cardiac output or hyperventilation
Type 3 Dizziness or Gait or Postural in-coordination	• Imbalance while standing or walking • Never in bed or when just sitting • Feeling that he may fall down or lose balance • Many neurological causes, as well as bilateral vestibular failure
Type 4 Dizziness or Psychogenic	• Vague lightness or heaviness or numbness in head or inability to think clearly • Close relation to fatigue or stress • Not looking like any of the earlier three sub-types • Sometimes patient may have type 1–3 dizziness, but not describe it appropriately • Never in bed or when just sitting • Feeling that he may fall down or lose balance • Many neurological causes, as well as bilateral vestibular failure

TABLE 17.2: **Common causes of the four types of dizziness**

Type of vertigo	Causes	
Type 1 or True vertigo	Peripheral • Benign positional paroxysmal vertigo • Vestibular neuritis • Meniere's disease	Central • Migraine • Stroke demyelination/tumor
Type 2 or Presyncope	• Postural hypotension • Vasovagal attacks • Hyperventilation • Low cardiac output states	
Type 3 or Loss of balance	Various neurological causes • Binswanger's disease • Parkinson's disease • Cerebellar • Myelopathy • Neuropathy Bilateral vestibular failure, e.g., ototoxicity	
Type 4 or Psychogenic	• Stress, anxiety, depression • Watch out for mild forms of type 1–3, or poor descriptions by anxious patients	

TABLE 17.3: **Triggers of dizziness**

On lying down or turning in bed	True vertigo
On getting up suddenly from sitting position	Faintness
Walking or turning	Loss of balance
When stressed or overworked	Psychogenic

TABLE 17.4: **Causes of true vertigo according to duration of spells**

Duration	Causes
Fraction of a second	Old vestibular deficit, e.g., old neuritis
Few seconds	Benign positional paroxysmal vertigo, migraine, rarely tumor or demyelination
Minutes	TIA, migraine
Hours	Meniere's disease, stroke, migraine
Days	Vestibular neuritis, stroke, migraine
Continuous	Usually psychogenic

Note: Migraine and psychogenic can cause any of the above!

OTHER IMPORTANT POINTS IN HISTORY

Triggers and Duration

It is very important to take into consideration factors that trigger or aggravate or relieve an attack, as well as the duration of individual attacks (Tables 17.3 and 17.4).

This may sometimes be more important and reliable than paying attention to the quality or type of dizziness. For example, irrespective of the "quality," brief attacks of dizziness brought on by looking up or down or turning in bed are likely to be due to BPPV.

A good social and medication history is also important, as several medications including aminoglycosides, diuretics, antidepressants, alcohol, and antipsychotics can lead to dizziness.

Many patients, especially older individuals, may have more than one kind of dizziness. Therefore, the question "how many kinds of dizziness do you have?" is often a useful question, since each variety of dizziness requires separate evaluation.

It is generally useful to ask about the first episode of dizziness and understand it first. One should not allow the patient to generalize and describe all his feelings of dizziness as one. For example, a person may get an attack of true syncope or BPPV, and subsequently suffer from psychogenic dizziness.

After the Rotatory Vertigo is Diagnosed

Once it is concluded that the patient has rotatory vertigo, it usually means she/he has a disorder of the vestibular system or its central connections. Thus, the second step is to differentiate peripheral from central vertigo.[2]

Peripheral vertigo appears to be more serious and may cause distressing symptoms, but is usually not really life threatening. Presence of ear symptoms like pressure or fullness, tinnitus or hearing loss, does point to a peripheral cause, but one needs to keep in mind anterior inferior cerebellar artery (AICA) territory ischemia or infarct, as this artery supplies both the labyrinth and parts of the cerebellum and brainstem (pons).

The severity of vertigo, unsteadiness, nausea, and vomiting are usually matching or concordant in peripheral disorders. Hence, an individual who has mild nystagmus will have mild unsteadiness and mild nausea, while a person who has gross nystagmus will have considerable vomiting and vertigo. If the patient has vomiting or ataxia out of proportion to the subjective feeling of vertigo, a central cause should be suspected.

Central vertigo can be deceptively mild and may have more variable symptoms. Accompanying central symptoms include the following: presence of any central symptoms like diplopia, dysarthria, dysphagia, dysphonia,

TABLE 17.5: **Differentiating central vertigo from peripheral vertigo**[2]

Features	Central vertigo	Peripheral vertigo
Illness	May appear deceptively mild	Patient may look very ill
Ataxia	More	Less
Feeling of vertigo	May be less	May be more
Tinnitus or deafness	Usually absent (except in anterior–inferior cerebellar artery ischemia)	May be present (not always)
Brainstem symptoms/signs diplopia, dysarthria, dysphagia, dysphonia, paresthesia, etc.	May be present (but not always)	Absent
Nystagmus	Unidirectional, mixed horizontal torsional, attenuated by visual fixation	Pure vertical, pure torsional, pure horizontal. Direction changing or dissociated

TABLE 17.6: **Causes of loss of balance or unsteadiness**

Area of brain	Etiology	Signs
Cerebral	Binswanger's disease, isolated gait apraxia	Mental change, dysarthria, urgency, shuffling gait
Basal ganglia	Parkinsonism	Hypokinesia, rigidity, tremor, reduced arm swing
Cerebellum	Cerebellar ataxia	Broad based gait, limb ataxia, dysarthria, eye signs
Spinal cord	Myelopathies	Spasticity, brisk reflexes, up going plantars, impaired position, and vibration at toes
Peripheral nerve	Neuropathies	Absent deep tendon jerks, impaired sensations
Vestibular	Bilateral vestibulopathy	Oscillopsia, only gait ataxia, head impulse positive bilaterally

dysesthesia, or limb ataxia, or weakness. These would clearly point to a central disorder. Significant headache usually implies either a central cause or vestibular migraine. However, more sinister causes like dissection of the vertebral artery are to be kept in mind (Table 17.5).

A DIFFERENT APPROACH TO THE PATIENT WITH ACUTE FIRST-TIME DIZZINESS

In a patient with acute first-time dizziness, we should use a different approach as outlined below:

TRIAGE

First identify whether there are obvious clinical "red flags" that point towards a more sinister cause for dizziness: (a) abnormal vital signs, (b) confusion or otherwise impaired mental state, (c) sudden, severe, or sustained head or neck pain, (d) worrisome neurologic symptoms (e.g., diplopia, dysarthria, and dysphagia), or (e) worrisome cardiovascular symptoms (e.g., chest pain, dyspnea, and syncope). If present, these need to be addressed in an appropriate and urgent manner (Table 17.6).

TIMING

Divide the remaining patients into those with transient or episodic (lasting seconds to hours), and those with persistent dizziness (lasting days to weeks).

TRIGGERS (for Patients with Transient Dizziness <24 Hours)

A search for history of triggers to identify benign or dangerous causes; in general, transient dizziness that is exertional or spontaneous is most likely to be caused by sinister disorders; other triggers (e.g., changes in head position) most often indicate benign causes; when possible, try to reproduce symptoms (e.g., Dix–Hallpike maneuver) during physical examination.

TELL-TALE SIGNS (for Patients with Persistent Dizziness >24 Hours)

In patients with acute vestibular syndrome, the head impulse nystagmus test of skew (HINTS) battery might be used to distinguish stroke from vestibular neuritis. We shall see about HINTS later in the chapter.[3,4]

EXAMINATION

Introduction

Usually, a systematic approach during history taking can point to the diagnosis; subsequently, the physician can tailor examination to confirm or rule out the first impressions. However, at times the history is inconclusive or inconsistent. In such cases, neuro-otological examination may still help to clinch the diagnosis. For example, in a patient with an inconclusive history of dizziness, a positive Dix–Hallpike test may confirm a diagnosis of BPPV; similarly a certain characteristic pattern of nystagmus may suggest a central disorder. Hence, all patients with vestibular symptoms must have a complete neurological examination including cranial nerves, vision, and hearing.

The most important part of the neuro-otological examination is the eye movement evaluation: nystagmus, the head impulse test (HIT), and positioning maneuvers as evidence in favor of BPPV, apart from evaluating saccadic and pursuit eye movements.

Sometimes, only subtle clinical signs can distinguish between benign and sinister causes of vertigo, even more useful than MRI or other investigations.

General Examination

Always check the pulse, blood pressure, both supine and standing, evaluate for anemia, and auscultate the heart, keeping in mind the possibility of general medical conditions causing dizziness (Box 17.2).

Examination of the Ears

One must examine hearing at the bedside by performing the tuning fork tests, including Rinne's and Weber's tests.

> **Box 17.2: Minimal physical examination in dizzy patients**
> - Check BP supine and standing
> - Check ears for discharge, zoster, perforation, fistula
> - Check for spontaneous nystagmus with and without visual fixation (Frenzel goggles)
> - Head impulse test
> - Dix–Hallpike test
> - Check smooth pursuit and saccadic eye movements
> - Check standing balance (Romberg)
> - Check gait, including tandem gait

The ear needs to be checked for herpes skin lesions, wax or any growth, or other lesions in the canal. It is easy to check the eardrums for perforation and also perform the Hennebert's sign by pushing on the tragus and external auditory meatus to observe if vertigo or nystagmus can be induced.

Assessment of Vestibular Functions: Vestibulo-ocular and Vestibulospinal Reflexes[5]

Vestibulospinal Reflexes

These test the influence of the vestibular system on the spinal cord. One checks past pointing, Romberg's and other tests of posture, and the various walking tests and the gait.

With an acute vestibular lesion, the patient often is tilted, sways, and may even fall toward the side of the lesion especially with eyes closed. This can be made more sensitive by standing on one's toes or in the tandem position (Sharpened Romberg's test).

Tandem walking with eyes open and eyes closed may show a tendency to fall to one side, but it may occur in cerebellar lesions as well.

The side toward which the patient falls in Romberg's test or tandem walking is not always reliable, especially in chronic lesions.

Stepping tests like Unterberger's test looks for a tendency for the patient to turn towards the affected ear, when asked to march in place with eyes open.

Tests for Nystagmus

Pathologic nystagmus is basically of three types, spontaneous, gaze evoked, or positional.
1. Spontaneous is seen with the eyes in the primary position, without any external stimulation, e.g., movement of head or surroundings.
2. Gaze-evoked is induced by changes in gaze positions, e.g., looking to the sides or up or down.
3. Positional is nystagmus that is not seen at rest or gaze, but seen only in certain positions of the head and body.

To look for pathologic nystagmus, one must examine for nystagmus and any changes with fixation, eye position, and head positions. Sometimes pathologic nystagmus may be brought out only after vibration or head shake or hyperventilation.

Spontaneous Nystagmus

Nystagmus when looking straight ahead and the head at rest is the hallmark of an imbalance in the vestibular system, either peripheral or central. It should always be examined with visual fixation eliminated also, e.g., by Frenzel goggles or a Video-Frenzel.

Peripheral vestibular spontaneous nystagmus is typically unidirectional, mixed horizontal and torsional, and gets suppressed or reduced when the patient is able to fixate a target. It gets worse on looking in the direction of the fast phase (Alexander's law). It may sometimes be seen only when visual fixation is eliminated.

Alexander's law refers to spontaneous nystagmus that occurs after an acute unilateral vestibular loss. Alexander's law states that in individuals with nystagmus, the amplitude of the nystagmus increases when the eye moves in the direction of the fast phase (saccade). It is manifested during spontaneous nystagmus in a patient with a vestibular lesion. The nystagmus becomes more intense when the patient looks in the quick-phase than in the slow-phase direction.

However, spontaneous central nystagmus may be purely vertical or pure torsional, may be direction changing, may not be affected by fixation or may get affected by change in the position of the head. Unlike that in peripheral vertigo, the nystagmus in central vertigo may not follow Alexander's law, that is, it may not get exaggerated with gaze in the direction of the fast component.

Vibration applied to the mastoid, head shaking, Valsalva's maneuver, or hyperventilation can bring out diagnostic features. For example, mild unilateral loss of vestibular function may be brought out by vibration or head shaking by the demonstration of a unidirectional horizontal nystagmus with slow component towards the affected ear. If a vertical nystagmus is elicited, it suggests a central disorder.

Gaze-evoked Nystagmus

It is always central and not peripheral. It changes direction with change in the gaze position. It may arise in the central nervous system (CNS) at various levels, or due to drugs or even due to neuromuscular junction abnormalities.

Symmetric gaze-evoked nystagmus can be seen in brainstem or cerebellar disorders or with toxic–metabolic conditions of the CNS.

Asymmetric gaze-evoked nystagmus implies a unilateral lesion of the brainstem or cerebellum, e.g., with acoustic neuromas.

Dissociated nystagmus, more in the abducting eye implies an internuclear ophthalmoplegia, e.g., in multiple sclerosis or stroke, but can also be seen in myasthenia or muscle disorders.

Paroxysmal Positional Nystagmus[6-8]

Sometimes one elicits nystagmus only when the patient moves into the supine, right lateral, and left lateral position or by the Dix–Hallpike maneuver (Fig. 17.1).

The most common nystagmus elicited by the Dix Hallpike maneuver is that of posterior canal type of BPPV. After a latency of about 3–10 seconds, there is an upbeating and torsional nystagmus beating towards the affected (downward) ear. It rarely lasts >30 seconds and tends to fatigue on repeated testing. It is associated with severe vertigo (Table 17.7).

Horizontal canal variants of BPPV show horizontal nystagmus elicited by turning the head to either side when lying supine (roll test). There are two types, apogeotropic and geotropic, depending on whether the nystagmus beats towards the downward ear (towards the earth) or away from it. This nystagmus tends to last longer than that of posterior canal BPPV and often there is nystagmus on either side, making it challenging to diagnose the side affected (Boxes 17.3 to 17.6).

Central disorders may also cause paroxysmal positional nystagmus, e.g., with lesions of the posterior fossa. It may not have a latent period, may not decrease in amplitude, may last longer, and may change in direction or may be purely vertical or downbeating. It may or may not be associated with vertigo and it may not fatigue on repeated testing.

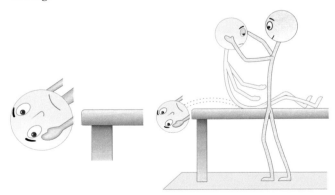

Fig. 17.1: Dix–Hallpike maneuver.

TABLE 17.7: **Types of nystagmus**

Types of nystagmus	Localization
Peripheral nystagmus	• Hallmark of labyrinthine disease, e.g., vestibular neuritis
Bruns nystagmus (asymmetric gaze evoked)	• Cerebellopontine angle tumors, e.g., acoustic neuroma • Focal cerebellar or brainstem lesions
Gaze-evoked nystagmus	• Brainstem or cerebellar lesions, e.g., degeneration • Drugs, e.g., sedatives, anticonvulsants
Upbeating	• Dorsal central medulla lesions, e.g., stroke, tumor, multiple sclerosis
Downbeating	• Cervicomedullary junction and midline cerebellum, e.g., chiari, cerebellar atrophy, stroke, demyelination
Pure torsional	• Syringomyelia and syringobulbia
Pendular	• Congenital • Acquired, e.g., in multiple sclerosis
See-saw	• Chiasmal lesions
Periodic alternating nystagmus	• Congenital • Acquired due to various pathologies
Persistent positional nystagmus	• Peripheral, e.g., apogeotropic benign positional paroxysmal vertigo • Central causes, especially, downbeating in cerebellar disorders

Box 17.3: Characteristic features of benign positional paroxysmal vertigo (BPPV)[6,7]

- The commonest vestibular disorder, with lifetime incidence of about 10%
- Annual incidence rate is about 1% of the population per year
- Depending on definition, vertiginous migraine might be commoner
- Definitely BBP is the commonest cause of positional vertigo
- Brief attacks of positional vertigo, triggered by change in head position, e.g., lying down, getting up, looking up or down, turning in bed
- May follow minor trauma, sometimes by months
- Other causes are after viral infections of ear, prolonged recumbency
- Very disabling entity affecting activities of daily living
- May get cured spontaneously over weeks
- Tends to recur 1–2 times or more in a year
- Diagnosis confirmed by maneuver and eliciting nystagmus
- Subtypes depending on canal(s) affected and location within canal
- Drugs are not the recommended treatment, though they give partial and temporary relief
- Can be easily treated by specific canalith repositioning maneuvers

Box 17.4: Lateral canal benign positional paroxysmal vertigo (BPPV)

- Not uncommon. About 10–20% of all BPPV
- Sometimes happens during repositioning of posterior canal BPPV
- Provoked by turning the head to either side in bed, whereas sitting up or lying down produces only minimal symptoms
- To test for lateral semicircular canal BPPV head is turned rapidly to either side with the patient lying supine
- Two variants the more common canalolithiasis with geotropic nystagmus, beating towards the ground, regardless of whether head is turned to left or right
- The rarer cupulolithiasis with apogeotropic nystagmus
- Often no latency and may last longer and so may suggest a central cause
- Nystagmus is purely horizontal
- Sometimes it is difficult to identify the affected ear
- Usually worse with head turned to the affected side in geotropic variety and the opposite side in apogeotropic
- Treated by different maneuvers like barbeque rolls or Gufoni maneuver

Box 17.5: Anterior canal benign positional paroxysmal vertigo (AC-BPPV)[8]

- Rare 1–2% maybe more
- Provoked by Dix–Hallpike positioning, to either side
- Straight head-hanging position is most sensitive
- Diagnostic positioning maneuver cannot identify reliably the side
- Nystagmus predominately downbeating with only a small torsional component that points to affected ear
- Repositioning needs different maneuvers, like reverse Epley

Box 17.6: Posterior canal benign positional paroxysmal vertigo

- Rare 1–2% maybe more
- Provoked by Dix–Hallpike positioning, to either side
- Straight head-hanging position is most sensitive
- Diagnostic positioning maneuver cannot identify reliably the side
- Nystagmus predominately downbeating with only a small torsional component that points to affected ear
- Repositioning needs different maneuvers, like reverse Epley

Persistent positional nystagmus remains as long as the provocating position is held. It can be seen in peripheral disorders, e.g., the cupulolithiasis variety of BPPV, e.g., apogeotropic lateral canal.

Central positional nystagmus of persistent type may be seen in disorders like a craniovertebral anomaly or a spinocerebellar degeneration, where it is usually of downbeating variety.

Use of Frenzel Goggles or a Video-Frenzel

The Frenzel goggles are of immense value in the examination of nystagmus, both spontaneously and with various maneuvers, e.g., Valsalva's maneuver may trigger a nystagmus in perilymph fistulas and superior canal dehiscence. The effect of tragal compression, loud sound, head shake, mastoid vibration, hyperventilation, as well as change in head position, can all be much better appreciated with these goggles.

Dynamic Visual Acuity

The patient's visual acuity is measured with the head still and then measured with the head passively rotated, first horizontally, then vertically, at a frequency of about 2 Hz. If one loses more than one line of acuity during such head shaking, the test is abnormal. Patients with a complete and acute loss of labyrinthine function may have a drastic drop in vision, up to five lines. One can do a rapid screening at the bedside by asking the patient to read a newspaper first with the head still and then shaking the head rhythmically from side to side. It is a useful test to do in a bedridden patient who is receiving aminoglycosides, to detect early vestibulotoxicity.

Skew Deviation

This is a vertical misalignment of the eyes/vertical divergence. It is not a common finding, but when seen, it usually indicates a central lesion.

Head-Impulse Test (Halmagyi and Curthoys)

This is a simple but grossly underutilized bedside test to identify significant unilateral or bilateral loss of vestibular function.

Intact vestibular function, with a good vestibulo-ocular reflex (VOR) keeps the eyes to maintain fixation and keep looking straight at the target despite a rapid head movement.

A patient with a peripheral vestibular deficit, especially bilateral, may complain of oscillopsia as his eyes cannot remain on the target whenever he moves his head.

To do the head impulse test or HIT, one grasps the patient's face and jaw in both hands and gives a small but fast head thrust to either side, while the patient is asked to keep his eyes open and fixed on the examiner's nose and avoid blinking (Fig. 17.2). If the VOR is normal, the patient's eyes remain fixed on the examiners nose. But if the VOR is impaired on one side, the eyes get dragged along and the patient has to make a corrective saccade to get the eyes back to look at the examiner's nose. This refixation saccade can be easily observed at the bedside and is a very important sign of significantly impaired vestibular function on the side to which the head is thrust.

The HIT is almost always positive, in moderate to severe paresis of vestibular function. It is almost always positive in acute vestibular neuritis, but is usually negative or normal in brainstem or cerebellar infarcts. Thus in the acute vestibular syndrome, the chances of a brainstem or cerebellar infarct are much more likely, if the HIT is negative.[9] The HIT is usually normal in Meniere's disease, BPPV, or migraine. It may be the only objective sign in bilateral vestibulopathy, e.g., due to aminoglycoside ototoxicity.

Caloric Test

The ideal test is done in both ears, with water at 30°C and 44°C. But one can do a rough semiquantitative caloric test, the so called 20-20-20-20 test. One irrigates 20 mL water at 20°C, for 20 seconds, keeping the patients head inclined up at 20°C and notes the duration of nystagmus on either side. The caloric test checks vestibular movements at slow acceleration (<0.5 Hz), while HITs it at fast acceleration (5–10 Hz). So, one might be abnormal when the other is normal. The caloric test in an alert patient can induce uncomfortable vertigo and vomiting and so, as a bedside test, has been largely replaced by the HIT.

We shall now briefly touch upon the salient features of the common disorders causing vertigo.

Vertiginous migraine can mimic any of these disorders, causing attacks lasting seconds, minutes, hours, or days (Table 17.8).

Brief attacks of vertigo lasting a few seconds may occur in BPPV apart from migraine (Box 17.7).

Not all paroxysmal positional vertigo is BPPV (Table 17.9).

Unprovoked attacks of vertigo lasting a few minutes suggest vertebrobasilar transient ischemic attacks (TIAs)

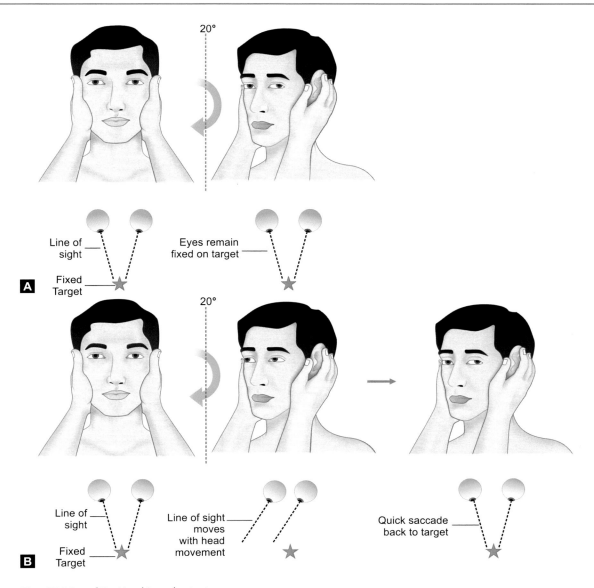

Figs 17.2A and B: Head impulse test.

TABLE 17.8: **Vertiginous migraine**

Vertiginous migraine probably the commonest cause of vertigo	
Features	**A chameleon: mimics all syndromes of vertigo**
• Any type of dizziness: true vertigo, nonvertiginous dizziness	• Meniere's disease with/without hearing loss
• Any duration	• Recurrent vestibular neuritis
• Any age but females more	• Intractable "BPPV"
• Migrainous headaches (maybe forgotten or missed or thought irrelevant)	• Vague chronic unsteadiness
• Nausea/vomit/photophobia/phonophobia may be present/absent	• Motion intolerance
• Common triggers like stress, hunger, travel	

Box 17.7: Benign positional paroxysmal vertigo: the commonest cause of vertigo (maybe after migraine)

- Often wrongly attributed to "spondylosis" or vertebrobasilar ischemia
- Brief attacks of positional vertigo: seconds to less than a minute
- Not really benign as leads to tremendous secondary anxiety, morbidity, and risk of falls
- Causes: idiopathic, ageing, trauma, prolonged recumbency, following vestibular neuritis
- History is almost diagnostic, but elicit and see nystagmus by Dix–Hallpike or roll test
- Posterior canal commonest: upbeating, torsional nystagmus
- Lateral canal 10–30%: horizontal nystagmus, geotropic, and apogeotropic varieties
- The most treatable cause of vertigo: sometimes almost "magical" cure
- Easily treated by particle repositioning maneuvers
- Different maneuvers for different canals
- Brandt–Daroff exercises if mild
- Almost never need drugs

TABLE 17.9: **Central positional vertigo**

Central positional vertigo	Causes
• Some atypical features unlike typical benign positional paroxysmal vertigo • Nystagmus without vertigo or only vertigo without any nystagmus seen (even on Frenzel) • Nystagmus has no latent period or persists, or does not fatigue on repeated testing • Downbeat, upbeat, or purely torsional • Other central symptoms, e.g., diplopia and dysarthria	• Migraine • Posterior fossa stroke or tumor or demyelination • Chiari malformation • Drugs

etc., even if there are no other brainstem symptoms. Sometimes, tinnitus and deafness may also occur in these TIAs, especially if the AICA territory is involved.

Attacks lasting hours may suggest Meniere's disease or stroke (Boxes 17.8 to 17.11).

Attacks lasting days usually occur in acute vestibular syndrome, caused by vestibular neuritis, but stroke may be the cause in up to 25% cases[3,4] (Box 17.12 and Table 17.10).

Box 17.8: Meniere's syndrome

Meniere's syndrome: typical tetrad not always present
- Attacks of vertigo: >20 minutes
- Fluctuating and progressive hearing loss
- Tinnitus: Typically low pitched, roaring, machine like
- Fullness in ear
- Not just any combination of tinnitus, deafness, and vertigo
- Often BPPV or vertiginous migraine with unrelated or non-significant hearing loss and tinnitus
- Must rule out vertiginous migraine, especially before doing any destructive therapy

Box 17.9: Vascular disorders causing dizziness or vertigo[9]
- Ischemia or TIAs in vertebrobasilar territory
- Infarcts: Anterior inferior cerebellar artery, posterior inferior cerebellar artery territory, cerebellar infarcts
- Cerebellar bleed

Box 17.10: Features of posterior inferior cerebellar artery (PICA) infarct (Wallenberg's syndrome)
- 2% of strokes, but commonest type of cerebellar infarct
- May cause only cerebellar infarct and mimic vestibular neuritis, especially medial PICA infarct
- 30% have a lateral medullary infarct too with dysphagia, palatal palsy, Horner's syndrome, impaired temperature, and pinprick sensation over body and face on same or opposite side
- Impaired visual vertical and tilt

Box 17.11: Features of anterior inferior cerebellar artery (AICA) infarct or ischemia
- Supplies labyrinth as well as brainstem and cerebellum. So may have tinnitus and deafness intermittently or permanent loss
- May also have impaired peripheral vestibular function, on HIT or caloric testing
- May have facial nerve palsy, facial numbness, and hemiparesis or numbness on the opposite side
- So ipsilateral hearing loss with or without tinnitus as well as a range of labyrinthine, brainstem, and cerebellar symptoms and signs
- The classic syndrome has ipsilateral facial palsy, hearing loss, tinnitus, trigeminal sensory loss, Horner's syndrome, and limb dysmetria with contralateral pain, and temperature sensory loss in limbs and trunk
- 30% may have episodes of acute auditory disturbance including transient or prolonged hearing loss with or without tinnitus
- Sudden onset of unilateral deafness
- The AICA infarcts often herald a basilar artery occlusion

TABLE 17.10: Diagnosis of stroke in acute vestibular syndrome[3,4]

HINTS to the diagnosis of stroke	

• History not reliable, e.g., age, absence of ear symptoms
• Absence of hard neurological signs and symptoms not reliable
• CT/MRI not reliable (MRI may miss in >10% even up to 3 days)
	• The HINTS battery is 100% reliable
	  ○ Subtle bedside eye signs
	• Even one means stroke
	  ○ Head impulse normal
	  ○ Direction changing nystagmus
	  ○ Presence of skew deviation

Box 17.12: Acute vestibular neuritis

• Acute onset vertigo, with nausea and vomiting lasting days
• Typical peripheral nystagmus (unidirectional horizontal rotatory)
• Unsteady gait, but able to walk unaided
• No cerebellar signs
• No diplopia/dysarthria
• No tinnitus/deafness
• Treatment 3–5 days of vestibular suppressants
• Steroids short course
• Ambulation and vestibular rehabilitation as early as possible
• 25% might be strokes (HINTS battery)
• If recurrent attacks, think of migraine

CONCLUSION

Dizziness and vertigo are very common symptoms. Most disorders can be diagnosed from history and a targeted examination. Systematic approach to history helps in narrowing down causes. Treat appropriately according to cause and not just "antivertigo" drugs. Use "antivertigo drugs" sparingly (not more than a few days). Remember stroke in first time attacks of vertigo (HINTS). Don't lose chance to do "magic" in benign positional paroxysmal vertigo. Vestibular migraine is probably the commonest cause of vertigo and is also very treatable. Vestibular rehabilitation is very useful in chronic cases, in recovery from vestibular neuritis and in ototoxicity. Don't confuse presyncope or balance disorders for vertigo.

REFERENCES

1. Kerber KA, Meurer WJ, West BT, et al. Dizziness presentations in U.S. emergency departments, 1995-2004. Acad Emerg Med. 2008;15(8):744-50.
2. Karatas M. Central vertigo and dizziness: epidemiology, differential diagnosis, and common causes. Neurologist. 2008;14(6):355-64.
3. Newman-Toker DE. Acute vestibular syndrome. http://content.lib.utah.edu/utils/getfile/collection/ehsl-dent/id/7/filename/5.pdf.
4. Kattah JC, Talkad AV, Wang DZ, et al. HINTS to diagnose stroke in the acute vestibular syndrome: three-step bedside oculomotor examination more sensitive than early MRI diffusion-weighted imaging. Stroke. 2009;40:3504-10.
5. Baloh RW, Kerber KA. Clinical neurophysiology of the vestibular system, 4th edition. Contemporary Neurology Series. New York: Oxford University Press; 2011.
6. Cakir BO, Ercan I, Cakir ZA, et al. What is the true incidence of horizontal semicircular canal benign paroxysmal positional vertigo? Otolaryngol Head Neck Surg. 2006;134(3):451-4.
7. Nakayama M, Epley JM. BPPV and variants: improved treatment results with automated, nystagmus-based repositioning. Otolaryngol Head Neck Surg. 2005;133:107-12.
8. Jackson LE, Morgan B, Fletcher JC Jr, et al. Anterior canal benign paroxysmal positional vertigo: an underappreciated entity. Otol Neurotol. 2007;28:218-22.
9. Edlow JA, Newman-Toker DE, Savitz SI. Diagnosis and initial management of cerebellar infarction. Lancet Neurol. 2008;7:951-64.

Chapter 18

Approach to Deafness

Anirban Biswas

INTRODUCTION

As per WHO estimates in India, there are more than 65 million people, who suffer from significant hearing impairment; the prevalence of deafness is about 6% in the Indian population by conservative estimates. These figures are from studies carried out more than a decade ago; current figures are not readily available, but as per the National Sample Survey Organisation (NSSO) survey, there are 291 persons per 1 lakh population who are suffering from severe-to-profound hearing loss (NSSO, 2001). Of these, a large percentage includes children between the ages of 0 and 14 years. It is known from published literature that the incidence of severe congenital deafness is about 3.5 per 1000 live births in India. An even higher percentage of our population suffers from milder degrees of hearing loss and unilateral (one-sided) hearing loss.

Deafness is the most common sensory handicap worldwide. An American survey had shown that in the year 2000, nearly 30 million Americans had a significant hearing impairment. Deafness not only impairs interpersonal communication skills but also induces significant psychological morbidity on the person. A deaf person is not only a burden to the society, the person is incapable of living a life of dignity, incapable of earning a livelihood, is mentally depressed as he cannot communicate, and is hence shunned by his peers and family members, and is (very unfortunately) looked down by the society as a social nuisance. Fortunately, however, hearing impairment is in most cases preventable and in all cases correctable if the deafness is detected and treated early. Deafness is such a common symptom that all

medical professionals need to have a grasp in the correct identification, (i.e., diagnosis) and in the management of hearing impairment. It is not always that the hearing impaired person will land up in a well-equipped ENT doctor's clinic, and often all sorts of physicians, such as general practitioners, family physicians, medical consultants, neurologists, pediatricians, pulmonologists, and gastroenterologists, have to handle patients presenting with deafness or other ear-related symptoms like tinnitus, i.e., a buzzing sound in the ear. Hence, a working knowledge for professionally and ethically managing the hearing impaired in accordance to current norms is essential. This chapter aims at updating the non-ENT specialists on the currently prevalent procedures of identifying, diagnosing, and managing the hearing impaired patients.

THE PRESENTATION OF DEAFNESS

Deafness can present in various forms. Examples of various case scenarios are given in the Box 18.1.

THE MECHANISM OF HEARING

The ear has three basic parts (Fig. 18.1):
1. The *external ear* that comprises of the auricle and the external auditory meatus collects the sound from the surroundings, amplifies some important frequencies especially the high frequency sounds, and conduct them to the eardrum.
2. The *middle ear* consists of the eardrum and three small bones that are connected together in the form of a chain. The function of the middle ear is to amplify the

Box 18.1: Case scenarios: The presentation of deafness

1. An old person may present to the family physician with the complaints that he is having difficulty in understanding when other people are speaking to him, or in listening to the TV, or while at the dinner table, he cannot make out what others are talking about. He has to raise the volume of the TV to an extent where others at home are being disturbed. He has been facing this difficulty for the last few years but now it is affecting his quality of life and he is being ridiculed by others.

2. A middle-aged lawyer comes with a complaint that he misses out some of the words that the judges tell him in a noisy court room, and this has often been a cause of professional embarrassment for him.

3. A banker presents to a medical consultant with the complaints that the previous night he had a bout of severe vertigo with vomiting, and since today morning he is unable to hear at all from his left ear. The vertigo is still persisting but lesser than the last night. He is extremely perturbed by this sudden deafness in his left ear and asks how soon he can get back his hearing. He is also worried if the right ear can also become totally deaf like the left one.

4. A young school teacher presents with the complaint that she is unable to follow when students from the last benches are communicating with her, she asks the doctor to examine her ears and tell her if she has any deafness or not. She goes on to say that some students have nicked-named her as the "deaf miss", and that other teachers and even students shout at her which is extremely embarrassing. She is feeling depressed and finding it impossible to pursue her profession.

5. A middle-aged active CEO of a pharma company presents to the neurologist saying that lately he is having difficulty in attending board meetings as he cannot make out what is being discussed when different persons are talking together and also complains of a buzzing sound in the ears. He also finds it extremely embarrassing at parties or other social gatherings as it difficult for him to understand others when there is a background noise. However, he does not have any problems within the four walls of his bedroom or during a one-to-one discussion in his office cabin.

6. A 7-year-old child is brought by the parents to the pediatrician with the complaint that the child is performing very well in all subjects except in spelling and dictation, and that the class teacher has sent a note to the parents to find out if the child has any hearing impairment.

7. A 5-year-old child is brought to the family physician as the child has not picked up speech and language skills like other children of his age. On further questioning by the doctor, the parents report that the child may not also be hearing properly.

8. A 4-month-old infant is brought to the neonatologist with the complaint that ever since the child had been admitted to the neonatal intensive care unit for pneumonia, the child has stopped responding to sounds and does not turn the head towards the source of the sound.

9. A newborn hearing screening test carried out on a just-born baby in the nursing home has revealed that the child probably has a hearing loss in both the ears. The entire family comprising of the parents, grandparents, and near relatives, lands up in the obstetrician's chamber ostensibly perturbed, and questions the obstetrician on the future line of management.

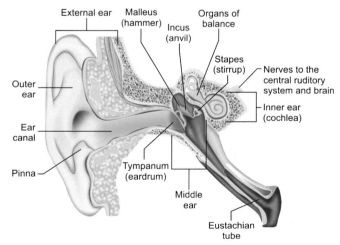

Fig. 18.1: The anatomy of the ear.

sounds, especially the low frequency sounds that have reached the eardrum, and then send the amplified sound into the inner ear. As sound impinges on the eardrum, the eardrum vibrates and this vibration is transmitted through the chain of the three small bones into the base of the inner ear such that the inner ear is mechanically stimulated.

3. The *inner ear* includes the cochlea and the nerve endings of the auditory nerve that pick up the neural impulses from the inner ear for sending them to the brain through the auditory nerve. The function of the cochlea is to convert the sound that is in the form of mechanical vibratory energy into electrical energy and stimulate the auditory nerve. The auditory nerve originates in the cochlea and traverses through a very complex pathway in the cranium and delivers the electrical impulses to the higher auditory pathways and nuclei in the brain where the impulses are processed and the meaning of the sound impulse decoded. Only after the impulse has been adequately processed in the brain (a process called central auditory processing) and decoded can we understand the meaning of the sound.

The mechanism of hearing is considerably complex. Any structural or functional problem in any portion of the various anatomical structures and processes that comprises the auditory system can result in hearing impairment. Depending on the structure/function of the auditory system that is damaged, the hearing loss can be categorized into the following four types:

1. *Conductive deafness*: This is caused by a disorder in the structure of the external ear or the middle ear (Fig. 18.2).

    The common causes of conductive deafness are elucidated in Box 18.2.

    In most cases, conductive deafness can be surgically corrected, and in some cases, even medical treatment helps.

2. *Sensorineural deafness:* This is caused by a disorder in the cochlea (when it is called sensory deafness), or in the auditory nerve (called neural deafness). The damage to the cochlea can be caused by numerous mechanisms, the commonest of which are degenerative changes induced by loud noise, ageing, ototoxic drugs, toxins, autoimmune disorders, etc. Occasionally, the cause remains unidentified when it is labeled as idiopathic sensorineural deafness.

3. *Mixed deafness:* This is a mixture of both sensorineural and conductive deafness;[1] i.e., both the external and/or middle ear and the inner ear/auditory nerve have been affected. Mixed deafness is commonly found

> **Box 18.2: The common causes of conductive deafness**
>
> The common causes of conductive deafness are atresia of the external auditory meatus, wax, or some foreign body in the external auditory meatus, perforation of the eardrum usually from infection (when it is called chronic/acute suppurative otitis media) or trauma to the ear, collection of fluid in the middle ear (termed as otitis media with effusion), stiffness or fixity of the bones in the middle ear that conduct the sound from the eardrum to the inner ear (commonest cause of which is a disease called otosclerosis in which the innermost bone becomes fixed and loses its pliability) or a discontinuity/breakage in the chain of the three bones inside the middle ear (called ossicular chain discontinuity).

in conditions like otosclerosis, advanced chronic suppurative otitis media (CSOM), sometimes after failed middle-ear surgeries, etc.

4. *Central deafness:* Also termed as the auditory processing disorder, it is believed to affect 2% of the normal population and is quite common in children.[2] Central deafness is caused by defects in the processing of the auditory impulses in the brain. Patients suffering from central deafness present with problems such as, an inability in understanding but not in hearing speech, especially in poor acoustic environments like noisy classrooms/restaurants. Many neurological conditions also result in central deafness.

How does the clinician identify the deafness, diagnose the cause of the deafness, determine the site of the pathology in the auditory system, and finally manage and treat the hearing impairment? It is not just enough to determine the type of deafness, i.e., whether the deafness is conductive/mixed/sensorineural or central, but also the specific cause of that particular type of deafness has to be identified as, without that a proper management is not possible. This is done by carrying out selected *clinical tests* and *investigations* to establish and confirm the nature and the cause of deafness.

CLINICAL TESTS (FIG. 18.3)

The clinical tests basically comprise of *otoscopy,* i.e., clinically examining the ear drum and the external auditory meatus, usually done by an otoscope; and some simple *hearing tests* carried out with tuning forks. Otoscopy reveals only the condition of the external auditory meatus and the eardrum, nothing beyond it, except in those patients with a large central perforation where parts of the middle ear can also be seen.

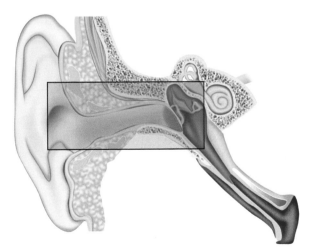

Fig. 18.2: Conductive deafness. The pathology in conductive deafness lies in the area from the outerpart of the external auditory meatus to the foot plate of stapes which is the innermost part of the middle ear as dipicted in the box.

An otoscope is an essential clinical instrument that all medical practitioners, pediatricians, and neurologists, in addition to ENT specialists must have.

An otoscope is a specially designed torch to visualize the external auditory meatus and the ear drum (Fig. 18.3). It shows whether the external auditory meatus is blocked by wax or any foreign body, and whether there is any deformity or perforation in the ear drum. Otoscopy is necessary not only for cases of conductive/mixed deafness that show some abnormality in the otoscopic findings (exception: otosclerosis where an intact normal ear drum is usually found) but in all patients presenting with deafness. One does not have to be an ENT specialist to use an otoscope; with a little practice, all clinicians should be able to use it effectively and efficiently.

A couple of tuning forks of the frequencies of 512 Hz and 1024 Hz must also be available with all clinicians who may be approached by patients suffering from hearing disorders (Fig. 18.4). For neurologists, tuning forks serve an additional purpose as tuning forks are also used to assess vibratory sense of the lower extremities. Tuning forks are used to determine the nature of deafness, i.e., whether the deafness is conductive/mixed/sensorineural in type. Central deafness cannot be identified by tuning fork tests and special audiological tests are necessary to identify it. The tuning fork tests include the Rinne's test, Weber's test, and the absolute bone conduction test (Fig. 18.5). In the Rinne's test, the tongs of the tuning fork are first hit on a hard rubber pad or on the elbow of the clinician and then held against the patient's ear such

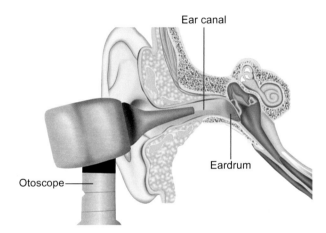

Fig. 18.3: Testing with an otoscope.

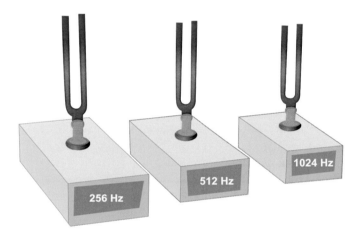

Fig. 18.4: Tuning forks.

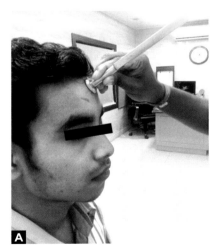
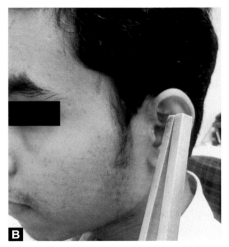

Figs 18.5A and B: Tuning fork tests. **(A)** Weber's test; **(B)** Rinnie's test.

that the upper end of the vibrating tongs is against the outer opening of the external auditory meatus. Next, the base of the vibrating tuning fork is placed on the most prominent part of the bone behind the auricle called the mastoid bone, and the patient's response to which of the two sounds is louder is ascertained. A patient with sensorineural deafness as well as subjects with normal hearing will hear the first sound louder than the second, i.e., the sound of the vibrating tongs of the tuning fork held against the hole of the ear will appear to be louder than the sound heard when the base of the tuning fork is placed on the bone behind the ear. Patients with conductive or mixed deafness will have just the opposite sensation, i.e., the sound heard when the base of the tuning fork is placed on the mastoid bone will be louder than the sound heard when the tongs are held against the ear. The Rinne's test is, hence, used to distinguish conductive/mixed deafness from sensorineural deafness or a normal hearing.

In the Weber's test, the tuning fork is first hit gently on a hard rubber pad or on the elbow of the clinician and then the base of the vibrating tuning fork is placed in the middle of the forehead and the patient is asked to determine on which side, the sound appears louder. In a conductive/mixed deafness, the sound appears louder in the deafer ear whereas in a sensorineural deafness the sound appears louder in the normal/better ear. If the patient has perfectly normal hearing on both sides or if there is an equal amount of sensorineural deafness in both ears, then the sound does not lateralize to any ear and the patient says that he is hearing the sound in the middle or sometimes equally in both ears.

In the absolute bone conduction test, the tuning fork is first hit on the hard rubber pad and then the base of the vibrating tuning fork is placed on the mastoid bone of the patient's ear just behind the auricle and the patient is asked to indicate as soon as the patient stops hearing the sound. Immediately, the base of the tuning fork is then placed on the same spot of the clinician's ear and the clinician has to find out whether he is able to hear the sound of the tuning fork or not. If the clinician has a normal hearing in his own ear (which he is supposed to know beforehand) then, in case the clinician can still hear the sound after the patient has stopped hearing it, it would indicate that the patient has a sensorineural deafness in the tested ear. If the clinician cannot hear the sound after the patient has stopped hearing it, then it would indicate that the patient has got normal hearing in the tested ear. The tuning fork tests are, thus, good clinical tests to distinguish between the different types of deafness and are a must for all clinicians who confront hearing-

impaired patients in their clinical practice. However, from the routine tuning fork tests, it is not possible to know the severity of deafness whether mild, moderate, severe, or profound, nor is it possible to know the cause of the deafness, i.e., if it is a conductive deafness or due to otosclerosis or CSOM or otitis media with effusion, but by supplementing the tuning fork tests with otoscopic findings an idea of the nature and the cause of deafness can be obtained in most patients.

INVESTIGATIONS IN A PATIENT PRESENTING WITH DEAFNESS

The primary and the most basic investigation necessary in a patient presenting with hearing impairment is the *pure tone audiometry test.* Other tests are advised depending on the findings of the pure tone audiometry test and the clinical examination. If it is a case of conductive or mixed deafness with the eardrum intact, then a *tympanometry* test is advised along with it.[2,3] If it is a sensorineural deafness, especially unilateral, then a brainstem-evoked response audiometry (BERA) for the site of the lesion must essentially be advised.[4] The clinician must be capable of interpreting the findings of the pure tone audiometry test, the tympanometry test, and the BERA test.

PURE TONE AUDIOMETRY TEST (FIG. 18.6)

This is the basic test that must be advised to all patients presenting with deafness provided the patient is over 5 years of age. It is a subjective test and is completely dependent upon the responses of the patient. If the patient responds incorrectly, the results of the test are bound to be erroneous. The test cannot be reliably carried out if the responses of the patient are not dependable as often happens in children below 5 years of age and in some difficult adults like malingering subjects or mentally unstable persons. The instrument used for testing hearing is called the audiometer, the test process as audiometry,

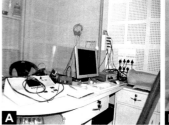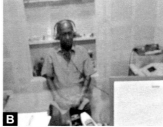

Fig. 18.6: The pure tone audiometry test.

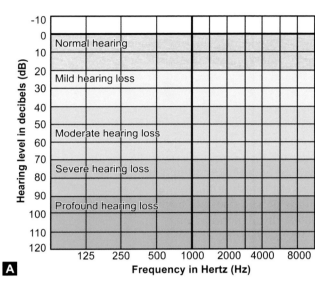

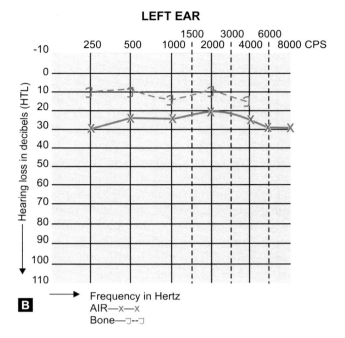

LEFT EAR

TONE AUDIOGRAM

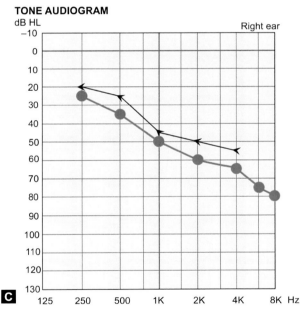

Figs 18.7A to C: **(A)** Intensity of the hearing loss. Hearing thresholds between –10 to 20 dB in all frequencies is considered as normal hearing i.e., no deafness; thresholds between 20–40 dB is considered as mild deafness/hearing loss, that between 40–70 dB as moderate deafness/hearing loss, between 70 and 90 dB as severe deafness/hearing loss and above 90 dB as profound deafness/hearing loss; **(B)** Normal hearing threshold. This audiogram is indicative of a normal hearing. The average air conduction threshold are all within 25 dB approxmately, the bone conduction threshold are all within 20 dB and the air bone gap is less than 20 dB; **(C)** Sensorineural deafness. This audiogram shows normal hearing thresholds in the low frequencies, mild to moderate deafness in the middle frequencies and moderate to severe deafness in the high frequencies.

and the test results plotted in a chart with the hearing threshold on the y-axis and the test frequencies on the x-axis is called the audiogram (Fig. 18.7). The audiometry test, if carried out properly by a reliable person, who may be a doctor (not necessarily an ENT doctor), audiologist, or a technician well-versed with the intricacies of audiometry test, informs the clinician about (1) the degree of hearing loss whether mild, moderate, severe, or profound and (2) the nature of the hearing loss, i.e., whether the deafness is conductive, sensorineural,

or mixed in type. From the audiometry report, the clinician can understand whether the pathology lies in the middle/external ear (conductive deafness) or in the inner ear/auditory nerve (sensorineural deafness), or in both the middle and inner ears (mixed deafness) along with the degree of hearing handicap. The adjoining figures (Figs 18.7 A to C) and the text below describe how the clinician can distinguish between conductive, sensorineural, and mixed deafness from the audiogram. From the audiometry test it is possible to determine the type or nature of deafness but not the cause, e.g., if it is a conductive deafness, whether it is caused by otosclerosis, or by CSOM, or by otitis media with effusion. Other tests like tympanometry along with the clinical findings need to be carried out to establish the etiology. Central deafness, however, cannot be identified by pure tone audiometry and pretty difficult and sophisticated tests are required to diagnose central deafness but fortunately, most patients do not seek medical advice for central deafness. Central deafness is considered as a diagnosis in those patients where pure tone audiometry test shows normal hearing but the patient complains of difficulty in hearing and understanding speech sounds in acoustically unfriendly environments such as noisy classrooms/courtrooms/ marketplaces. There are not many centers that are equipped enough and have the requisite manpower to reliably carry out tests for central deafness.

INTERPRETING THE PURE TONE AUDIOMETRY TEST

The pure tone audiometry shows the hearing threshold by air conduction and bone conduction. Hearing threshold is defined as the minimum sound in decibels (dB) that a subject can hear at each individual frequency. The hearing threshold is marked in 5 dB steps and the test is carried out between 0 dB and 100 dB for all practical purposes. So, if there is a point plotted in the audiogram of the left ear in the frequency of 1,000 Hz at 30 dB, it means that the hearing threshold for sounds of 1,000 Hz is 30 dB and implies that this person can hear only sounds above 30 dB in intensity and does not hear sound below this level. There are two points plotted at each frequency, one representing the hearing threshold by air conduction and the other by bone conduction. Air conducted sounds enter the ear through the external ear, pass through the ear drum, then through the middle ear and finally reaches the inner ear, whereas bone conducted sounds reach the inner ear directly through the skull and does not traverse the external and middle ear. In pure tone audiometry, the hearing threshold is tested both by air conduction as well as by bone conduction and both air conduction hearing thresholds as well as bone conducted hearing thresholds are plotted in the audiogram. The gap in dB between the air conduction thresholds and bone conduction thresholds is called the air-bone gap.[2] The frequencies routinely tested in pure tone audiometry test are 250 Hz, 500 Hz, 1,000 Hz, 2,000 Hz, 4,000 Hz, and 8,000 Hz. Though the range of human hearing is 20–20,000 Hz, the pure tone audiometry test assesses for hearing of speech

frequencies only that range from 250 to 8,000 Hz. As human speech sounds are all between 250 to 8,000 Hz, testing the hearing acuity between 250 to 8,000 Hz usually suffices as the main purpose of hearing is to hear other humans speaking. But for special purposes, e.g., for hearing and appreciating music one needs to have good hearing in the high frequencies. To test the hearing in the high frequencies, i.e., above 8,000 Hz a high frequency audiometry tests required. This test evaluates hearing acuity between 8,000 and 20,000 Hz. For a person to have a hearing impairment in any frequency, the hearing threshold at that frequency by air conduction has to be anything between 30 dB and 100 dB. So, if a patient has a hearing threshold of, say, 20 dB at 2,000 Hz, it means that the person does not have any hearing impairment at 2,000 Hz by air conduction.

a. *Normal hearing:* The air conduction hearing threshold for all the tested frequencies should be <30 dB, preferably 0–25 dB, and the bone conduction threshold levels between 0 dB and 20 dB, preferably 0–15 dB.

b. *Conductive deafness;* The air conduction hearing threshold level should definitely be above 30 dB, the bone conduction level below 20 dB in all frequencies, and the average air bone gap should not be <20 dB (Fig. 18.8).

c. *Sensorineural deafness:* The air conduction hearing threshold level should be above 35 dB, the bone conduction hearing threshold level above 20 dB and above, and the air bone gap should be <20 dB, i.e., between 0 dB and 20 dB.

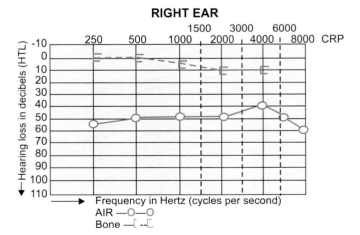

Fig. 18.8: Conductive deafness. The bone conduction thresholds are within normal limits (within 20 dB) in all frequencies; the air conduction gap is more than 20 dB. Hence this is a conductive deafness. As the average air conductive thresholds is approximately 50–55 dB, this is moderate degree of deafness.

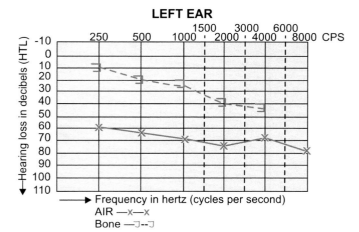

LEFT EAR

Frequency in hertz (cycles per second)
AIR —x—x
Bone —Ɔ--Ɔ

Fig. 18.9: Mixed deafness. This is mixed deafness as the bone conduction thresholds are mostly above the normal range of 20 dB, the air conduction thresholds are all much above the normal range of 25 dB and the air bone gap is more than 20 dB. In mixed deafness there is both a sensorineural component (bone conduction thresholds above 20 dB) as well as a conductive component (air-bone gap above 20 dB). As the average air conduction thresholds are in the range of 65–70 dB, this is a moderate to severe deafness.

d. *Mixed deafness:* The air conduction hearing threshold level should be above 30 dB, the bone conduction level above 20 dB, and the air bone gap should be >25 dB (Fig. 18.9).

As pure tone audiometry is the basic hearing test and needs to be done in all patients presenting with hearing impairment, all clinicians must be well versed in interpreting the audiogram. As already mentioned, the pure tone audiometry test is a subjective test and is possible only in reliable and cooperative patients above 5 years of age. In other patients where responses are not reliable, objective tests of hearing like BERA for threshold estimation and the auditory steady-state response (ASSR) test are performed as results of these tests are not dependent on the subject's responses.

IMPEDANCE AUDIOMETRY (FIG. 18.10)[5]

This is not a test for determining hearing acuity; it does not evaluate the hearing threshold and hence how much the patient hears in different frequencies cannot be ascertained from the impedance audiometry test. The impedance audiometry test is indicated in patients suffering from conductive or mixed deafness, i.e., if the patient on clinical tuning fork test has been found to have a conductive deafness (bone conduction better than air conduction), or if the pure tone audiometry test has shown an air-bone gap

above 20 dB. It is an objective test and is not dependent on the subject's responses and hence can be carried out in all types of patients including very young patients. This test helps to distinguish between the different types of conductive deafness that is whether the deafness is caused by otosclerosis or otitis media with effusion or ossicular chain discontinuity or due to a perforation in the ear drum.[5] However, if clinically the patient is found to have a perforated eardrum then the impedance audiometry test is not of any additional help except if the clinician is interested in knowing the status of the Eustachian tube function. The best use of impedance audiometry is therefore in patients having conductive or mixed deafness with an intact ear drum.[2] The acoustic reflex and Eustachian function tests that are an integral part of impedance audiometry are for more specialized diagnostic purposes and is outside the scope of this chapter.

BRAINSTEM-EVOKED RESPONSE AUDIOMETRY (FIG. 18.11)

This is an objective test and is used primarily for two purposes viz. (a) determination of site of lesion in sensorineural deafness, the test is mandatory if the sensorineural deafness is unilateral or if there is a unilateral tinnitus and (b) objective estimation of the approximate hearing threshold in difficult to test subjects in whom a subjective pure tone audiometry cannot be reliably done such as infants and some difficult to test adults.[1]

In the BERA test, a reasonably loud sound is presented to the ear and the electrical activity generated in the brain as the impulse passes through the auditory pathway between the cochlea and the midbrain is monitored and recorded by an electrode placed on the vertex or on the forehead. The recording is obtained as a graph ideally with five peaks, each peak being generated by one particular anatomical structure that acts a relay station in the auditory pathway between the cochlea and the midbrain. Each of these peaks are obtained at intervals of roughly 1 ms. If there is a defect in any part of this complex neural pathway that conducts the sound from the cochlea to the higher centers in the brain, there is a delay in the corresponding peak by noting which the clinician can pinpoint the site of lesion in the brain.

The five relay stations in the auditory pathway from where the five wave-peaks of the BERA graph orginate are (a) Wave I is generated from the distal most part of the auditory nerve, i.e., the cochlear end of the auditory nerve, (b) Wave II is generated from the proximal part of the

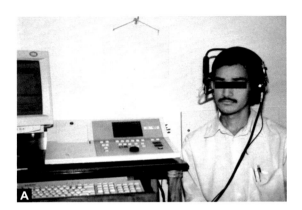

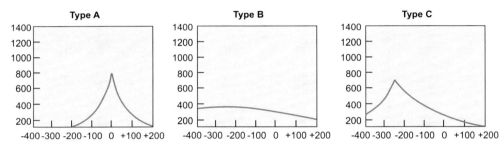

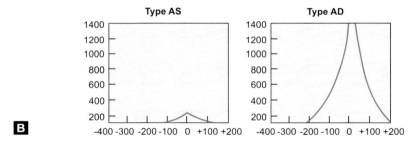

Figs 18.10A and B: Impedance audiometry test and the different types of tympanometric graphs.

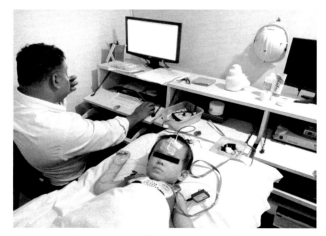

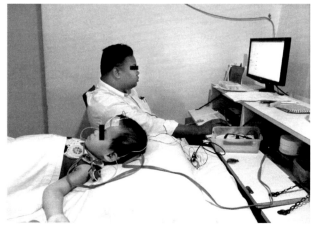

Fig. 18.11: Brainstem-evoked response audiometry.

auditory nerve, (c) Wave III is generated from the cochlear nucleus in the brainstem, (d) Wave IV is generated from the superior olivary complex and (e) Wave V is generated from the lateral lemniscus - inferior colliculus area of the brainstem. So if there is an abnormal delay (above 2.4 ms) between wave I and wave III we suspect a lesion between the cochlea and the cochlear nucleus, i.e., in the auditory nerve. Normally it should have been to 2 ms. Similarly a delay of more than 2 ms between wave III and V suggests a rostral brainstem lesion. The BERA for site of lesion test is of immense value to neurologists and also to ENT specialists and pediatricians. It helps in the early diagnosis of disorders like acoustic neuroma, multiple sclerosis and auditory neuropathy. Acoustic neuroma is a benign tumor in the brain that originates from the nerve sheath of the vestibular nerve. Acoustic neuroma should be ruled out in all cases of sensorineural deafness and since acoustic neuroma is usually (but not always) a

unilateral pathology, a BERA test for site of lesion should essentially be requested for in all patients presenting with unilateral sensorineural deafness.[2] Auditory neuropathy is usually bilateral and occurs due to degenerative/functional changes in the auditory nerves. It induces a very poor understanding of speech sounds and BERA for site of lesion combined with tests like otoacoustic emission test are required (Fig. 18.12) for diagnosis.

The BERA test is also used as already mentioned for evaluating the hearing threshold level in some patients. For evaluating the hearing threshold it is only the peak V that is significant. The other four peaks in BERA graph are not very helpful in evaluating hearing thresholds. In the BERA for threshold test, the BERA is recorded at progressively lower intensities till the peak V completely disappears. The minimum intensity of sound presented below which no wave V is recorded is known as the BERA threshold. The average hearing threshold level is about

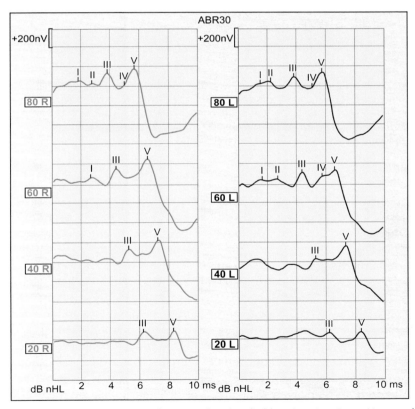

Fig. 18.12A: The brainstem-evoked response audiometry for threshold estimation in a 41-year-old male subject. This patient had presented to the doctor feigning deafness. The subjective pure tone audiometry test suggested severe deafness bilaterally. The pressure of wave V even at 20 dB indicated that the patient has normal hearing and that he is malingering. Objective hearing tests like BERA and ASSR are often required in adults too.

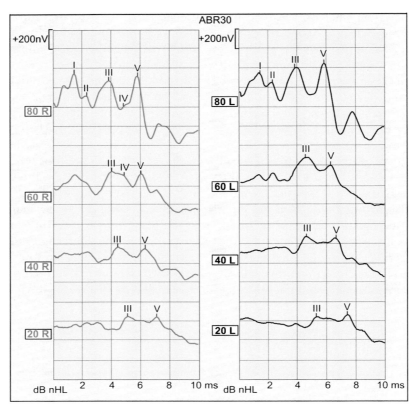

Fig. 18.12B: BERA for threshold estimation done in a 5-year-old mentally retarded child. The presence of an identifiable wave V even at 20 dB stimulation suggests normal hearing. BERA test can be done with click sounds and also with pure tone sounds called tone-pips. Though not specifically mentioned in this printout, the BERA test was done using click sounds. BERA test done with click sounds are indicative of hearing threshold in the 2000–4000 Hz range. Hence from this BERA tracing it may be inferred that the child has normal hearing at 2000–4000 Hz range.

10 dB below the BERA threshold. The BERA for threshold estimation is a very reliable and objective mode of ascertaining the hearing threshold.

Though, the basic hearing tests are pure tone audiometry, impedance audiometry, and the BERA test, there are other tests of hearing, e.g., otoacoustic emission test (OAE) and ASSR test (Fig. 18.13). The OAE test is a screening test and is usually carried out on infants and neonates to verify whether the subject has normal hearing or if there is any hearing impairment.[2] It is a quick test and is very popular for neonatal hearing screening. The ASSR test does not have much neurological diagnostic significance. It is basically done to objectively evaluate the hearing threshold at some specific frequencies and is a very good test to evaluate frequency specific hearing threshold objectively in infants and difficult to test children. Another test related to hearing disorders is the electrocochleography (ECochG) test. ECochG is best used to confirm Ménière's disease. Through the Glycerol test is also used to confirm Ménière's disease the sensitivity of electrocochleography is higher as a diagnostic tool for Ménière's disease. ECochG test should be asked for in all patients suspected to have Ménière's disease.

Though deafness is one of the commonest sensory disoders, the nature and intensity of the deafness can be very well documented in all cases right from newborns to the old and infirm patients subjectively and/or objectively. The cause of the deafness can be ascertained in most cases also. Treatment is available for most if not all patients of deafness either by medical or surgical means or by other modalities like hearing aids and cochlear implants. Except for some cases of central deafness, deafness can be corrected in practically all patients if diagnosed in treated early and rationally.

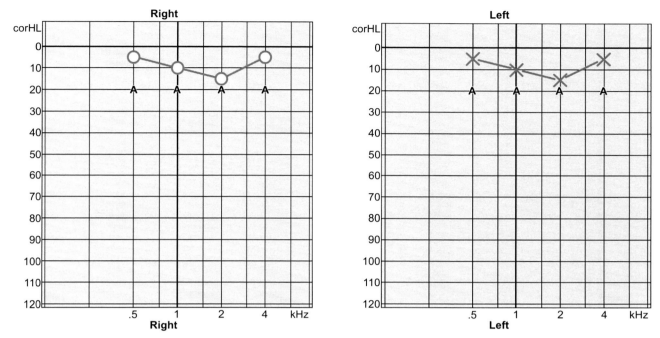

Fig. 18.13: An ASSR showing normal hearing threshold at 500 Hz, 1,000 Hz, 2,000 Hz, and 4,000 Hz. This frequency specific hearing thresholds have been obtained objectively, i.e., without the patient having to subjectively respond to the test sound signals. ASSR provides the opportunity of evaluating the hearing threshold at different frequencies without the patient having to subjectively respond to the test sound unlike the pure tone audiometry test. This is a very big advantage and is the only way to ascertain the freqency specific hearing thresholds in difficult to test patients like infants and children and also in some difficult adults like mentally unstable patients or in malingerers who feign deafness.

REFERENCES

1. Biswas Anirban. (2015). Clinical Audiovestibulometry for Otologists and Neurologist. 5th ed. Chapter 1. Bhalani Medical Book House, Mumbai, India.
2. Biswas Anirban. (2009). Clinical Audiovestibulometry for Otologists and Neurologist. 4th ed. Chapter 2. Bhalani Medical Book House, Mumbai, India.
3. Roeser RJ, Valente M, Hosford-Dunn H. Audiology Diagnosis. 2nd ed. 2007.
4. Musiek FE, Geurkink NA. Auditory brainstem response and central auditory test findings for patients with brain stem lesions. Laryngoscope. 1982;92:891-900.
5. Jerger J. Clinical experience with impedance audiometry. Arch Otolaryngol. 1970;92:311-24.
6. Katz Jack. Handbook of Clinical Audiology. 7th ed. Wolters Kluwer. 2015.

Chapter 19

Approach to a Patient with Neurogenic Dysphagia

Kiran Bala, Shaily Singh, Preeti Singla

INTRODUCTION

Swallowing is a complex process in which food (liquid/solid) reaches the stomach from oral cavity. This can be viewed as three-stage process:

Stage 1—voluntary oral preparatory phase leading to formation of a bolus.

Stage 2—pharyngeal phase (deglutition reflex) leading to propulsion of the food bolus into esophagus and preventing its entry to the air passage/nose.

Stage 3—esophageal phase leading to transfer of bolus into the stomach.

Neural structures involved in normal swallowing.[1-3]

1. Bolus preparation (cranial nerves V and VII).
2. Bolus propulsion (cranial nerves X and XII).
3. Palatal elevation (cranial nerves X).
4. Apposition of the true and false vocal cords and of the arytenoids against the base of the epiglottis (cranial nerves X).
5. Upward and forward movement of the hyoid and larynx (cranial nerves V, VII, C1-3) enhances airway protection and pulls open the relaxed upper esophageal sphincter.
6. Breathing is centrally inhibited during the swallow (deglutition apnea)? Brainstem reflex.[4]
7. Central pattern generator (nucleus ambiguus and the nucleus of the tractus solitarius under various peripheral and supranuclear controls).[5-7]
8. Cerebral cortex (primary motor, inferior frontal gyrus, insula) modulates the above mechanisms.[8-10]
9. Basal ganglia and cerebellum probably assist the cerebral cortex.

Dysphagia or difficulty in swallowing either refers to the difficulty someone may have with initiating a swallow (usually referred to as oropharyngeal dysphagia) or to the sensation that food and/or liquids are somehow hindered in their passage from the mouth to the stomach. (Usually referred to as esophageal dysphagia.) Dysphagia, therefore, is the "perception" that there is an impediment to the normal passage of swallowed material.

In view of the multiple structures working during the process of swallowing, structural, or functional dysfunction at the level of any of these may lead to neurogenic dysphagia.

Neurogenic causes of dysphagia predominantly affect the oropharyngeal phase; however, it rarely may be caused by disorders of esophageal innervation, thus affecting the esophageal phase.

PRESENTING COMPLAINTS

On the basis of the structures affected, in a case of dysphagia, the following features may be found:

- Oral dysfunction—drooling, food spillage, sialorrhea, difficulty initiating a swallow, piecemeal swallows, and dysarthria.
- Pharyngeal dysfunction—"food getting stuck" immediately upon swallowing, postnasal regurgitation, coughing, or choking during food consumption and dysphonia.
- Esophageal dysfunction—onset of symptoms several seconds after initiating a swallow. Frequently point to the suprasternal notch or behind the sternum when asked to localize.

Patients with neurogenic dysphagia typically present with difficulty in swallowing, which is usually more for liquids than solids. Difficulty in swallowing might not be the presenting symptom especially in patients with mild or moderately severe neurogenic dysphagia. However, direct questioning often reveals that they have been avoiding certain foods that they found difficult to chew or swallow. They often change their diet to include softer foods to facilitate swallowing. Weight loss may be the first complaint in some cases. Drooling, especially in the sitting up posture, results, both from hypersalivation and difficulty in deglutition. Choking, coughing, throat clearing, or change in voice may suggest aspiration. Micro aspiration, where the patient does not manifest with these complaints, occurs commonly in the recumbent position, especially during sleep. Recurrent chest infections may be the presenting complaints in these patients. Occasionally interrupted sleep may be the only indication of swallowing difficulties. Pain during swallowing is generally not a feature of neurogenic dysphagia.

A careful medical history and physical examination is essential but not always sufficient to distinguish dysphagia due to mechanical causes from neurogenic dysphagia. This has to be supplemented by special investigations often.

SYMPTOM ANALYSIS

Asking a few questions can help the clinician to arrive at the possible etiology for dysphagia.
1. How was the onset—acute/chronic?
2. How was the progression—static/gradually progressive/rapidly progressive?
3. What was the course—fluctuating/constant?
4. More to solids/liquids?
5. Painful/Painless?
6. Associated features—choking, nasal regurgitation, and speech changes?

In case of dearth of information clinically, patients should be evaluated by an ENT specialist as conditions like tumors in the tongue base and hypopharynx, large anterior cervical osteophytes, and other retropharyngeal pathology[11,12] upper or lower esophageal sphincter dysfunction, esophageal reflux and its complications,[13] and external compression of the esophagus (enlarged left atrium, aberrant subclavian artery, retrosternal goitre) may all present as progressive dysphagia with an apparently normal examination.

ONSET OF SYMPTOMS

Acute—Almost Always Neurogenic in Origin

- Acute stroke is complicated by dysphagia in about 25–42% of all cases.[14] Dysphagia in these patients is usually associated with hemiplegia due to lesions of the brain stem or the involvement of one or both hemispheres. Dysphagia, in the absence of other neurological symptoms and signs has been reported in patients with lacunar infarcts in the periventricular white matter[15] and after discrete vascular brain stem lesions.[16] Unilateral lesions in the lowest part of the precentral gyrus and the posterior part of the inferior frontal gyrus may be associated with severe dysphagia unassociated with any buccolingual apraxia, speech impairment, or local paresis.[17]

Dysphagia was commonly found (29% of cases) in another large stroke series when patients were assessed on the day of admission and were found to have a negative effect on outcome independent of other factors associated with stroke severity.

Subacute

- *Guillain-Barré syndrome (GBS):* Cranial nerve involvement is reported in 45–75% of patients of GBS and pharyngeal weakness is the second most common after facial weakness. The history of preceding prodromal illness accompanied by flaccid limb weakness that generally precedes the dysphagia, suggests GBS. Electrophysiology further supports the diagnosis.
- Dysphagia without limb weakness may occur as part of polyneuritis cranialis, an entity described in the early twentieth century.[18,19]
- *Myasthenic crisis:* Dysphagia is a frequent symptom in myasthenia gravis and it eventually occurs in 15–40% of patients with the generalized form.[20,21] However, it may present as the sole manifestation of the disease.[22] Diagnosis in these patients may be difficult, especially if acetylcholine receptor (AChR) antibodies are negative or if there is not a clear clinical response to anticholinesterase. In addition to dysphagia, patients with disorders of the neuromuscular junction often have dysphonia and dysarthria. A proper clinical history to suggest fluctuations and a battery of investigations may clarify the picture.
- *Diphtheritic neuropathy:* Neurological complications occur in up to 15% of patients with diphtheria and

typically begin with paralysis of soft palate and impaired pharyngeal sensation causing dysphagia. Paralysis of pupillary accommodation with preserved light reflex suggests the diagnosis in such a scenario.

- *Polymyositis/dermatomyositis*: Dysphagia may be the presenting complaint as the swallowing difficulties occur early in these disorders and are severe. Weight loss, aspiration, and chest infections follow. Associated facial weakness, neck weakness, and systemic features contribute to the diagnosis.
- *Drugs*: The mechanisms implicated in drug induced dysphagia are diverse, dose dependent, and usually reversible.
  a. Sedatives and hypnotics depress the level of consciousness and interfere with the oropharyngeal phase of swallowing.
  b. Dopaminergic agents may cause orofacial dyskinesia that affects the preparation of the food bolus and its delivery to the pharynx.
  c. Neuroleptic drugs delay the initiation of the swallow reflex, sometimes in the absence of obvious extrapyramidal features.
  d. Botulinum toxin causes dysphagia due to inhibition of neural transmission at the neuromuscular junction. This adverse effect is seen in 10–28% patients with spasmodic torticollis treated with botulinum toxin and may cause dysphagia. This is usually mild and transient, lasting 10–14 days and usually occurs in patients receiving large doses of botulinum.

Chronic

- *Basal ganglia disorders*: Parkinson's disease patients may have dysphagia, usually a late feature but sometimes it may occur in the early stages and may even be the presenting symptom in some cases. More than 80% of patients with Parkinson's disease have dysphagia but, as a rule, this is mild and has little or no effect on the patient's nutritional status. However, in about 10% of parkinsonian patients with dysphagia, the symptoms are severe and this generally correlates with the severity and duration of the disease. Drooling is an indication of bradykinesia of the oropharyngeal musculature. Other parkinsonian syndromes, like multisystem atrophy (MSA), progressive supranuclear palsy results in similar, but usually more severe symptoms.
- *Motor neuron disease*: A study on dysphagia in motor neuron disease (MND) revealed that moderate or severe swallowing difficulty was present in 89% of those whose disease had presented as bulbar palsy, in 45% of those in whom the disease began many months before as progressive muscular atrophy, and in 29% of those with amyotrophic lateral sclerosis.[23] In these patients features suggestive of anterior horn cell and/pyramidal tracts supplemented with electrophysiology will clinch the diagnosis. However, not all the patients with an abnormal video fluoroscopy picture had swallowing difficulties.[23]

- *Myopathies*: Although in theory any muscular disorder may present with impairment of swallowing, abnormalities of deglutition tend to predominate in some types of muscle disease. These include certain muscular dystrophies such as oculopharyngeal muscular dystrophy, myotonic dystrophy, and rare patients in the advanced stages of Duchenne muscular dystrophy. Inflammatory disorders such as polymyositis, dermatomyositis, and inclusion body myositis can involve the muscles of deglutition. Certain metabolic myopathies, particularly mitochondrial myopathies, may present with impairment of swallowing.

PROGRESSION AND COURSE

- *Static and improving*: This type of dysphagia is usually seen in stroke patients and drug induced dysphagia, which improve with the stroke recovery or on discontinuation of the offending agent.
- *Intermittent/fluctuating*: Typically seen with myasthenia gravis and other myasthenic syndromes. Dysphagia developing late while taking a meal usually suggests myasthenia.
- *Rapidly progressive*: Seen in inflammatory myopathies, GBS, and infective etiologies involving local sites.
- *Slowly progressive*: Degenerative disorders such as MND, extrapyramidal syndromes.

Pain upon swallowing (odynophagia) can result from local inflammation, infection, or malignancy. Pain on swallowing (odynophagia) is not a symptom of neurogenic dysphagia and is commonly seen in cases of esophagitis, usually secondary to candida infection.

ASSOCIATED FEATURES

A history of dry mouth or dry eyes may indicate inadequate saliva/tear production. Anticholinergics, antihistamines, and certain antihypertensive agents can reduce salivary flow. Sjögren's syndrome should also be considered in such cases.

- Changes in speech may provide important clues, and often implicate neuromuscular dysfunction.
- Hoarseness or a weak cough may represent vocal cord paralysis.
- Slurred speech may indicate weakness or incoordination of muscles involved in articulation and swallowing.
- Dysarthria and nasal speech or regurgitation of food into the nose may represent weakness of the soft palate or pharyngeal constrictors.
- The combination of hoarseness, dysphonia (difficulty or pain while speaking), and nasal speech accompanying dysphagia is associated with the muscular dystrophies.

FUNCTIONAL DYSPHAGIA

Functional dysphagia is a diagnosis of exclusion in patients with dysphagia who have undergone a complete diagnostic evaluation without evidence of a structural abnormality or motility disturbance.

Recommended diagnostic criteria include at least 12 weeks of a sense of solid and/or liquid foods sticking, lodging, or passing abnormally through the esophagus, with symptom onset at least 6 months prior to diagnosis; and the absence of gastro esophageal reflux and motility disorders such as, scleroderma and achalasia.

Symptoms of dysphagia may be intermittent or present after each meal, and may be difficult to distinguish from dysphagia caused by mechanical or motility disorders. These patients pose a diagnostic and therapeutic dilemma since management options are limited (Box 19.1).

Box 19.1: Quick Checklist for assessment of a case of suspected Neurogenic Dysphagia

- Level of consciousness
- Head/neck posture and mobility (e.g., tracheostomy, neck lines, neck surgery)
- Breathing and effectiveness of cough (e.g., control of respiratory cycle, inspiratory and expiratory capacity, pulmonary function, laryngeal function)
- Neurological factors [e.g., spasticity, rigidity, weakness (central or peripheral), sensory loss, movement disorder, incoordination, loss of voluntary control, exaggeration of oropharyngeal, and laryngeal reflexes]
- Accompanying symptoms (vertigo, nausea, neuralgic pain, syncope)
- Gastro-esophageal function (e.g., acid reflux disease)
- Psychological and social factors (e.g., confidence, embarrassment, fear)
- Medication (e.g., anticholinergic drugs, neuroleptic medication, benzodiazepines)

ASSESSMENT OF A CASE OF DYSPHAGIA

Assessment comprises of the following:
1. Local examination
2. Investigations
   a. Direct laryngoscopy
   b. Indirect laryngoscopy
   c. Endoscopy.

It goes as a rule that patients presenting with dysphagia alone, without accompanying neurological symptoms or signs, should be evaluated by an ENT expert to rule out mechanical causes of dysphagia. There are several exceptions to this rule; however, ENT problems presenting as dysphagia are beyond the scope of this chapter.

LOCAL CLINICAL EXAMINATION

This is the first step in assessment of a patient with neurogenic dysphagia. This comprises of the following:
1. *Inspection of the oral cavity*: Inspection of oral cavity is done to look for obvious pathologies like enlarged tonsils/adenoids/candidiasis/pseudomembrane.

   Local examination can reveal food residues in the mouth or secretions pooled in the oropharynx either due to hypokinesis of swallowing (as in parkinsonism) or facial/bulbar muscular weakness.
2. Examination of cranial nerves 5, 7, 9, 10, 12, including gag reflex.
   - Both IX and X cranial nerves have motor and sensory functions and can be assessed together by checking for gag reflex.
     ○ Pharyngeal or gag reflex is tested by stimulating the posterior pharyngeal wall, tonsillar area, or base of the tongue with a long handle swab stick. The response is tongue retraction associated with elevation and constriction of the pharyngeal musculature.
     ○ Whereas a truly absent gag reflex may impair the ability to eject a bolus from the pharynx back into the mouth, its role in causing dysphagia is unclear.
     ○ Reduced voluntary palatal oropharyngeal movement with brisk reflex responses is seen in pseudo bulbar palsy.
     ○ It is not clear whether the bedside sensory examination can reliably distinguish IXth and Xth nerve lesions but lack of posterior wall pharyngeal sensation is reported to have prognostic implications in stroke.[24]

- *XII nerve examination*: A unilateral XIIth nerve lesion causes the tongue to deviate to the healthy side on retraction (unopposed action of styloglossus), and the affected side on protrusion (genioglossus).

3. Assessment of articulation and resonance (Nasality):
   - Volitional cough may be feeble due to a depressed consciousness level or respiratory or laryngeal weakness.
   - "Bovine" cough suggests vocal cord paresis.
   - Breathing may be stridulous (MSA, laryngeal dystonia), obstructed (laryngeal or pharyngeal occlusion), or abnormal in pattern (respiratory dyskinesia).
   - Patients with corticobulbar lesions may exhibit impaired voluntary control of facial movements, cough, and respiration while retaining emotional or reflex responses.
   - Dyskinesia or dystonia of the throat, face, jaw, and head and neck may be important clues to the underlying neurological disorder for e.g., Whipple's disease, celiac disease with encephalopathy, and multi system atrophy.

4. The presence of dysphagia and its severity can be assessed bedside by observing the patients during trial swallows. Swallowing behavior can be observed while the subject is taking food and fluids of different consistencies under "normal" everyday conditions. Some patients attempt to compensate for their swallowing difficulties by taking small, frequent drinks during the meal in order to "washdown" the food bolus.

SWALLOW TEST

This simple bedside measurement of the swallowing speed has been suggested as a diagnostic test for neurogenic dysphagia.[25] Qualitative water swallow tests have proved useful for dysphagia screening[26-28] and have been extended to include a quantitative element.[29-31]

Test Procedure

- The patient is made to sit upright and is given 150 mL of cold water to drink.
- This test consists of measuring the speed with which the patient drinks 150 mL of water. A swallowing speed of <10 mL/s suggests the presence of dysphagia.

Interpretation

- Reduced capacity and volume per swallow are interpreted as compensatory mechanisms to reduce the risk of laryngeal penetration or aspiration.
- Cough, wet hoarse voice, or breathlessness are evidence of decompensation.
- The presence of a palatal, gag, or pharyngeal reflex is not functionally equivalent to swallowing reflex and does not guarantee of a safe swallow and its absence is not a reliable indicator of an impaired swallow.

INVESTIGATIONS

1. *Videofluoroscopy:* It is considered the gold standard for the evaluation of dysphagia. If silent aspiration is considered likely, the possibility can be pursued with videofluoroscopy under supervision. This study is done in the radiology department. Patient is given different foods and drinks mixed with barium. The barium makes the food and liquid show up on the X-ray. The X-ray machine is only turned on while the patient swallows so that the patient does not get too much radiation.
   Advantages: It permits the observation of the oral preparatory phase, the reflex initiation of swallowing, and the pharyngeal transit of the food bolus.
   Disadvantage: Not suitable for repeated assessments because of the undesirable frequent exposure to radiation and the cost of the procedure.

2. *Fiberoptic nasal endoscopy:* This procedure consists of introducing an endoscope through the nose into the nasopharynx and placing the tip just above the soft palate. The patient is then given food and drink colored with a dye, and before and after swallowing pharyngeal pooling is observed.
   Advantage: Nasal endoscopy is a reliable method for assessing dysphagia and the risk of pulmonary aspiration.
   Disadvantages: Special expertise is necessary to carry out the procedure and to interpret its results.

3. *Pulse oximetry*
   Principle: Aspiration of food or fluid in the airways causes reflex bronchoconstriction that leads to ventilation-perfusion mismatch. The resulting oxygen desaturation of arterial blood can be readily measured with pulse oximetry. In a recent study, pulse oximetry predicted aspiration or the lack of it in 81.5% of stroke patients with dysphagia.[32]

Advantages: Noninvasive, quick, and repeatable but its results must be interpreted with caution in smokers and in those with chronic lung disease.
4. *Esophageal manometry:* It enables measurements of the intraesophageal pressure gradient and is useful in the evaluation of dysfunction of the cricopharyngeus muscle and abnormalities of esophageal motility.

REFERENCES

1. Donner MW, Bosma JF, Robertson DL. Anatomy and physiology of the pharynx. Gastrointest Radiol. 1985;10:196-212.
2. Logemann JA. Swallowing physiology and pathophysiology. Otolaryngol Clin North Am. 1988;21:613-23.
3. Dodds WJ, Stewart ET, Logemann JA. Physiology and radiology of the normal oral and pharyngeal phases of swallowing. AJR Am J Roentgenol. 1990;154:953-63.
4. Miller FR, Sherrington CS. Some observations on the bucco-pharyngeal stage of reflex deglutition in the cat. Q J Expl Physiol. 1916;9:147-86.
5. Miller AJ. Deglutition. Physiol Rev. 1982;62:129-84.
6. Jean A. Brainstem control of swallowing: localisation and organisation of the central pattern generator for swallowing. In: Taylor A (Ed). Neurophysiology of the Jaws and Teeth. New York: McMillan; 1990. pp. 294-321.
7. Miller AJ. The search for the central swallowing pathway: the quest for clarity. Dysphagia. 1993;8:185-94.
8. Hamdy S, Aziz Q, Rothwell JC, et al. The cortical topography of human swallowing musculature in health and disease. Nat Med. 1996;2:1217-24.
9. Urban PP, Hopf HC, Connemann B, et al. The course of cortico-hypoglossal projections in the human brainstem: functional testing using transcranial magnetic stimulation. Brain. 1996;119:1031-8.
10. Daniels SK, Foundas AL. The role of the insular cortex in dysphagia. Dysphagia. 1997;12:146-56.
11. Artenian DJ, Lipman JK, Scidmore GK, et al. Acute neck pain and dysphagia due to tendinitis of the longus colli: CT and MRI findings. Neuroradiology. 1989;31:166-9.
12. Hughes TA, Wiles CM, Lawrie BW, et al. Dysphagia and sleep apnea associated with cervical osteophytes due to diffuse idiopathic skeletal hyperostosis. J Neurol Neurosurg Psychiatry. 1994;57:384.
13. Singh S, Stein HJ, DeMeester TR, et al. Nonobstructive dysphagia in gastroesophageal reflux disease: a study with combined ambulatory pH and motility monitoring. Am J Gastroenterol. 1992;87:562-7.
14. Kidd D, Lawson J, Nesbitt R, et al. Aspiration in acute stroke: a clinical study with videofluoroscopy. Q J Med. 1993;86:825-9.
15. Celifarco A, Gerard G, Faegenburg D, et al. Dysphagia as the sole manifestation of bilateral strokes. Am J Gastroenterol. 1990;85:610-3.
16. Buchholz DW. Clinically probable brain stem stroke presenting as dysphagia and nonvisualised by MRI. Dysphagia. 1993;8:235-8.
17. Meadows JC. Dysphagia in unilateral cerebral lesions. J Neurol Neurosurg Psychiatry. 1973;36:853-60.
18. Van Bogaert L, Maere M. Les polyradiculonevritescraninnesbilaterales avec dissociation albumino-cytologique: forms craniennes des polyradiculonevrites du type GuillaineetBarre. Belge Neurol Psychiatrie. 1938;38:275-81.
19. Munsat TL, Barnes JE. Relation of multiple cranial nerve dysfunction to the Guillain-Barre syndrome. J Neurol Neurosurg Psychiatry. 1965;28:115-20.
20. Ertekin C, Yuceyar N, Aydogdu I. Clinical and electrophysiological evaluation of dysphagia in myasthenia gravis. J Neurol Neurosurg Psychiatry. 1998;65:848-56.
21. Huang MH, King KL, Chien KY. Esophageal manometric studies in patients with myasthenia gravis. J Thorac Cardiovasc Surg. 1988;95:281-5.
22. Llabrés M, Molina-Martinez F, Miralles F. Dysphagia as the sole manifestation of myasthenia gravis. J Neurol Neurosurg Psychiatry. 2005;76:1297-300.
23. Leighton SE, Burton MJ, Lund WS, et al. Swallowing in motor neurone disease. J R Soc Med. 1994;87:801-5.
24. Kidd D, Lawson J, Nesbitt R, et al. Aspiration in acute stroke: a clinical study with videofluoroscopy. Q J Med. 1993;86:825-9.
25. Nathadwarawala KM, Nicklin J, Wiles CM. A timed test of swallowing capacity for neurological patients. J Neurol Neurosurg Psychiatry.1992;55:822-5.
26. Gordon C, Langton HR, Wade DT. Dysphagia in acute stroke. BMJ. 1987;295:411-4.
27. DePippo KL, Holas MA, Reding MJ. The Burke dysphagia screening test; validation for its use in patients with stroke. Arch Phys Med Rehabil. 1994;75:1284-6.
28. Kidd D, Lawson J, Nesbitt R, et al. The natural history and clinical consequences of aspiration in acute stroke. Q J Med. 1995;88:409-13.
29. Ertekin C, Aydogdu I, Yuceyar N. Piecemeal deglutition and dysphagia limit in normal subjects and in patients with swallowing disorders. J Neurol Neurosurg Psychiatry. 1996;61:491-6.
30. Nilsson H, Ekberg O, Olsson R, et al. Quantitative assessment of swallowing in healthy adults. Dysphagia. 1996;11:110-6.
31. Hughes TA, Wiles CM. Clinical measurement of swallowing in health and in neurogenic dysphagia. Q J Med. 1996;89:109-16.
32. Collins MJ, Bakheit AM. Does pulse oximetry reliably detect aspiration in dysphagic stroke patients? Stroke. 1997;28:1773-5.

Chapter 20

Evaluation of Acute Headache

Rakesh Shukla

INTRODUCTION

Headache is a ubiquitous complaint and is one of the most common medical reasons for neurological consultation. In general, headaches can be grouped into two broad diagnostic categories.

Primary headaches are those headaches where there is no cause identifiable on examination or investigation and where a diagnosis is made by recognizing the pattern, e.g., migraine, cluster headache, and tension-type headache.

Secondary headaches are those headaches where there is a definite underlying cause identifiable on examination or investigations, e.g., brain tumor, meningitis, and subarachnoid hemorrhage (SAH). Patients belonging to both categories can present with acute headache.[1]

It has been suggested that patients attend the emergency department (ED) because of headache for three distinct reasons: (a) they may have experienced a severe headache, for the first time unlike any previous one, (b) they may have associated features that cause concern (altered mental state, fever, focal neurological signs), (c) or they may be at the end of their tether with recurrent headaches that are unresponsive to treatment.[2-4]

MAGNITUDE OF THE PROBLEM

Headache accounts for nearly 2–3% of all visits to the ED.[2,5-7] A prospective study of 137 consecutive patients with severe headache of sudden onset presenting in the ED of a university hospital gave an incidence of 43 per 100,000 per year.[8] In the National Hospital Ambulatory Medical Care Survey (2006), headache was the fourth most common reason for adult patients (15 years and older) to visit the ED, third most common reason among women and seventh most common reason among men. Two-thirds of the visits were for a primary headache disorder.[9] About 90% of patients had a primary headache, and the vast majority of those presenting with a secondary headache had a benign cause. In fact, only 2% of the visits to the ED with acute headache were due to a serious underlying cause. In a prospective study of 3799 patients seen over 3 months in the ED, primary headaches were seen in 86.3%, secondary headaches in 6.4%, cranial neuralgias in 1.6%, and no precise diagnosis could be made in 5.7% of cases. Amongst primary headaches, migraine accounted for 60.9% of cases, episodic or chronic tension-type headache 20.6%, while 5% came for cluster headache, mostly not previously diagnosed. Sinusitis was the most frequent cause of secondary headache (1.7%), followed by post-traumatic headache (1.5%), and cerebrospinal fluid (CSF) hypotension (0.6%). Vascular disorders were detected in only 0.5%, while the rest (3.1%) were due to miscellaneous causes including brain tumors.[10]

It can be difficult to differentiate a primary headache from a secondary headache on the basis of clinical features alone. Certain clinical characteristics such as sudden onset, older age, and marked severity increase the probability of finding an underlying cause.[11] In a case–control study of 468 patients, who presented to a metropolitan ED with chief complaint of headache, nearly 4% were found to have an intracranial pathology. Acute onset, occipitonuchal location, presence of associated symptoms, and age 55 years or older, were independent predictors of the presence of intracranial pathology.[12]

Clinical Vignettes

The following clinical scenarios illustrate the situations where a neurologist has to deal with a patient having acute headache (Case vignettes). The resolution of these case scenarios is discussed later (*see* page 238).

In the above mentioned situations, the patient and their family members as well as the doctor are concerned about a serious underlying cause. Distinguishing between primary and secondary headaches is essential for the safe and effective management of patients with acute headache. A favorable response to analgesics/triptans should not be used to exclude a serious secondary cause of headache. In a recent report, 7 out of 18 studies found that 46/103 patients (44%) described a significant or complete resolution of secondary headache from medications such as antiemetic and nonsteroidal anti-inflammatory drugs (NSAIDs).[13]

APPROACH TO ACUTE HEADACHE

A systematic approach is extremely important for correct diagnosis of acute headache (Fig. 20.1). The first step is to exclude a secondary headache and for that one has to keep in mind certain red flags in history and examination. Once that has been done the patient needs to be categorized into a primary headache disorder. In most instances an accurate diagnosis of the patient's headache can be made by obtaining a thorough headache history and performing a focused clinical examination.[14-21] The applicability of the International Classification of Headache Disorders (ICHD) in ED was assessed in a

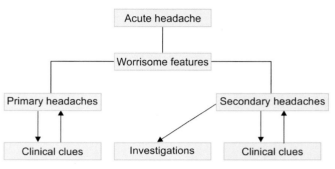

Fig. 20.1: Diagnostic evaluation of a patient presenting with acute headache.

recent study by performing a structured interview and medical record review of 484 patients with nontraumatic headache by two emergency medicine investigators independently. A high level of interobserver agreement was seen for both primary (91%) and secondary (94%) headaches. However, a specific ICHD diagnosis could not be assigned for more than one-third of acute headache patients.[22]

HISTORY

The approach to history given in Box 20.1 facilitates the generation of a differential diagnosis and preliminary classification of the headache type based on the criteria established by the International Headache Society (IHS).[1] An attempt to elicit these features should be part of every headache evaluation since the cost of mistaking a serious disease for another migraine or sinus headache can be devastating. Of note, however, a patient with an

---

CASE VIGNETTES

1. A 15-years-old boy presented with history of sudden onset severe holocranial headache with vomiting for 3 days. There was no photophobia, phonophobia. He had no history of fever, trauma, motor weakness, sensory loss, bladder, and bowel complaint, vision loss, cranial nerve involvement. Neurological examination was normal except for neck rigidity. Vitals were normal.

2. A 40-years-old man nonhypertensive presented with sudden onset severe bursting headache located in the frontal as well as occipital region of 2 days duration, associated with vomiting, photophobia, and phonophobia. The vitals were normal, patient was drowsy, meningeal signs were present, and there was right supranuclear VII nerve palsy with right hemiparesis (power-2/5 MRC grade), plantars were bilateral flexor.

3. A 48-years-old man practicing as ENT surgeon presented with a 7-day history of the left frontal headache, moderate to severe in intensity lasting for 7–8 hours, without any photophobia, phonophobia, vomiting. He had enteric fever 2 weeks prior to this. Vitals-normal, no positive findings on general and neurological examination.

4. An elderly lady presented with two episodes of headache in the last 1 month, which were moderate to severe in intensity, holocranial, reaching maximum intensity in one hour and lasting for 6–8 hours associated with vomiting, photophobia, and phonophobia. Past history of migraine like headache for 10 years was present. She had been operated for hip fracture that was complicated by foot drop with sensory loss in lower limb. Neurological examination was normal except the right foot drop with sensory loss and absent right ankle jerk.

Box 20.1: Questions to be asked in history to a patient with headache

- Is this your first or worst headache? How bad is your pain on a scale of 1–10 (1 means not too bad, and 10 means very bad)? Do you have headache on a regular basis? Is this headache like the ones you usually have?
- What symptoms do you have before the headache starts? What symptoms do you have during the headache? What symptoms do you have right now?
- When did this headache begin? How did it start (gradually, suddenly, other)?
- Where is your pain? Does the pain seem to spread to any other area? If so, where?
- What kind of pain do you have (throbbing, stabbing, dull, other)?
- Do you have other medical problems? If so, what?
- Do you take any medicines? If so, what?
- Have you recently hurt your head or had a medical or dental procedure?

TABLE 20.1: Red flags "SNOOP" suggestive of secondary headaches

Systemic symptoms	Myalgia, fever, malaise, weight loss, jaw claudication
Neurological symptoms	Focal or abnormal physical findings, confusion, impaired level of alertness, or consciousness
Onset	Sudden, abrupt, split-second (thunderclap)
Age	New onset and progressive headache, especially in middle age (> 50 years)
Previous headache history	First, worst, or different (change in attack frequency, severity, or clinical features)

Box 20.2: Possible causes of thunderclap headache

- Subarachnoid hemorrhage
- Orgasmic (coital) headache
- Exertional headache
- Benign cough headache
- Intracranial cysts and tumors
- Intracerebral hemorrhage
- Hypophyseal apoplexy
- Migraine
- Sphenoid sinusitis
- Arterial dissection
- Sinus thrombosis
- Segmental reversible vasospasm

acute severe headache may be extremely sick and so unable to give a good history or to cooperate fully in the examination.

If a patient complains of a headache that is worst ever (unusually severe) or first ever, even if it resembles a migraine headache (throbbing pain associated with nausea, vomiting, photophobia, phonophobia) further investigations should be undertaken to exclude intracranial conditions such as SAH, meningitis, encephalitis, raised intracranial pressure, stroke, arterial dissection (carotid or vertebral), and venous sinus thrombosis. If the headache is new (hours-months) or different from previously diagnosed headaches, there are several features, which should raise red flags and signal a possibility of a serious underlying disease.[23,24] The red flags for that one must always "snoop" are listed in Table 20.1.

Questions should be asked about the time and nature of headache onset (e.g., gradual, sudden, and subacute). The term thunderclap headache is used for a severe headache, which reaches its peak intensity within 30 seconds. This kind of headache may herald a potentially life-threatening SAH but most patients have a benign condition. There are no pathognomonic symptoms or signs that enable a reliable clinical differentiation between SAH and non-SAH forms of thunderclap headache.[25,26] The possible causes of thunderclap headaches are listed in Box 20.2.

In a prospective study of 102 patients with acute severe headache who were alert on admission and had no focal deficits, aneurysmal SAH (ASAH) was present in 42 patients, nonaneurysmal perimesencephalic hemorrhage (PMH) in 23 patients and nonhemorrhagic benign-thunderclap headache (BTH) in 37 patients. Headache developed almost instantaneously in half the patients with aneurysmal rupture and in two-thirds of patients with benign-thunderclap headache. Female sex, the presence of seizures, a history of loss of consciousness or focal symptoms, vomiting, or exertion increases the probability of ASAH, but these characteristics are of limited value in distinguishing SAH from benign-thunderclap headache. Aneurysmal rupture should be considered even if focal signs are absent and the headache starts within minutes.[27]

It is important to determine the location of a patient's pain and whether the pain radiates to another area. Cluster headaches are strictly unilateral, whereas tension-type headaches are usually band-like and bilateral. Migraines generally begin unilaterally but may progress to involve the entire head. Pain along the distribution of an artery may suggest temporal arteritis, and pain along the distribution of the trigeminal nerve is a feature or may be a sign of trigeminal neuralgia. Eye pain may suggest acute glaucoma.

A recent psychological stress such as discord in the family, recent bereavement, marital disharmony, stress at work place, or job loss should be enquired. However, an organic pathology should not be missed by placing too much emphasis on the presence of stress factors, especially when the patient presents with acute headache.

It is important to review any medications that patient may be taking, as a search of the online Physicians Desk Reference, 54th edition, yielded >1,000 references to medications with headache as a side effect. Prescription and "over the counter" medications (especially caffeine-containing analgesics) have been implicated as triggers for drug rebound and nonspecific headaches. Many patients do not regard "over-the-counter" drugs as "real medications" because they are not prescribed, and will not mention them unless asked for. Contrary to common belief, herbal remedies are not always harmless. When dealing with mysterious headaches in any age group, but especially the elderly, it is often useful to have the patient stop taking any medication that is not absolutely necessary.

Headache subsequent to trauma may signify a post-concussive disorder, although intracranial hemorrhage should always be suspected. Migraine and cluster headaches may be triggered by head trauma. Headache has been associated with common medical procedures (e.g., lumbar puncture, rhinoscopy, and dental procedures - tooth extraction).

Headache is a common neurological complaint among women of child bearing age. Although, most headaches are not attributable to an intracranial pathologic lesion, some headaches may herald ominous diagnoses, including eclampsia, stroke, tumor, SAH, or cerebral venous thrombosis (CVT). In a consecutive series of 63 pregnant women, emergent neuroimaging including noncontrast computed tomography (NCCT) and magnetic resonance imaging (MRI) brain revealed an underlying headache etiology in 27%, including CVT, reversible posterior leukoencephalopathy, pseudotumor, and intracerebral hemorrhage. The odds of having intracranial pathologic lesion were 2.7 times higher in patients with abnormal neurological examination.[28]

A postural relationship of headache suggests intra-cranial hypotension. The causes of headache that wakes up the patient from sleep are listed in Box 20.3.

Box 20.3: Relationship between headache and sleep

- Headache as the result of disrupted nocturnal sleep or the underlying process, which disrupts sleep.
  - Obstructive sleep apnea syndrome or nocturnal hypoxia/hypercarbia
  - Restless leg syndrome/periodic leg movements of sleep
  - Psychophysiological insomnia
  - Chronic pain syndrome of fibromyalgia
  - Depression/anxiety
- Primary headache disorders that occur during nocturnal sleep
  - Migraine
  - Cluster headache
  - Chronic paroxysmal hemicranias
  - Hypnic headache

EXAMINATION

The primary purpose of the physical examination is to identify causes of headaches. The examination should target areas identified as abnormal during the headache history. The general physical examination should include vital signs, fundoscopic, and cardiovascular assessment; and palpation of the head and face. A complete neurological examination is essential, and the findings must be documented. The examination should include mental status, level of consciousness, cranial nerve testing, pupillary responses, motor strength testing, deep tendon reflexes, sensation, pathologic reflexes (e.g., Babinski's sign), cerebellar function and gait testing, and signs of meningeal irritation (Kernig's and Brudzinski's signs). Particular attention should be given to detecting problems related to the optic, oculomotor, trochlear, and abducens nerves (cranial nerves II, III, IV, and VI, respectively). Box 20.4 lists the suggested central nervous system (CNS) examination that should be performed in the ED.

Box 20.4: Suggested brief central nervous system examination for patients presenting with headache

- Fundoscopy
- Eye movements
- Binocular visual fields to confrontation
- Pupillary responses and Horner's syndrome
- Facial weakness
- Romberg's sign
- Tandem gait
- Drift of outstretched hands
- Finger-nose test
- Finger dexterity
- Tendon reflexes and plantar responses

INVESTIGATIONS

If serious pathology is suspected or the diagnosis remains unclear, investigations are indicated.[29-32] Investigations are necessary when the patient complains of worst headache ever, new onset headache, change in pattern of headache, onset of headache with exertion (more suggestive of SAH or raised intracranial pressure), reduced alertness or cognition, neck not perfectly supple (implying meningeal irritation, or any abnormality on examination [including fever]), or worsening under observation. On the other hand, investigations are not required when all of the following are present: previous identical headaches, intact alertness and cognition, supple neck, normal neurological examination, normal vital signs (including temperature), and the headache is improving under observation.[33] The indications of a CT/MRI are listed in Box 20.5.

The American College of Emergency Physicians has guidelines on the evaluation and management of adult patients presenting to the ED with acute nontraumatic headache (Box 20.6).

Currently, recommended guidelines are based on clinical experience rather than evidence-based data derived from prospective studies, e.g., many HIV experts and consensus groups have recommended a contrast CT scan of head for "HIV-infected patients with neurological symptoms including headache". However, a recent study shows that this may not always be correct. Patients with preserved cellular immunity and without neurological examination findings, seizures or altered mental status can perhaps be managed conservatively with analgesics and clinical follow-up. A history of prior HIV opportunistic complications, altered mental status and focal abnormality on neurological examination are

---

Box 20.5: Indications for computed tomography/magnetic resonance imaging scan

- Acute, extremely severe headache (thunderclap headache)
- Headache that is not similar to previous headaches
- Headache or vomiting on awakening
- Unvarying location of headache
- Extremes of age
- Altered mental status (even if intoxicated)
- Associated focal neurological signs, papilledema, meningeal signs
- HIV-infected patients with neurological symptoms including headache
- Presence of ventriculo-peritoneal shunt
- Presence of neurocutaneous syndrome

Box 20.6: The American College of Emergency Physicians guidelines on the evaluation and management of adult patients presenting to the emergency department (ED) with acute nontraumatic headache[34]

- Patients presenting to the ED with headache and new abnormal findings in a neurological examination (e.g., focal deficit, altered mental status, altered cognitive functions) should undergo emergent [noncontrast computed tomography (CT) head]
- Patients presenting with new sudden onset severe headache should undergo an emergent head CT
- In patients presenting to the ED with sudden onset, severe headache and a negative noncontrast head CT scan result, lumbar puncture should be performed to rule out subarachnoid hemorrhage

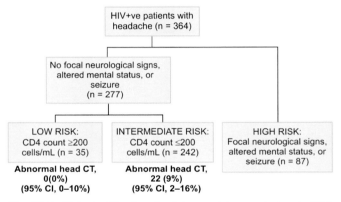

Fig. 20.2: Risk stratification for intracranial mass lesion in HIV-infected patients with headache.

---

all independent predictors of abnormal head CT. Seizures and CD4 cells <200/mL approached but did not reach statistical significance in a multivariate predictive model (Fig. 20.2).[35]

Neuroimaging is the most sensitive diagnostic tool in patients with headache. The first choice of investigation is usually a CT or an MRI scan. There is virtually no place for plain radiography of the skull in a patient with headache. The choice between CT and MRI depends on several factors such as the need to identify hemorrhage (CT preferred); the need to evaluate the posterior fossa (MRI preferred); easy accessibility (CT more readily available); and cost (CT is less expensive). Although, older American Academy of Neurology practice parameters for nonacute headache (i.e., headache present for at least 4 weeks) could find no evidence that MRI was superior to CT,[36] a recent evidence-based review from the European Federation of the Neurological Societies (EFNS) task force recommends MRI and not CT for appropriate patients with nonacute headache.[37]

An MRI helps to delineate the pituitary and parasellar regions, the posterior fossa, craniocervical regions, facial and retropharyngeal regions, and has the advantage of studying the vasculature without contrast injection. An MRI/MR venography (MRV) should be performed in all patients with recent headache progressive or thunderclap with normal CT scan and CSF examination to exclude cortical venous sinus thrombosis as headache may be the only manifestation of CVT. The MRI scan also helps more in the identification of other conditions that may present with headache.

The CT scan is underutilized for the diagnosis of sinusitis or sinus-associated headaches, particularly when there is a suspected frontal, ethmoidal, or sphenoidal sinusitis. It is also important to bear in mind that a significant number of serious causes of headache cannot be visualized by CT scanning or may be easily overlooked (Table 20.2). A high index of suspicion is, therefore, indicated, and appropriate diagnostic studies or gadolinium-enhanced MRI may be necessary depending upon the underlying cause.

Lumbar puncture is useful for assessing the CSF for blood, infection, and cellular abnormalities. It is also important for documenting abnormalities of CSF pressure that might be related to headache. Headaches are associated with a low CSF pressure (<90 mm of H_2O as measured by manometer) and elevated CSF pressure (>200–250 mm of H_2O). Headaches related to CSF hypotension include those caused by post-traumatic leakage of CSF (i.e., after lumbar puncture or CNS trauma). Headaches related to CSF hypertension include those associated with idiopathic intracranial hypertension and CNS space occupying lesions (i.e., tumor, infections, mass, hemorrhages).

TABLE 20.2: "CT-negative" causes for headache

Vascular	Tumor
Cerebral venous sinus thrombosis	Posterior fossa tumor
Arterial dissection	Infiltrative glioma
CNS vasculitis	Pituitary tumor
Temporal arteritis	Leptomeningeal cancer
Isodense subdural hematoma	
Infections	**Other**
Encephalitis	Pseudotumor cerebri
Meningitis	Low-pressure headache

Transcranial doppler and extracranial duplex scanning should be conducted if the clinical picture indicates a possible carotid or vertebral artery dissection. However, these two examinations can be strictly normal, particularly in the purely cephalalgia forms, either when the dissection affects only small segments of the arteries or when it does not lead to a significant arterial stenosis. The diagnosis must then be verified by MRI with MR angiography (MRA).

Conventional cerebral angiography is indicated in acute headache in two situations. Documented SAH in which angiography must be conducted by an intra-arterial method to diagnose a possible ruptured aneurysm. In sudden and severe headache which is nonregressive and when all preceding examinations are normal it may also show string and beads of a reversible acute cerebral angiopathy that can present with one or more episodes of thunderclap headache even when the CT scan, LP, and MRI are normal.

The National Headache Foundation reports that electroencephalography (EEG) has "not been shown to effectively identify headache subtypes or headaches caused by structural defects. Hence, the routine use of EEG in the evaluation of headache is not warranted."

It is important to remember that in the evaluation of headache, the investigations that a patient is subjected to are not without risk. In susceptible individuals, there is a small risk of anaphylaxis and renal insufficiency after contrast administration. Incidental findings (brain infarcts, cerebral aneurysms, and benign primary tumors) detected on MRI may provoke worry, fear, and often additional investigations. Nephrogenic systemic fibrosis is a rare complication of MRI studies in which a gadolinium containing contrast agent is given to individuals with impaired renal function.[32]

The sequencing of investigations in a given patient depends on the probable diagnosis. A CT scan without contrast is the neuroimaging study of choice in the detection of acute SAH with a high initial sensitivity.[38] The probability of recognizing aneurysmal hemorrhage on CT is maximum on day zero (95%), going down to 50% at week one, and becoming almost zero at 3 weeks.[39] A CT scan without contrast medium followed by lumbar puncture, if the scan is negative, is preferred to rule out SAH within the first 48 hours. A negative CT scan and a negative lumbar puncture do not completely rule out SAH because it may take hours for blood to enter the CSF after hemorrhage. If a relatively recent hemorrhage is suspected, the CSF should be evaluated for xanthochromia. It is recommended that the lumbar puncture should not be performed until at least 12 hours after the onset of symptoms to be able to detect xanthochromia (by spectrophotometer) in 100% of cases.[40,41] When clinical suspicion for intracranial aneurysm is high and initial imaging and CSF studies are nondiagnostic, further imaging via MRA or CT angiography (CTA) should be considered. The sensitivity of MRA for the detection of intracranial aneurysm ranges from 69 to 100%. Sensitivity improves with increasing aneurysm size, reaching values >95% when aneurysm is 6 mm or larger. Although, CTA has been studied less extensively, it is thought to have a detection rate of 85–98%.[32] A CSF manometry followed by gadolinium enhanced MRI of the brain should be done if spontaneous intracranial hypotension is suspected. Whether this should be preceded by an imaging study or not is controversial. Some clinicians believe that when meningitis is suspected, and there is neither papilledema nor focal abnormality to suggest an intracranial space occupying lesion, then it is incorrect to waste time obtaining CT or MRI, and lumbar puncture should be resorted swiftly. However, others might differ with this approach. In the presence of papilledema or raised intracranial pressure, an imaging study has to be done prior to a lumbar puncture.

RESOLUTION OF SCENARIOS

In the first scenario, head CT scan showed perimesencephalic hemorrhage, there was no midline shift. A CTA and digital subtraction angiography (DSA) (four vessels) was normal (Fig. 20.3).

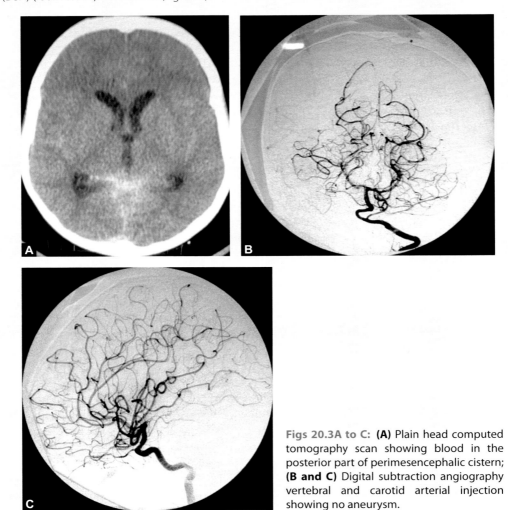

Figs 20.3A to C: **(A)** Plain head computed tomography scan showing blood in the posterior part of perimesencephalic cistern; **(B and C)** Digital subtraction angiography vertebral and carotid arterial injection showing no aneurysm.

Continued

Continued

In the second scenario a NCCT head revealed SAH with blood in the left sylvian fissure (Fig. 20.4A). A DSA revealed normal arterial and capillary branching pattern, but venous phase revealed nonpacification of superior sagittal sinus, transverse sinuses, and inferior sagittal sinus, and multiple collaterals. A MRV [3D Time of flight (TOF) technique] confirmed thrombosis in various sinuses as described above (Figs 20.4B and C). Patient was put on anticoagulants for 1 year. Repeat MRV showed near complete recanalization of all previously thrombosed venous channels. This patient also presented with a thunderclap headache with SAH on CT scan where no aneurysm was detected on angiography. However, MRV confirmed cortical venous sinus thrombosis. An SAH as a sole presentation of CVT is rare with only a few case reports.[42,43]

In the third scenario, CT and MRI including MRV were normal. The headache subsided in a few weeks with symptomatic treatment and did not recur over the next 3 months. So, the patient was categorized as headache attributed to infection.

In the fourth scenario, head CT scan showed a calcified rounded lesion in the left frontal region attached to the calvarium, which did not show any enhancement on contrast injection. There was no edema or midline shift (Fig. 20.5).

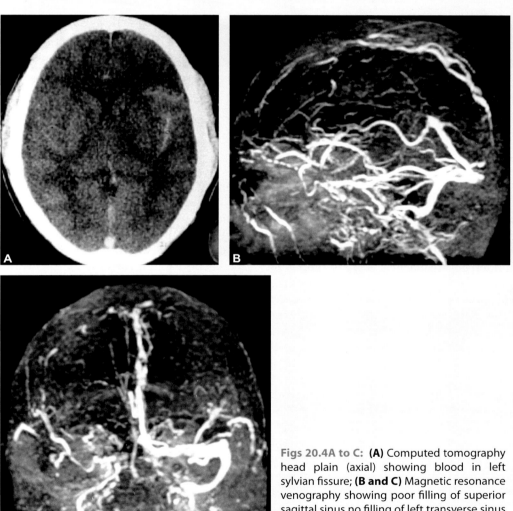

Figs 20.4A to C: (A) Computed tomography head plain (axial) showing blood in left sylvian fissure; **(B and C)** Magnetic resonance venography showing poor filling of superior sagittal sinus no filling of left transverse sinus and large number of collaterals.[42]

Continued

Continued

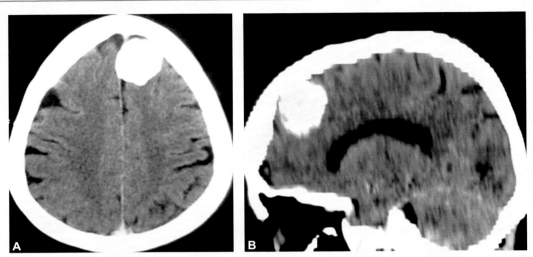

Figs 20.5A and B: Head computed tomography scan axial and sagittal films showing a round hyperdense lesion in the right frontal lobe without any contrast enhancement.

CAUSE OF ACUTE HEADACHE

Subarachnoid Hemorrhage

Cerebrovascular aneurysms are present in 2% of the population. An ASAH is a devastating illness with mortality rates approaching 50% and substantial morbidity. Thunderclap headache (TCH) is the classic presenting symptom of ASAH. A SAH is present in ~25% of patients with thunderclap headache. Further, arrival by ambulance, age ≥40 years, complaint of neck stiffness or pain, onset with exertion, vomiting, witnessed loss of consciousness, and raised blood pressure are strongly and reliably associated with SAH and 50% of patients with SAH present with TCH without other symptoms. In a community based, prospective study, 70% of patients with SAH presented with headache alone, and without loss of consciousness or focal symptoms. Typically, a SAH headache lasts for a few days. Although, more rapid resolution may occur, it is highly atypical for the headache to last <2 hours.[44] Cortical SAH, in which the blood is located over the cerebral convexities rather than near the circle of Willis, should be differentiated from ASAH. Two small case series of cortical SAH found that none were due to aneurysm. Cortical SAH may be associated with TCHs, reversible posterior leukoencephalopathy, vasculitis, cerebral venous sinus thrombosis, abscess, and cavernoma.

Unruptured Intracranial Aneurysm (Sentinel Headache)

Patients with a SAH frequently describe a distinct unusually severe headache with subsequent recovery in days or weeks preceding a diagnosed ASAH. The headache is often referred to as a warning or sentinel headache and is thought to represent a "warning leak" from the weakened walls of an aneurysm. Alternatively, the pain of sentinel headache may be due to structural changes in the arterial wall that occur prior to aneurysmal rupture.

CORTICAL VENOUS SINUS THROMBOSIS

Headache is the most common symptom of cortical venous sinus thrombosis, occurring in over 80% of patients. The headache may be diffuse or localized, persistent, worse on recumbency, and aggravated by Valsalva maneuver. Approximately, 15–30% of patients with cortical venous sinus thrombosis present with isolated headache in the absence of seizures, papilledema, altered level of consciousness, and focal neurologic symptoms or signs. Suspicion for cortical venous sinus thrombosis should be high in patients who are in the peripartum state, have a known or suspected hypercoagulable state, or are dehydrated.

CERVICAL ARTERY DISSECTION

Spontaneous carotid and vertebral artery dissections are frequently associated with headache. Head or neck pain is present in >70% of cervical artery dissections. In one-third to one-half of cases, headache precedes other symptoms, often by days or weeks. Headaches are described as severe in 75% and are located ipsilateral to the dissected artery. Dissection usually leads to ischemia in the distribution of the artery involved, it is often accompanied with lower cranial nerve palsies, visual field defects, cerebellar signs, amaurosis fugax, Horner's syndrome, and sensory-motor deficits. A history of preceding trauma to the neck, chiropractic neck manipulation, or whiplash injury from a roller coaster ride, increase the suspicion for dissection.

REVERSIBLE CEREBRAL VASOCONSTRICTION SYNDROME

This refers to a group of disorders characterized by reversible, segmental, cerebral vasospasm, which was precariously referred to as benign angiopathy of the CNS or migrainous vasospasm. The proposed diagnostic criteria for reversible cerebral vasoconstriction syndrome (RCVS) include, (1) clinical presentation with TCH with or without additional neurological symptoms or signs, (2) no evidence of ASAH, (3) normal or near-normal CSF, (4) angiographic documentation of multifocal segmental cerebral artery vasoconstriction, and (5) reversal of vasoconstriction within 12 weeks of onset.

Reversible cerebral vasoconstriction syndrome is not rare, as suggested by a prospective study in which 67 patients were seen at a single institution over 3 years. The typical patient is a woman aged between 20 and 50 years. The condition RCVS should be differentiated from primary angiitis of the CNS. The most helpful clinical feature in the distinction is the acuteness of onset of headache and other clinical manifestations. Patients with primary angiitis of the CNS do not present with TCH, with the exception of the rare ruptured intracranial aneurysm associated with vasculitis.[45]

POSTERIOR REVERSIBLE ENCEPHALOPATHY SYNDROME

Reversible posterior leukoencephalopathy is due to vasogenic edema, which preferentially affects the white matter of the posterior cerebral hemispheres. It occurs in association with acute hypertension, with selected immunosuppressants, and eclampsia/preeclampsia. There is a substantial overlap between posterior reversible encephalopathy syndrome (PRES) and RCVS in terms of triggers (hypertension, eclampsia), presentation, and neurological sequel.

SPONTANEOUS INTRACRANIAL HYPOTENSION

Positional headache that is exacerbated by the upright posture and improves upon lying down is the most common presenting symptom of spontaneous intracranial hypotension (SIH). It is a condition of low CSF volume and/or pressure caused by CSF leaking from a dural defect, most commonly in the thoracic region. A history of recent lumbar puncture, epidural injection, spinal surgery, lifting a heavy object, coughing, and sports activities or motor vehicle accident suggests a persistent traumatic CSF leak. Headaches are located anteriorly or posteriorly but may also be holocephalic. Approximately, 15% of patients with SIH present with TCH. Spontaneous CSF leaks may occur through weak meningeal diverticula or weak dural and may be associated with connective tissue disorders such as Marfan's syndrome or Ehlers–Danlos syndrome. Thus, a family history of these diseases and physical examination indicators of connective tissue pathology (e.g., arachnodactyly, hyperextensible joints) should be sought.[46]

PITUITARY APOPLEXY

Pituitary apoplexy refers to hemorrhage or infarction of the pituitary gland, usually in the setting of a pituitary adenoma. A TCH is the most common presenting symptom and may be associated with nausea/vomiting, ophthalmoplegia, diminished visual acuity, reduction in visual fields, and altered mental status. The risk factors include, pregnancy, general anesthesia, bromocriptine therapy, and pituitary irradiation.

PITFALLS IN THE DIAGNOSIS OF ACUTE HEADACHE

There are several pitfalls in the evaluation and diagnosis of acute headache.

1. *Headache is only a symptom.*

   It is not possible to differentiate a primary and secondary headache disorder on the basis of headache characteristics alone as our current understanding of headache suggests that there is a common pathway for pain regardless of the underlying etiology. Even the criteria for the diagnosis of primary headache disorders require that secondary causes of headache are excluded by history, physical examination, and if necessary relevant investigations. One must remember that according to the IHS classification, a first episode of severe headache cannot be classified as migraine or tension-type headache as the diagnostic criteria require multiple episodes with specific characteristics (more than nine episodes of tension-type headache and more than four episodes for migraine without aura). Although, patients with primary headache disorders will have their first attack at some point, the diagnosis cannot be made definitely at that time.

2. *A diagnosis of migraine and tension-type headache does not mean that there cannot coexist other causes of headache.*

A 20-year-old girl presented with severe, holocranial, throbbing headache with vomiting and photophobia of one-week duration. She gave a history of migraine with aura for five years. Her mother was also suffering from migraine. Patient's neurological examination was normal. Her CT head showed solitary IV ventricular NCC with noncommunicating hydro-cephalus (Fig. 20.6A). Endoscopic cyst removal was unsuccessful, so a third ventriculostomy was done followed by a course of albendazole. Contrast head

CT scan 10 days after surgery showed normal sized IV ventricle with hyperdense cyst (Fig. 20.6B). There was no recurrence of her migraine attacks during the six month follow-up.[47]

3. *Errors in the diagnosis are often due to omissions in history and physical examination.*

A 50-year-old doctor, convalescing at home, two weeks after an acute MI and taking nitrates, had severe throbbing headache in the left temporal region associated with vomiting. He had past history of migraine without aura for 25 years. Vitals were normal, neurological examination was normal. He was advised paracetamol and domperidone. However, the headache did not subside completely. The next morning he developed slight ptosis of left eye and by evening developed a total III nerve palsy. Head CT scan confirmed the diagnosis of SAH.

4. One must keep in mind, other, unusual causes of headache (Fig. 20.7) before labeling the patient to be suffering from a psychiatric disorder.

5. Repeat imaging should not be delayed if it is indicated.

6. Response to treatment does not exclude a secondary headache disorder.

Some patients of SAH who are considered to be having migraine in the ED do respond to triptans. These patients should not be denied neuroimaging.

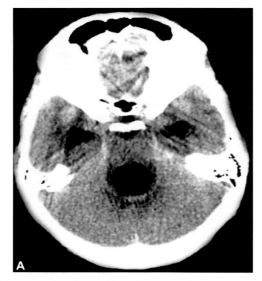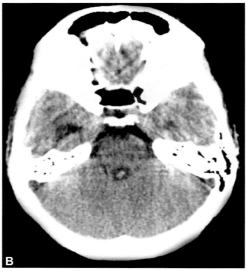

Figs 20.6A and B: (A) Contrast head computed tomography (CT) scan (axial) showing dilated IV ventricle with hyperdense IV ventricular cyst; **(B)** Contrast head CT scan (axial) done 10 days after endoscopic III ventriculostomy showing normal size IV ventricle with hyperdense cyst.[47]

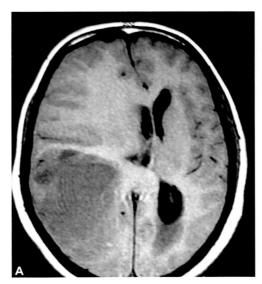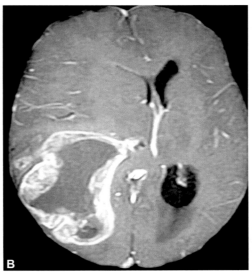

Figs 20.7A and B: (A) Magnetic resonance imaging (MRI) brain (axial) T_1 weighted image showing large mass in the right parieto-occipital lobes with mass effect and midline shift; **(B)** Contrast MRI brain (axial) showing peripheral linear enhancement of mass lesion.

CONCLUSION

A patient with acute headache poses a challenge to the physician as well as the health care system. On a case by case basis, the challenge for the physician is to make a correct diagnosis that will serve as the foundation for appropriate therapy, while on a larger societal scale it collectively challenges the healthcare system to assess the need for diagnostic resources. Unlike in other areas of medicine where investigative technologies have overtaken the need for detailed history taking, one still has to master the art of history taking in order to arrive at the right diagnosis of the headache disorder. The process of history taking is time consuming, but it is an art that needs to be perfected by practice. History taking is all about entertaining the RIGHT suspicions, asking the RIGHT questions in the RIGHT sequence to arrive at the RIGHT diagnosis, and initiate the RIGHT treatment within the RIGHT time-frame.[48] The following aphorism is still true today: "Neurology has always relied upon good clinical skills, and while we should embrace new technology where appropriate, let us not forget that in many situations, particularly headache, clinical skills are all we need. Missing SAH is bad enough, but randomly investigating every headache patient is equally bad medicine".[2]

REFERENCES

1. Headache Classification Committee of the International Headache Society (IHS). The International Classification of Headache Disorders, 3rd edition (beta version). Cephalalgia. 2013;33:629-808.
2. Davenport R. Acute headache in emergency department. J Neurol Neurosurg Psychiatry. 2002;72(Suppl 2):33-7.
3. Friedman BW, Lipton RB. Headache emergencies: diagnosis and management. Neurol Clin. 2012;30:43-60.
4. Robertson CE, Black DF, Swanson JW. Headache in the emergency department. In: Roos KL (Ed). Emergency Neurology. New Delhi: Springer ; 2013. pp. 1-32.
5. Locker T, Mason S, Rigby A. Headache management—are we doing enough? An observational study of patients presenting with headache to the emergency department. Emerg Med J. 2004;21:327-32.
6. Cerbo R, Villani V, Bruti G, et al. Primary headache in emergency department: prevalence, clinical features, and therapeutical approach. J Headache Pain. 2005;6:287-9.
7. Goldstein JN, Camargo CA Jr, Pelletier AJ, et al. Headache in the United State emergency departments: demographics, work-up and frequency of pathological diagnosis. Cephalalgia. 2006;26:684-90.
8. Landtblom AM, Fridikriksson S, Boivie J, et al. Sudden onset headache: a prospective study of features, incidence and causes. Cephalalgia. 2002; 22:354-60.
9. Pitts SR, Niska RW, Xu J, et al. National hospital ambulatory medical care survey: 2006 emergency department summary. Natl Health Stat Report. 2008;7:1-38.
10. Valade D. Headache presenting to a casualty service: four year experience at an emergency headache centre. Rev Neurol. 2005;16:729-31.
11. Locker TE, Thompson C, Rylance J, et al. The utility of clinical features in patients presenting with non-traumatic headache: an investigation of adult patients attending an emergency department. Headache. 2006;46:954-61.

12. Ramirez-Lassepas M, Espinosa CE, Cicero JJ, et al. Predictors of intracranial pathologic findings in patients who seek emergency care because of headache. Arch Neurol. 1997;54:1506-9.
13. Pope JV, Edlow JA. Favourable response to analgesics does not predict a benign etiology of headaches. Headache. 2008;48:944-50.
14. Clinch CR. Evaluation of acute headaches in adults. Am Fam Physician. 2001;63:685-92.
15. Ward TN, Levin M, Phillips JM. Evaluation and management of headache in the emergency department. Med Clin North Am. 2001;85:971-85.
16. Sridharan R. Approach to acute headache. Ann Indian Acad Neurol. 2002;5:29-32.
17. Shukla R. Evaluation of acute headache. In: Prabhakar S, Singh G (Eds). Reviews in Neurology. Chandigarh: Continuing Medical Education Program of Indian Academy of Neurology: 2007. pp. 159-81.
18. Matharu MS, Schwedt TJ, Dodick DW. Thunderclap headache: an approach to a neurologic emergency. Curr Neurol Neurosci Rep. 2007;7:101-9.
19. Edlow JA, Panagos PD, Godwin SA, et al. Clinical policy: critical issues in the evaluation and management of adult patients presenting to the emergency department with acute headache. Ann Emerg Med. 2008;52:407-36.
20. Ceppi M, Willi C, Hugli O, et al. Guidelines for the diagnostic evaluation of patients presenting in emergency for an acute non-traumatic headache. Rev Med Suisse. 2008;4:1741-6.
21. Nallasamy K, Singhi SC, Singhi P. Approach to headache in emergency department. Indian J Pediatr. 2012;79:376-80.
22. Friedman BW, Hochberg ML, Esses D, et al. Applying the International Classification of Headache Disorders in the emergency department: an assessment of reproducibility and the frequency with which a unique diagnosis can be assigned to every acute headache presentation. Ann Emerg Med. 2007;49:409-19.
23. Dodick DW. Diagnosing headache: clinical clues and clinical rules. Adv Stud Med. 2003;3:87-92.
24. Vincent MB. Red flags in the diagnostic process. In: Martelletti P, Steiner TJ (Eds). Handbook of Headache–Practical Management. New Delhi: Springer International Edition; 2013. pp. 211-25.
25. Evans RW, Davenport RJ. Benign or Sinister? Distinguishing migraine from subarachnoid hemorrhage. Headache. 2007;47:433-5.
26. Ju YE, Schwedt TJ. Abrupt-onset severe headaches. Semin Neurol. 2010;30:192-200.
27. Linn FH, Rinkel GJ, Algra A, et al. Headache characteristics in subarachnoid haemorrhage and benign thunderclap headache. J Neurol Neurosurg Psychiatry. 1998;65:791-3.
28. Ramchandren S, Cross BJ, Liebeskind DS. Emergent headaches during pregnancy: correlation between neurologic examination and neuroimaging. Am J Neuroradiol. 2007;28:1085-7.
29. Evans RW. Headaches. In: Evans RW (Ed). Diagnostic Testing in Neurology. Philadelphia: WB Saunders Company; 1999. pp. 1-20.
30. Masdeu JC, Drayer BP, Anderson RE, et al. Atraumatic isolated headache—when to image. American College of Radiology. ACR appropriateness criteria. Radiology. 2000;215 (Suppl):S487-93.
31. Sempere AP, Porta-Etessam J, Medrano V, et al. Neuroimaging in the evaluation of patients with non-acute headache. Cephalalgia. 2005;25:30-5.
32. De Luca GC, Bartleson JD. When and how to investigate the patient with headache. Semin Neurol. 2010;30:131-44.
33. Edmeads J. Challenges in the diagnosis of acute headache. Headache. 1990;30:537-40.
34. American College of Emergency Physicians Clinical Policies Sub-committee on Acute Headache. Clinical policy: critical issues in the evaluation and management of patients presenting to the emergency department with acute headache. Ann Emerg Med. 2002;39:108-22.
35. Gifford AI, Hecht FM. Evaluating HIV-infected patients with headache: who needs computed tomography? Headache. 2001;41:441-8.
36. Silbertstein SD. Practice parameter: evidence based guidelines for migraine headache (an evidence based review). Report of the Quality Standards Subcommittee of the American Academy of Neurology. 2000; 55:754-62.
37. Sandrini G, Friberg L, Janig W, et al. Neurophysiological tests and neuroimaging procedures in non-acute headache: guidelines and recommendations. Eur J Neurol. 2004;11:217-24.
38. Webb S, Bone I, Lindsay K. The investigation of acute severe headache suggestive of probable subarachnoid haemorrhage: a hospital based study. Br J Neurosurg. 2003;17:580-4.
39. van Gijn J, van Dongen KJ. The time course of aneurysmal haemorrhage on computed tomograms. Neuroradiology. 1982;23:153-6.
40. Vermeulen M, Hasan D, Blijenberg BG, et al. Xanthochromia after sub-arachnoid haemorrhage needs no revisitation. J Neurol Neurosurg Psychiatry. 1989;52:826-8.
41. Alons IM, Verheul RJ, Ponjee GA, et al. Optimising blood pigment analysis in cerebrospinal fluid for the diagnosis of subarachnoid haemorrhage–a practical approach. Eur J Neurol. 2013;20:193-7.
42. Shukla R, Vinod P, Prakash S, et al. Subarachnoid haemorrhage as a presentation of cerebral venous sinus thrombosis. J Assoc Physicians India. 2006;54:42-4.
43. Shukla R, Vinod P, Gupta RK, et al. Recanalisation of cerebral venous thrombosis in a patient presenting with subarachnoid haemorrhage. JIACM. 2007;8:173-5.
44. Perry JJ, Stiell IG, Sivilotti ML, et al. High risk clinical characteristics for subarachnoid haemorrhage in patients with acute headache: prospective cohort study. BMJ. 2010;341:c5204.
45. Tan LH, Flower O. Reversible cerebral vasoconstriction syndrome: an important cause of acute severe headache. Emerg Med Int. 2012:303152, doi: 10.1155/2012/303152.
46. Brodley SA, Park N, Renowden S, et al. Unusual cause of sudden onset headache: spontaneous intracranial hypotension. Emerg Med Australas. 2005;17:520-3.
47. Shukla R, Paliwal VK, Jha D. Solitary fourth ventricular neurocysticercosis presenting as status migrainosus. Headache. 2006;46:169-73.
48. Ravishankar K. The art of history–taking in a headache patient. Ann Indian Acad Neurol. 2012;15:S7-S14.

Chapter 21

Chronic Headache

K Ravishankar, Meghna Bhatnagar

INTRODUCTION

Chronic headache (CH) is a problem commonly encountered in medical practice. It can cause significant pain and disability and lead to disruption in quality of life for the patient. Diagnosing the underlying cause can often be quite challenging, and management of these patients is often fraught with frustration. This chapter attempts to outline a logical approach to patients who present with CH. Terminologies have been clarified and etiological conditions have been detailed.

At the outset, we would like to clarify that the terms chronic daily headache (CDH) and CH are used synonymously and interchangeably in this chapter and essentially refer to the same type of headaches. The common feature of both these terms is the "chronicity." As mentioned in the first International Headache Society Classification of Headache Disorders–ICHD1, CDH or CH includes conditions that present with headache lasting for >15 days per month for at least 3 months.[1] It is important to note that although the 2004 revised International Headache Society Classification of Headache Disorders–ICHD2 includes many conditions that can present with CH, it still does not specifically embrace the term CDH. Furthermore, in ICHD-2, the term "chronic" has been used inconsistently, and conveys different inferences when used with reference to migraine, tension-type headache, and cluster headache.[2]

Although, the term CDH was first coined to essentially describe primary headaches that occurred on a daily or near-daily basis,[3] the terms "CH" and "CDH" have been used here to include both primary and secondary headache disorders. Primary CDHs are those chronic headaches, where clinical examination, and investigations are normal and where diagnosis is arrived at through pattern-recognition based on experience and expertise. These account for approximately 95% of all chronic headaches and contribute significantly to headache burden. Secondary CDHs are those where an abnormality is revealed on examination or investigation. These form a much smaller percentage of chronic headaches seen in practice, but since, they could be due to an underlying life-threatening cause, they need to be diagnosed, and treated with high priority.

The foremost goal therefore of a physician faced with a patient having chronic headache is to rule out an underlying secondary cause. One has to look for the presence of subtle clues that may be indicative of an underlying secondary headache disorder and accordingly investigate and plan further treatment. The warning signs that may be indicative of a secondary cause for chronic headache have been listed in Box 21.1.[4]

Box 21.1: Red flags should suggest the possibility of an underlying secondary headache disorder

- New onset of chronic headache
- Onset of chronic headache after the age of 50
- Prolonged chronic headache with side-locked features
- Chronic headache with papilledema, progressive visual changes
- Chronic headache with neurological deficit
- Chronic headache with memory impairment/confusion/drowsiness

Box 21.2: Secondary headaches that can present with chronic headache

- Intracranial space occupying lesions
- Cerebrovascular disease—cerebral venous sinus thrombosis/arteriovenous malformations/giant cell arteritis
- Altered cerebrospinal fluid (CSF) dynamics (spontaneous CSF leak/idiopathic intracranial hypertension/secondary intracranial hypertension)
- Infective causes—extra or intracranial infections or sinusitis
- Post-traumatic headache
- Cervical spine abnormalities
- Temporomandibular joint disorders
- Medication overuse headache
- Other miscellaneous causes

Given any of the above clinical scenarios, the physician should investigate further and rule out the possibilities that have been listed in Box 21.2.[4]

Secondary causes of chronic headache that may be overlooked because of their occasional atypical presentation include intracranial hypertension without papilledema, cerebrospinal fluid (CSF) hypovolemia without postural variation, Chiari malformation type I without Valsalva maneuver-induced headache, cervicogenic lesions, space occupying lesions without localizing signs. Some metabolic, systemic, and endocrine conditions can also give rise to chronic headache. If there is a suspicion of any of the above causes of secondary CH, then we need to manage further on the lines discussed below.

By and large, however, most of the cases of CH that are seen in practice are primary CH. For convenience of diagnosis, primary CHs are subdivided into two broad groups based on the duration of the attack of headache. They could either be short-lasting where the headache comes on a daily basis for 3 or more months, but each episode lasts for <4 hours or long-lasting, which includes daily headaches for 3 months or more but with episodes that last longer than 4 hours.

The entities included in the short-lasting group are as follows:
- Chronic cluster headache
- Chronic paroxysmal hemicrania (CPH)
- Short-lasting unilateral neuralgiform headaches with conjunctival injection and tearing (SUNCT syndrome)
- Hypnic headache syndrome (HHS).

The long lasting primary chronic group includes:
- Chronic migraine
- Chronic tension-type headache (CTTH)
- Hemicrania continua
- New daily persistent headache (NDPH).

The diagnostic features of headaches that are included under these two broad headings are outlined below.

SHORT-LASTING PRIMARY CHRONIC DAILY HEADACHE

Chronic Cluster Headache

Cluster headache is a prototype trigeminal autonomic cephalalgia (TAC), characterized by severe ocular/temporal pain along with the presence of cranial autonomic features like lacrimation and rhinorrhea. It is said to be chronic, if attacks occur for more than a year, and the remission period lasts for less than a month. Cluster headache attacks have a seasonal periodicity and differ from other TACs, in terms of the duration of individual attacks.[5] There could be 5–8 attacks in a 24 hours period, lasting for anywhere between 30 and 180 minutes and more in the night after rapid eye movement sleep.

Chronic Paroxysmal Hemicrania

Chronic paroxysmal hemicrania (CPH) is a severe, unilateral headache, seen more commonly in women. Individual attacks last for 10–30 minutes, recur several times in a day, and are associated with cranial autonomic features.[5] Chronic paroxysmal hemicrania is more easily diagnosed by its exquisite response to indomethacin.

Although the pathogenesis of CPH is not completely understood, it is associated with raised levels of calcitonin gene related peptide and vasoactive intestinal peptide. These correlate with trigeminovascular and cranial sympathetic activation respectively. The symptoms of CPH are mediated by the trigeminal autonomic reflex. This is a brain stem connection between trigeminal nerve and the facial nerve parasympathetic outflow. Extratrigeminal distribution of pain in CPH is due to the caudal extension of trigeminal nucleus caudal to C1–2.[5]

Short-lasting Unilateral Neuralgiform Headaches with Conjunctival Injection and Tearing

The SUNCT syndrome includes strictly unilateral, severe, neuralgiform attacks that occur around the distribution of the ophthalmic division of the trigeminal nerve. There is severe burning, stabbing, sharp pain in the periorbital region, and the duration of each episode can vary from 5 to 240 seconds. It is associated with conjunctival injection, lacrimation, and is more common among males.[6]

Hypnic Headache Syndrome

This chronobiological disturbance causes headache in the elderly population exclusively during sleep. Pain is moderate, generalized, and without associated symptoms. It lasts for less than an hour and occurs at the same time each night.

Its pathogenesis involves the suprachiasmatic nucleus, which modulates the endogenous circadian rhythm. This sends afferent and efferent projections to the periaqueductal grey and aminergic nuclei. The latter are the most important structures for pain modulation. With advancing age, the function of the hypothalamic–pineal axis reduces, and melatonin that is the main neurotransmitter lessens or disappears completely. This may account for the nocturnal periodicity of headache attacks.[6]

LONG-LASTING PRIMARY CHRONIC DAILY HEADACHE

Chronic Migraine

This term refers to migrainous headaches that occur for >15 days/month, for at least 3 months, out of which, migraine features must be present for at least 8 days/month, and there should not be any associated history of medication overuse. Alternatively, it can be defined as headache for >15 days/month in a patient with a past history of migraine. It usually begins as episodic migraine, which later becomes continuous.[7] The term "transformed migraine" was formerly used for this clinical presentation.[3] As the frequency of attacks increase, associated migrainous features like photophobia, phonophobia, and nausea become less frequent and less severe. The headache may acquire characteristics of tension-type headache.[3] There are risk factors that facilitate this transformation. Box 21.3 lists the risk factors that can facilitate the worsening of episodic to chronic migraine.[7]

Patients with chronic migraine can sometimes present in a puzzling manner. In such situations, it becomes necessary for them to undergo imaging in order to rule out serious underlying causes of headache. There are specific indications when patients of chronic migraine must undergo imaging. Box 21.4 lists these indications.[8]

Some recent theories regarding the pathogenesis of chronic migraine center around impaired descending inhibition from higher pain-modulating centers enhanced ascending facilitation or neuronal hyper excitability,

---

Box 21.3: Risk factors that can facilitate the worsening of episodic to chronic migraine

- Attack frequency of >4 per month
- Life stressors
- Excess caffeine consumption
- Female gender
- Prior history of episodic migraine
- Low education/socioeconomic background
- Medications like containing compounds like narcotics, ergotamines
- Traumatic brain injury
- Snoring/sleep apnea/sleep disturbance
- Medication overuse
- Obesity

Box 21.4: Indications for imaging in patients with features of chronic migraine

- Confusional states
- Unusual, prolonged, or persistent aura
- Increasing frequency or severity of attacks or a change in the usual migraine profile
- Persistent headache on the same side
- Post-traumatic migraine

---

resulting in a reduced threshold for trigeminovascular neuronal activation. Factors that are likely to influence the progression of migraine are genetic predisposition, persistent or recurring noxious stimuli (extrinsic or intrinsic), trigeminal or cervical pathology, repetitive, and persistent migraine attacks leading to persistent central sensitization, and deposition of iron in central antinociceptive structures.[7]

Due to the unbearable nature of pain, most patients with chronic migraine overuse analgesics and end up with medication overuse headache (MOH). Patients of chronic migraine also have an increased incidence of comorbidities like sleep disorders, fatigue, other pain and gastrointestinal complaints, and psychiatric disorders.[9]

Chronic Tension-type Headache

This is an ill-defined syndrome. It is a "featureless" headache, because its only symptomatology is pain in the head.[10] The pain lasts for hours or is continuous with >2 of the following symptoms: pain of pressing nature/tightness in the head, mild or moderate in severity, bilateral in location, and not aggravated by routine physical activities.[11] Increased pericranial tenderness may be elicited on manual palpation.[10]

Chronic tension-type headache has its origin in episodic tension-type headache. Psychiatric comorbidities play a very important role in the development of CTTH. This results in a temporary change in central pain control mechanisms and increased nociception from strained muscles.

Hemicrania Continua

This is an unremitting, unilateral, side-locked headache of moderate intensity with exacerbations of severe pain lasting for hours to days, and is more common in women. The pain is steady and nonthrobbing and may be associated with autonomic features. It is typically present for 24 hours a day for 7 days of the week. This entity should not be confused with cluster headache. Ipsilateral foreign body sensation in the eye/ocular pain and a superimposed stabbing headache are often reported. Hemicrania continua is typically responsive to indomethacin therapy. This may be a strong criterion for diagnosing HC.

New Daily Persistent Headache

This is a new-onset chronic headache with features of CTTH as per the ICHD-2 (2004).[2] It develops into a daily pattern within 3 days of onset and lasts for at least 3 months. The striking feature of NDPH is the mode of onset. Patients are often able to recall the exact date of onset of the headache. All patients of NDPH must undergo neuroimaging to rule out underlying secondary conditions. NDPH can also present with headache that has migrainous features.

Having described in brief, the features of the different primary CH, let us now look at the features of some important secondary causes of chronic headache.

Medication Overuse Headache

Increased analgesic intake is a known causative factor in the development of chronic headaches.[12] The term "MOH" was introduced for the first time, in ICHD-2 (2004).[2] This term implies chronic headache that is associated with regular overuse of acute headache medications for >3 months. "Regular overuse" would mean administration of ergot, triptan, opioid, or butalbital for >10 days/month, other nonopioid analgesics for >15 days/month or a total exposure of all acute drugs for >15 days/month. Although

this is included under secondary headaches in ICHD-2, it has a close association with primary CDH. Prophylactic medications used in the treatment of primary chronic headache are more likely to be effective, if medication overuse headache is first dealt with successfully.

It is important to note that only patients of headache, who overuse analgesics, develop this headache. This disorder is not seen in patients, who use painkillers for other comorbidities. Besides the process of central sensitization in its pathogenesis, fluorodeoxyglucose positron emission tomography scans have demonstrated reversible metabolic changes in pain processing structures and persistent orbitofrontal hypofunction in migraineurs with MOH.[12]

Cervicogenic Headache

Headaches of cervical origin are caused by abnormalities of various neck structures—the synovial joints, ligaments, muscles, tendons, nerve roots, and the vertebral artery. These headaches are often posterior in location.[11] The ICHD-2 accepts three varieties of headaches that are attributable to disorders of the neck.[2]
- Headache attributable to cranial dystonia
- Cervicogenic headache
- Headache attributed to retropharyngeal tendinitis.

Cervicogenic headache is usually unilateral, but may also be bilateral. This headache may be confused with tension-type headache or migraine without aura. A single attack can last for few hours to a few weeks. Initially, the headache is episodic. Later on, it becomes chronic and fluctuating. Generally, there is a limitation of neck movement or a mechanical precipitation of attacks. A positive response to anesthetic blockade is a must in the diagnosis of cervicogenic headache. There is no characteristic radiological abnormality that is pathognomonic of cervicogenic headache (Box 21.5).

Box 21.5: Established causes of cervicogenic headache
• Chiari malformation type I
• Traumatic subluxation of the upper cervical vertebrae
• Ankylosing spondylitis of the upper cervical spine
• Retropharyngeal tendinitis
• Osteomyelitis of the upper cervical vertebrae
• Tumors of the craniovertebral junction and upper cervical spine
• Paget's disease of the skull with a secondary basilar invagination
• Craniocervical dystonias

Low CSF Volume Chronic Headache

The most common clinical manifestation of low CSF volume is headache. This may be orthostatic, may not be throbbing, and most commonly is bilateral. It is present when the patient is upright and is relieved in the recumbent posture. It may be localized to the frontal or occipital regions. It is a holocephalic headache, though there have been patients with a headache that began as a focal/unilateral pain and then evolved into a holocephalic headache due to the continued upright posture of the patient. These headaches are often worsened by Valsalva type maneuvers. The CSF shows opening pressures are low.[13]

The two causative disorders for low CSF volume headaches are spontaneous intracranial hypotension and cerebrospinal fluid leaks. These are best diagnosed by magnetic resonance imaging (MRI) of the head/spine. The features that are visible on MRI of the head in case of low CSF volume headaches are listed below.[13]

1. Diffuse pachymeningeal enhancement
2. Descent/sinking of the brain, obliteration of the prepontine or perichiasmatic cisterns, crowding of the posterior cranial fossa, descent of the cerebellar tonsils similar to Chiari malformation type I.
3. Flattening of the optic chiasm
4. Enlargement of the pituitary (may mimic pituitary hyperplasia/tumor)
5. Subdural fluid collections.

The following features may be seen on MRI of the spine in case of low CSF volume headaches.

1. Spinal pachymeningeal enhancement
2. Meningeal diverticula
3. Identification of the level of leak
4. Extra arachnoid fluid collections often seen across several levels.

Raised CSF Pressure Chronic Headache

There are a variety of disorders that can cause raised CSF pressure headache. According to CSF pressure recording studies, it is the rate of change of CSF pressure, rather than the absolute value of raised CSF pressure that is an important causative factor in headaches. Frequently, headaches of raised intracranial pressure are associated with nausea, vomiting, and nuchal rigidity. The pain is usually dull, generalized, and nonthrobbing. Common causes of raised CSF pressure headache are listed below.[14]

Headache secondary due to brain tumor

Infratentorial tumors are more common in children. In contrast, supratentorial tumors are more common in adults and usually manifest with headache, seizures, or other focal neurological deficit. Occasionally, headaches may not even be present, even if the tumors are large. When headache is ipsilateral to the tumor and examination reveals papilledema, it is of great value in localization of the tumor.

Headache secondary to hydrocephalus

Headache secondary to hydrocephalus may be episodic and may have migraine-like features. Pain is more often localized to the occipital region. It may be present on awakening, and may worsen with Valsalva maneuver. In adults, hydrocephalus may be accompanied by gait difficulty or urinary incontinence. Imaging in hydrocephalus may reveal enlargement of the ventricular system proximal to the blockade.

Headache in idiopathic intracranial hypertension

Idiopathic intracranial hypertension is characterized by raised intracranial pressure. It manifests as headache, with no localizing signs, normal CSF, and papilledema. Rarely, papilledema may be absent. The headache is holocranial, unilateral, and may be worsened by Valsalva maneuver. There may even be pain on eye movement or radicular pain down the neck and shoulder. This condition is best diagnosed by MRI that can visualize the venous sinuses with a 2D time of flight (TOF) magnetic resonance venography (MRV) to rule out cerebral venous thrombosis.

Headache in cerebral venous thrombosis

Cerebral venous thrombosis is characterized by headache, papilledema, seizures, and may be associated with focal neurological deficits. The headache is nonspecific and often diffuses. It may be localized to any region of the head and neck. Its severity can range from a slight discomfort to intense pain. It can be intermittent, associated with nausea or vomiting, and may thus resemble migraine attacks. It has a subacute onset and progresses over 2 days to a month. It is commonly diagnosed by 2D TOF MRV, contrast enhanced computed tomography (CT) venography, and digital subtraction angiography.

Post-traumatic Headache

This is a headache arising within 7 days of traumatic brain injury, which is characterized by features of both migraine and tension-type headache. Most often, it is caused by mild traumatic brain injury. Studies have found a cumulative effect of head injury on the genesis of post traumatic CDH.

WORK UP OF A PATIENT WITH CHRONIC HEADACHE

Armed with knowledge of underlying possibilities and information about "subtle clues," after a complete neurological examination, one is able to rule out most chronic secondary headaches, and decide which patients will need further workup. Comprehensive examination of a headache patient will include, evaluation of the head and neck, careful otorhinolaryngologic and ophthalmic checkup, testing for tenderness over paravertebral muscles, temporomandibular joints, paranasal sinuses, occipital nerves, and/or thickening of temporal vessels, noting the range of cervical movements and listening for a "bruit."

The best investigation for most chronic headache patients is a gadolinium-enhanced MRI scan. It is far superior to CT scan, especially for the evaluation of the leptomeninges, dura, craniocervical junction, and posterior fossa. Listed below are the lesions that may be missed on CT scan and where a gadolinium enhanced MRI is indispensable.[15]

1. Meningitis (viral, bacterial, carcinomatous) and encephalitis
2. CNS vasculitis
3. IIH without papilledema
4. Bilateral isodense subdural hematoma
5. Ethmoidal or sphenoidal sinusitis
6. Infiltrating glioma
7. Temporal arteritis
8. Some aneurysms/vascular malformations
9. Some posterior fossa/craniocervical lesions
10. Venous sinus or cortical vein thrombosis

CONCLUSION

Chronic headaches are generally thought of as challenging and difficult to treat. They form a large part of the neurologist's outpatient workload. But with a systematic approach as outlined here and based on sound knowledge of underlying causes, knowing what to look for and when, it is possible to diagnose and treat most patients with chronic headache.

REFERENCES

1. Headache Classification Committee, International Headache Society. Classification and diagnostic criteria for headache disorders, cranial neuralgia and facial pain. Cephalalgia. 1988;8(Suppl 7):1-96.
2. Headache Classification Committee, International Headache Society. The international classification of headache disorders, 2nd edition. Cephalagia. 2004;24(Suppl 1):1-160.
3. Mathew NT, Stubits E, Nigam MP. Transformation of episodic migraine into daily headache: analysis of factors. Headache. 1982;22(2):66-8.
4. Sobri M, Lamont AC, Alias NA, et al. Red ags in patients presenting with headache: clinical indications for neuroimaging. Br J Radiol. 2003;76:532-5.
5. Boes CJ, Pareja JA. Chronic Paroxysmal Hemicrania. Chronic Daily Headache for Clinicians. BC Decker; 2005. pp. 81-8.
6. Matharu MS, Goadsby P. Short-Lasting, Unilateral, Neuralgiform Headache Attacks with Conjunctival Injection and Tearing (SUNCT) Syndrome. Chronic Daily Headache for Clinicians. BC Decker; 2005. pp.89-104.
7. Halker RB, Hastriter EV, Dodick DW. Chronic daily headache: an evidence-based and systematic approach to a challenging problem. Neurology. 2011;76(7 Suppl 2):S37-43.
8. Evans RV. Diagnostic testing for chronic daily headache. Curr Pain Headache Rep. 2007;11(1):47-52.
9. Lainez MJ. Chronic headaches: from research to clinical practice. J Headache Pain. 2005;6(4):175-8.
10. Fumal A, Schoenen J. Chronic Tension-Type Headache. Chronic Daily Headache for Clinicians. BC Decker; 2005. pp. 57-64.
11. Pascual J. Headache due to cervical disease–Clinical Implications. Chronic Daily Headache for Clinicians. BC Decker; 2005. pp. 145-54.
12. Couch JR. Update on chronic daily headache. Curr Treat Options Neurol. 2011;13:41-55.
13. Mokri B. Low Cerebrospinal Fluid Volume Headaches. Chronic Daily Headache for Clinicians. BC Decker; 2005. pp. 155-66.
14. Santiago ME, Corbett JJ. Raised Cerebrospinal Fluid Pressure Headache. Chronic Daily Headache for Clinicians. BC Decker; 2005. pp. 167-82.
15. Purdy RA. Diagnostic Evaluation of Chronic Daily Headache. Chronic Daily Headache for Clinicians. BC Decker; 2005. pp. 13-20.

Chapter 22

Approach to Ataxia of Limbs and Gait

Achal K Srivastava, Mohammed Faruq

INTRODUCTION

The term ataxia denotes "out of ordered voluntary movements (A-taxis')" and ataxic disorders exhibit imbalance and incoordination in walking, targeted limb movements, eye movements, and speech.[1] Cerebellar ataxia either as a predominating feature or as an associated sign with other primary neurological events has been described in over 500 neurological disorders. The diagnosis of ataxic disorders is clinically challenging due to wide variability in the symptoms and signs. Ataxia can occur due to aberrations in cerebellum, its afferent or efferent connections and in isolation as a consequence of sensory neuropathy. Diagnostic delineation of the exact etiology involves obtaining a meticulous history from the patient as well as close associates, complete family history, extensive neurological examination and a battery of paraclinical tests comprising of biochemical profiling, neuroimaging, and electrophysiological studies. In this chapter we have focused on describing in brief the semiology of ataxic disorders and the approach to an ataxic patient when it presents as the chief complaint in the neurology clinic.

Anatomy: Connections, Deep Nuclei, and Vascular Anatomy

According to Jansen, anatomically, the cerebellum is grossly divided into three main lobes by two fissures, a primary fissure, which separates anterior lobe from rest of the cerebellum and a posterior fissure separating posterior lobe from flocculonodular lobe. Larssell proposed a lobular architecture of cerebellar hemispheres comprising lobule I–X arranged rostrocaudally. Anterior lobe contains lobule I–IV, lobule V–1X constitute posterior lobe, and flocculonodular is lobule-X. Lobule-VII is the largest with crus-I, crus-II, and crus-VIIb lobules. Functionally, according to Dow, based on nerve fiber projection, cerebellum is organized mediolaterally into vermis and paravermis (spinocerebellum, paleocerebellum), lateral hemispheres (corticopontocerebellar projections, neocerebellum), and flocculonodular lobe (vestibulo-cerebellar projection, archecerebellum) (Fig. 22.1).[1]

The afferent innervations of the cerebellum pass through peduncular system of nerve bundle organizations. The key areas of brain to which cerebellum is connected are inferior olivary complex, pons, spinal cord, and vestibular nuclei. The three peduncles, superior cerebellar peduncle (brachium conjectivum — ventral spinocerebellar tract, and tactocerebellar tracts), middle cerebellar peduncle (brachium pontis — pontocerebellar tracts), and inferior cerebellar peduncle (restiform body — olivocerebellar tracts, spinocerebellar tracts, vestibulospinal tracts, cuneocerebellar tracts, and reticulocerebellar tracts) are the input system carrying afferent system. The vermis and intermediate zones (spinocerebellum) receive afferents from spinal cord/inferior olives/vestibular nuclei, whereas lateral hemispheres receive from the cerebral cortex (Fig. 22.2).

The efferent systems of the cerebellum are projection of fibers from cerebellar deep nuclei. The deep nuclei of the cerebellum from mediolaterally are fastigial nucleus, interpositus nuclei (globus and emboliform nuclei), and dentate nuclei. The projections from spinocerebellum

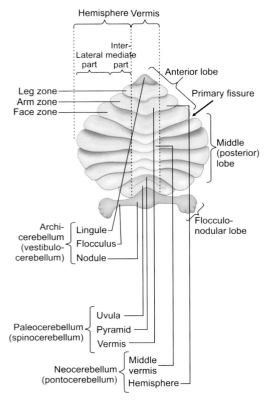

Fig. 22.1: Functional subdivisions of cerebellum.

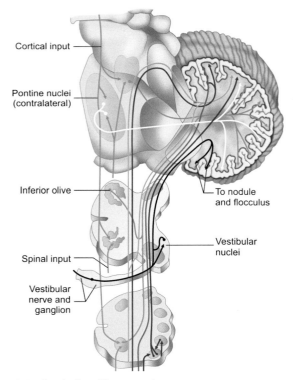

Fig. 22.2: Cerebellar afferent pathways.

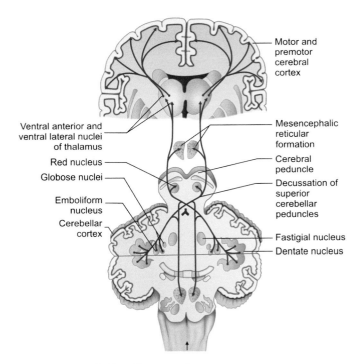

Fig. 22.3: Cerebellar efferent pathways.

internally end in fastigial and interpositus nuclei. From fastigial nuclei, efferent projections are targeted to the vestibular nuclei, and reticular nucleus bilaterally. It also sends fibers to the ventrolateral nucleus (VLN) of the thalamus, which controls the cells of origin of ventral corticospinal tract in the motor cortex. The interpositus nucleus sends its output to the magnocellular portion of red nucleus, reticular nuclei, and VLN of thalamus, which controls origin of the lateral-CST. The dentate nuclei projects mainly to the thalamus, inferior olivary complex, and parvocellular portion of red nucleus. The spinocerebellum basically controls balance, gait, and limb movements. The neocerebellum controls planning, learning, and related activities[1] (Fig. 22.3).

Vascular Supply of the Cerebellum

The vascular branches of vertebral and basilar arteries constitute the arterial supply of the blood to the cerebellum. Three main arteries, superior cerebellar artery (SCA, originates from superior part of the basilar artery), anterior inferior cerebellar artery (AICA, from proximal segment of the basilar artery), and posterior inferior cerebellar artery (PICA from vertebral artery). SCA supplies anterior lobe, deep nuclei, and superior cerebellar peduncle along with pons. AICA supplies middle portion of the cerebellum including middle cerebellar peduncle, inferior cerebellar peduncle, flocculonodular lobe, and ventrolateral portion of the pons. The PICA supplies inferior portion of the vermis, posterior lobe of the cerebellum, and dorsal medulla. Three groups of veins, superior, anterior, and posterior vein carry the venous drainage of the cerebellum.[1]

The main role of this functional arrangement of the cerebellum is to maintain posture, balance, and smooth activity of motor function. The central part of the cerebellum (median and intermediate) has a key role in maintaining balance while sitting and walking. The anterior lobe lesions produce postural sway of high-velocity and low-amplitude anteroposteriorly and postural tremors. Lesions of vestibulocerebellum (flocculonodular lobe) produce postural sway of low frequency and high amplitude without directional preference. The lesion of the intermediate lobe has little effect on balance on erect posture but has stronger influence on directionality of limb movements, coordination of the activity of agonist and antagonist muscles to bring precision in the target reaching movements of the limbs. Lateral cerebellar region has little influence on posture and balance, but it is important for complex motor activity requiring planning, anticipatory motor adjustments, and movements requiring visual guidance.

MAJOR SYMPTOMS AND SIGNS OF CEREBELLAR ATAXIA

Ataxia of Lower Limb, Gait, and Posture

The gait abnormality in cerebellar ataxia resembles walking impairment in acute alcohol intoxication. In the early stages, the patient notices problems such as imbalance, lateral swaying of the body upon walking on narrow path, crowded places, and while performing acts requiring skilled movements, e.g., cycling, climbing stairs, etc. In more advanced stages, the patient walks with wide base gait even with support with corrections and errors. On examination, patient sways when asked to walk straight on a 10 m walk and associated with wide-based stance of the feet, on natural stance feet are placed wide apart >20 cm. Ataxia can be elicited in patients even earlier on performing tandem gait or a one foot stance. Heel–shin test provokes tremor in limb movement, decomposition, and lateral movement while sliding the heel on shin. Posture abnormality, truncal tremor, head tremor on maintained erect posture on standing or even

during sitting position may be observed.[2] In midline cerebellar lesions, patient may perceive ataxia of central axis involving the trunk or head. The oscillation may be felt in anteroposterior or lateral sway. Ataxia of stance can be observed while allowing patient to stand on 1 ft or with feet together or tandem stance with eyes open and eyes closed. One can also observe flexion–extension rhythmic movements of the feet. The eye closure in cerebellar lesion may lead to the worsening of ataxia of stance (Rhomberg's sign) but less pronounced than seen in sensory ataxias.

Kinetic Dysfunction in Upper Limb in Ataxic Disorders

Deregulation in rate, rhythm, and force of contraction of voluntary muscle groups in the upper limb produces symptoms, i.e., hand shaking on sustaining posture during object holding, e.g., a glass of water, or a cup of tea. The patient often reports change in hand writing and tremor while reaching an object or while performing skilled activities, e.g., buttoning and unbuttoning or eating with spoon. In clinics, upper limb incoordination can be elicited by finger–nose testing, finger–finger testing, examiner's finger chasing movements, dysdiadochokinesia (abnormal rapid alternating hand movements).

Intention Tremor

This term refers to a characteristic cerebellar sign that results from impairment of synergism of agonistic and antagonistic muscle activity toward precision of a goal directed task by limbs. It is characteristically observed while allowing patient to perform finger–nose test, finger chase test, or heel–shin test. The tremulousness of finger movements increases in amplitude at the end of the movement or while reaching the target. It can also be observed throughout the range of the movement. Tremor is more observed in proximal joints and increases upon adding weight (increasing inertia) to the moving limbs.

Action Tremor

These tremors are observed while keeping limbs outstretched against the gravity. In upper limbs, cerebellar lesions may produce moderately severe tremor during finger–finger test, hand–hand test, or in outstretched hands. Tremors may involve distal as well as proximal joints. These tremors may also be observed in lower limbs.

Advanced progressive cerebellar lesions may lead to complexly looking tremors involving whole of the body with kinetic, action, and axial components together resembling tremors of cerebellar outflow tract lesions, e.g., rubral tremor/wing-beating seen in Wilson's disease, midbrain stroke, and multiple sclerosis.

Dysdiadochokinesia

Impairments in rapid and repetitive movements of hand is termed as adiadochokinesia or dysdiadochokinesis. These abnormal movements can be elicited while rapid supination–pronation alternating movements of forearm or tapping one hand (with dorsum and palmar) onto other hand on palm. Impairment in rhythm, regularity, and elbow sway can be noticed. In addition, abnormality of rhythm can be observed by successive tapping movements of index finger and thumb.

Speech Disturbances

The key abnormality in cerebellar speech (dysarthria) is imprecise articulation, phonation, variable loudness, and irregular intervals between syllables. The dysarthric speech in ataxic patients is slurred with uncontrolled volume, pitch, and irregular pause between syllables. There is disarticulation of syllables with distortion of vowels creating slurred speech, impaired control over breathing during speech lead to bursting loudness, and equal stress and prolonged pause make speech of the scanning type.

Oculomotor Abnormalities

Topographically, oculomotor impairment in cerebellar disorders is the result of a lesion in the dorsal vermis, flocculonodular, or the fastigial region. The observed abnormalities include nystagmus, fixation abnormality, impaired saccades, and pursuit movements. Nystagmus is observed when gaze is fixed at 30° from midline, and a fast phase of the nystagmus is seen toward direction of gaze. Down-beating nystagmus is also observed in some ataxic conditions and that is characterized by fast phase of nystagmus toward down gaze in primary position of eyes. Saccadic intrusions and square wave jerks are eye movement fixation abnormalities seen in cerebellar disorders. The saccadic movements are hypermetric or hypometric upon alternating movement toward examiner's finger placed on temporal visual field of the patient.

Other Associated Symptoms and Signs

Apart from ataxia of gait and limbs, other symptoms are also variably experienced by the patients, and they include dizziness, headache, cognitive abnormalities, symptoms of autonomic dysfunction, and dysphagia. Among extraneurological manifestations, signs, and symptoms with the specific subtype of ataxias may be observed due to muscular involvement, cardiac dysfunction, mental retardation, hypogonadism, and radiosensitivity.

Hypotonia

In cerebellar lesions more often in children, reduced resistance to passive movement can be observed in peripheral muscles and joints. Proximal musculatures are more affected than distal compartments. The association of pendular reflexes in cerebellar ataxia is observed due to hypotonic muscles. Apart from muscular hypotonia, posterior fossa malignancies affecting cerebellar hemisphere can give rise to condition called cerebellar seizures.[1]

Cerebellar Mutism

This condition, primarily affecting the speech has been observed in children (nearly in 25%) who have undergone posterior fossa surgery for tumor, trauma, or other causes. In postoperative period, a latency to develop mutism is observed that may range from hours to days. It follows a phase of mutism, which resolves spontaneously with time period ranging from days to several months. After recovery from mutism, residual affliction to language disorders in the form of dysarthria or language disturbances and behavioral and emotional changes can be seen. A possible explanation for cerebellar mutism has been hypothesized to be resulting from disjunction of cerbrocerebellar connection (from the dentate nuclei to cerebral cortex) or direct injury to the cerebellum).[3]

Cognitive Incoordination

As similar to the motor control neural circuitary, cerebellum also makes connection with the cerebral cortex to regulate various cognitive, and behavioral tasks. The connection of cerebellum via thalamus with lateral prefrontal cortex has been assigned the task of controlling cognitive tasks. The executive function refers to the coordinated activity of various cognitive functions to accomplish a particular goal. In addition, lateral cerebellar cortex has been shown to be involved in learning and memory. The cerebellar cortex is involved in procedural learning (motor skills and habits), conditional (associative learning), and perceptual learning.[1] The main connections of learning, e.g., conditional eye-blink response is mediated via coordinated activity of mossy fibers (conditional response), climbing fibers (unconditional response) and their coordination centers like, pontine nuclei, inferior olive, and cerebellar nuclei. In cerebellar lesion/disorders having onset at the late age have shown to impair the deficits in learned psychomotor behaviors (e.g., cognitive decline, executive function, depression, anxiety, restlessness, and other psychiatric symptoms), whereas genetic/developmental-ataxias having onset at the childhood age or juvenile age show impairment of learning and executive functions.[1,4]

LESION SYMPTOMS MAPPING OF ATAXIC FEATURES

The loss of any afferent or efferent connections to cerebellum, essentially, can manifest as ataxia. In general, focal and lateralized lesions of the cerebellum produce ipsilateral signs, whereas symmetrical deficits are observed in neurodegenerative forms of cerebellar lesions. The medial and intermediate zones of the cerebellum take control of posture and gait through spinovestibular and corticospinal connections, respectively. The midline lesions of the cerebellum lead to truncal ataxia or imbalance, titubation, dysarthria, and oculomotor impairments. The affection of upper vermial region leads to low-amplitude and high-frequency oscillations, whereas the lower vermial lesion produces high-amplitude and low-frequency oscillations. Lesions of intermediate zone produce decomposition and dysmetria in limb movements. The dentate nucleus controls the reaction time, whereas interpositus nuclei control reflex activity of the moving limb by inhibiting antagonistic muscles. The paravermal area controls speech articulation with intrinsic and extrinsic connection with supplementary motor area, Broca's area, and superior cerebellum. The lower cerebellum with basal ganglia and thalamus control executive speech.[5] Lesions in the lateral cerebellar hemisphere lead to loss of tuning in rate, rhythm, and force of contraction of voluntary muscles and is responsible for signs, i.e., dysmetria, decomposition, action tremor, dysdiadochokinesia, and rebound phenomenon. Flocculous and parafloccular nodules with vestibular nuclei control eye movements. Cerebrocerebellar system is involved in motor adaptive

> **Box 22.1: Definition of terms**
>
> **Glossary**
>
> Dysmetria—This term is used to define the movement abnormality while target reaching maneuver repeatedly. When a patient with cerebellar ataxia is asked to perform fast and accurate movements toward a target (finger–nose test), either of the two errors may be noticed hypermetria; where the test finger's movement pass the point of targets (overshoot) and it fails to reach the target in first effort (undershoot). With a series of correction movements finger finally touches the target with imprecision.
>
> Dyssynergia—Cerebellar damage leads to asynchronization of movements involving multiple joints for a complex motor task.
>
> Isometrataxia—Cerebellar lesions are often associated with impairments in generation of stable force particularly requiring hand muscles. This can be elicited by asking patient to hold examiner's thumb laterally with his finger and thumb exerting constant pressure.

phase of learning tasks as exemplified by Serial Reaction Time Task (SRTT) impairment. The lobules IV–VI are involved with disgust, happiness, and sad behaviors.[6] Ataxia as a symptom may also arise due to involvement of abnormality of various regions across peripheral or central neural axis. The loss of afferent tract, i.e., dorsalspinocerebellar tracts can present as isolated ataxia of gait in absence of sensory clues, clinically known as sensory ataxia. Romberg's sign (swaying posture upon eye closure) is observed primarily in sensory ataxia and often may be associated with the cerebellar degeneration. In addition, damage to frontopontocerebellar tracts may lead to frontal lobe ataxia. Vestibular lesions may have manifestation of vertigo, ataxia, and rotary nystagmus. Lesions of lateral medulla and inferior cerebellum can manifest as ataxia and vertigo together. Vestibular paresis can present as ataxia of gait without vertigo (nonvertiginous ataxia) commonly associated with drug induced causes (streptomycin toxicity). Lesions of anterior thalamus can produce transient ataxia of limbs contralateral to the side of the lesion (Box 22.1).

TYPES OF ATAXIAS: CENTRAL OR PERIPHERAL

The basis of ataxia (of gait) may lie in central or peripheral nervous structure disorders. Broadly, ataxia (of gait) may have central origin (cerebellar or frontal lobe lesion) or peripheral (proprioceptive inputs or vestibulopathies) lesion. The distinction between these could be made by careful observation of ataxic gait, associated signs, and pattern of progression. The key abnormalities of these ataxia types are depicted in Table 22.1. The disruption of

TABLE 22.1: Clinical description of type of ataxia (central or peripheral)

Feature	Cerebellar ataxia	Sensory ataxia	Frontal ataxia
Base of support	Wide-based	Narrow base, looks down	Wide-based
Velocity	Variable	Slow	Very slow
Stride	Irregular, lurching	Regular with path deviation	Short, shuffling
Romberg's sign	+/−	Unsteady, falls	+/−
Heel–shin	Abnormal	+/−	Normal
Initiation	Normal	Normal	Hesitant
Turns	Unsteady	+/−	Hesitant, multistep
Postural instability	+	+++	++++
Falls	Late event	Frequent	Frequent

frontal lobe connection to the cerebellum (probably the frontocerebellar tracts) may produce gait difficulties. The basic differences from typical cerebellar ataxia can be made by the absence of heel–shin incoordination, speech slurring, nystagmus, and normal upper limb movement coordination. The typical gait abnormalities observed in frontal lobe ataxia are wide-based gait, with frequent fall, short shuffling of gait, and apraxic component. The ataxia due to lesion of sensory afferent nerve fibers (dorsal spinocerebellar tracts) is called sensory ataxias. The causes of sensory ataxias described are diabetes, familial sensory neuropathy, drugs (cisplatin, paclitaxel etc.), pyridoxine toxicity, and others. The characteristic hallmark of the sensory ataxia is the presence of Rhomberg's sign (eye closure worsens the ataxia). The base of the gait observed is normal with high-stepping nature and moderate degree of postural instability. Sparing of speech, no nystagmus, normal heel–shin test differentiate it from cerebellar ataxia. Vestibular ataxia have predominant affection of balance difficulty while erect stance is accompanied by prominent vertigo. Speech is relatively spared. There could be presence of other signs and symptoms, which may point toward peripheral vestibulopathy (head-impulse test, caloric irrigation-induced nystagmus). Association of episodic ataxias (EAs) responding to acetazolamide, migrainous headache points toward the central vestibulopathy (Box 22.2).

Box 22.2: Etiological classification of ataxia

A. Cerebellar ataxia
  I Acquired or idiopathic cause
     Toxins and drug induced: Alcohol, anticonvulsants, anti-cancer drugs, etc.
     Autoimmunity associated: Multiple sclerosis, gluten ataxia, ataxia with anti-GAD antibodies, paraneoplastic cerebellar degeneration
     Infection mediated: Postviral infection cerebellitis, enteric fever, adeno/retroviral, malaria, prions
     Degenerative progressive: Multiple system atrophy-C, Idiopathic late onset cerebellar ataxia
  II Genetic causes
     Autosomal dominant cerebellar ataxias: Spinocerebellar ataxia type 1-31, SCA36, episodic ataxia type1 and 2
     Autosomal recessive cerebellar ataxias: Friedreich's ataxia, ataxia telangiectasia, etc
     X-linked ataxia: Fragile X tremor ataxia syndrome
     Ataxia with mitochondrial inheritance: Myoclonic epilepsy with ragged red fibers, Neuropathy, ataxia, and retinitis pigmentosa, Kearns-Sayre Syndrome
     Nonprogressive developmental disorders: Cayman ataxia, Joubert syndrome
B. Sensory ataxia: Peripheral neuropathy, Miller Fisher syndrome, autoimmunity to myelin-associated glycoprotein linked peripheral neuropathy
C. Frontal ataxia: Frontal lobe lesions—infarct, hemorrhage, tumors

DIAGNOSTIC APPROACH TO ATAXIA

The initial evaluation of ataxia comprises of meticulous history taking by determining the family history, age of onset of ataxia, tempo of the disease progression, and concurrent use of drugs, and alcohol or toxin exposure. In addition, history of symptoms apart from ataxia should be obtained. During neurological examination, a detailed survey of distribution of deficits should be undertaken including symmetry of signs (symmetric or asymmetric), type of ataxia (sensory or motor), and presence of ataxia plus signs. Based on history evaluation and neurological examination, appropriate paraclinical investigations can be sought comprising of electrophysiological examination (nerve conduction studies, electroencephalogram, visual evoked potentials (VEP), brainstem auditory. evoked responses (BEAR), and autonomic function tests), radiological investigations [plain computed tomography head, magnetic resonance imaging (MRI) and single-photon emission computed tomography (SPECT)],